BRAIN BUILDERS!

A LIFELONG GUIDE TO SHARPER THINKING, BETTER MEMORY, AND AN AGEPROOF MIND

RICHARD LEVITON

Reward Books
a member of
Penguin Group (USA) Inc.
New York

This book is reference work based on research by the author. The opinions expressed herein are not necessarily those of or endorsed by the publisher. The directions stated in this book are in no way to be considered as a substitute for consultation with a duly licensed doctor.

✦ Reward Books
a member of Penguin Group (USA) Inc.
375 Hudson Street
New York, NY 10014
www.penguin.com

Library of Congress Cataloging-in-Publication Data

Leviton, Richard.
Brain Builders! : a lifelong guide to sharper thinking, better memory, and an age-proof mind / Richard Leviton.
p. cm.
Includes bibliographical references and index.
ISBN 0-13-303611-1 (cloth)—ISBN 0-13-303603-0 (paper)
1. Brain—Aging. 2. Alzheimer's disease—Prevention. 3. Intellect. 4. Nootropic agents. 5. Memory. I. Title.
QP376.L46. 1995 95-32233
153—dc20 CIP

Printed in the United States of America

20 19 18 17 16 15

CONTENTS

CHAPTER 4

INTRODUCTION

USE YOUR BRAIN: THE 7 BRAIN BUILDERS! SECRETS

There is no reason in the world why when you get older you have to lose any of your brain power. It's true that public attention in recent years has focused on such dramatically miserable examples of brain power decline as Alzheimer's disease. And you often see images of the elderly as frail, forgetful, even occasionally amnesiac. Now, as a huge chunk of the population—the baby boomers, born between 1946–1964—approaches their fifties with a preliminary vista of their own old age, people are beginning to ask: "Do I have to lose my brain power just because I'm aging?"

The answer that this book emphatically gives is this: Not at all. You can start today to reclaim your natural brain power and ageproof your brain so you never lose any more. Brain power decline as you age may be common, but it is not inevitable. It's more a matter of taking the correct *preventive* steps earlier in your life so that what is a possibility never becomes a reality. Studies show that at least 20–30 percent of the elderly—people in their eighties—when they take brain power tests perform as well as people in their thirties and forties, an age that many consider to be a brain power peak.

DON'T SURRENDER A SINGLE IQ POINT TO OLD AGE

Scientists who study the elderly tend to focus on only a very small percentage (about 6–15 percent) who are technically frail and in a mental decline; but then they too often take their results from studying this group and project it onto the population at large.

But the other 85–94 percent of the elderly population doesn't fit into this group of diminished brain power. Perhaps you might lose some of your mathematics abilities once you hit your seventies; studies show men tend to score about 33 percent lower on math tests in their mid-seventies than they did in their fifties; and a further decline to about 50 percent occurs between the fifties and eighties. But you can always use a pocket calculator.

On the other hand, an 80-year-old man's ability to read a map correctly, which is about visual orientation, declines only by 16 percent. Other areas of brain power that can slip in old age include inductive reasoning, understanding verbal meaning, and word fluency. But then, many other aspects of your physical body are declining too as you age, especially if you haven't made a lifelong habit of using them—exercising, keeping fit, and using your brain. Using your brain, it turns out, is probably the most vital thing you can do to ensure that you'll keep most of your functional IQ well into your old age.

Use your brain—this is the key, scientists and gerontologists are discovering. There seem to be certain fundamentals by which you can almost tell how someone's brain power will weather getting old. Among them:

- Keep your verbal fluency and level of reading comprehension in trim.
- Keep your mental interests, both professional and personal, keen and well practiced.
- Keep your mental attitude flexible, open, ready to be challenged.
- Try to always learn new things, visit new places, entertain new ideas.
- Live or associate with people who share these habits of mind.

If your spouse is particularly brainy, count your blessings; you could almost say the IQ will rub off just from being close.

A recent study of 1,300 men and women in their mid-seventies gave a clear idea of what it takes to keep your brain power as you age. First, stay in good physical health because you need a sound and fit body to support a sound and fit brain. Exercise regularly and strenuously and keep your pulmonary function in top order. Your brain needs all the oxygen and nutrients your circulatory system can send it.

Second, keep your intellectual interests and activities alive in your years after school. Study subjects and master them; the sense of mastery or personal mental competence is vital to the ability to maintain your usable IQ into old age. Let your neurons know who's in charge; there'll be no early retirement for the brain chemicals of intelligence.

Third, your brain power is *trainable*. Men and women in this study took a special 5-hour brain-training seminar to hone their skills in spatial orientation and inductive reasoning, which are the two areas of brain power in which the elderly most typically tend to decline. About 40 percent of those in this class showed higher scores, similar to how they performed 14 years earlier.

Even when this same group entered their eighties, their scores after taking the brain-training class were still strong, showing little evidence of mental decline. Those who had not taken the classes fared quite poorly in the brain power tests. The clear lesson of these studies is this: Use your brain!

THE 3-POUND UNIVERSE IS YOUR MOST VALUABLE POSSESSION

Your brain, or what scientists like to call the "3-pound universe," is the next frontier in human development. Your brain contains an estimated 100 billion neurons, or nerve cells, and is capable of outstanding feats of computation and information processing. Despite this wealth of potential brain power, most people use no more than about 4–10 percent of their *possible* brain capacity. The good news is that this is easily changed.

You can increase your brain power dramatically once you know the smart ways to strengthen your mind—the brain building secrets. Acquiring greater brain power is not so difficult, but it will require a little training on your part, and that means you have to know all the smart ways to have more brain power on demand. This book gives you 86 smart ways to build your brain power in the form of 86 Brain Building Secrets.

In 1989, the U.S. government dedicated the 1990s as the Decade of the Brain. Now, as the 1990s progress, the emphasis is on rapid information processing as a way of life and business. So you need an edge in this data-rich environment; you want ways to maximize your brain's potential. It used to be physical fitness, but now the search is on for *brain fitness*, and it's booming. You need to think faster, sharper, more efficiently, and more creatively; you need to learn quicker, deeper, more thoroughly; and you cannot afford to forget anything.

Today, if your brain is sluggish, it could disqualify you from the brain power marketplace. Brain fitness has clearly become a job asset. Computers may have made every aspect of modern life easier, but they've also reset the pace of the mind at a much higher notch. Today, your work often demands ever-faster speeds from your brain. And why not? Why shouldn't you speed along at top brain power using some of that untapped 90–96 percent of your natural brain strength?

ADDING MORE BRAIN "MUSCLE" FOR SUPERSMARTNESS

Maximum brain performance is a birthright you are entitled to claim. But what is brain power? Brain power means alertness, concentration, perceptual speed, learning, memory, problem solving, and creativity—in sum, what scientists call *cognition*. Brain power means your ability to respond to the world, understand it, even reshape it through your creativity and intelligence.

Often, when you are honest with yourself, don't you feel you could do much better if only you had more intelligence, more brain power "muscle"? And at the same time, say you are now in a highly productive midlife plateau, don't you want more brain power, not less—and don't you want to keep *all of it* into your mentally fit old age? That's why BRAIN BUILDERS! is for you.

There are numerous books on brain power and mental fitness in the bookstores, but then there are also hundreds of cookbooks, too. Having a good idea for a casserole or building IQ is fine, but it doesn't in itself guarantee a good cookbook or brain power building strategy.

Too often, brain power books put the cart before the horse; that means they give you step 7 before you have mastered steps 1 through 6. They have you doing complicated memory techniques before you've even worked on your attitude about being smart. They ignore certain key factors in your life-style, diet, and physical health that can be undermining all your efforts to build brain power. And they forget to show you how to use your life-style, diet, habits, and other factors to support your effort to smarten up.

BRAIN BUILDERS! gives you all seven steps in their correct order. Building something in the right order is the key to success in any venture like this. That's what distinguishes BRAIN BUILDERS! from all the rest. It shows you how to build your brain power in the right and natural order. That's what the seven BRAIN BUILDERS! secrets are all about.

BRAIN BUILDERS! Secret One is *Believe Your Brain*. This means you must start believing that it is possible to gain more brain power. The secret is really your attitude. It sounds paradoxical, but the secret to claiming the power of your mind is to believe you have this power in the first place, even before you see any proof of it. So you need to believe in your brain and in your ability to gain more mastery of it.

BRAIN BUILDERS! Secret Two is *Free Your Brain*. This is an area often overlooked. There are many key factors in the way you live that directly interfere with the full expression of your natural brain power. In other words, you may be far smarter than you are capable of acting because of certain obstacles that drain your brain but can be removed.

These include stress, depression, alcohol use, dietary style, inadequate nutrition, chronic constipation, brain allergies, even the contents of your house. When you correct these factors, then you free your brain to start developing itself.

BRAIN BUILDERS! Secret Three is *Get in Rhythm with Your Brain*. Your brain has its own natural rhythms of activity and rest, as does your body. You can use these to your advantage in this brain-building program. Here you will learn techniques and exercises to develop attention and focus, to prime your memory muscles, and to determine the best times for brain activity.

BRAIN BUILDERS! Secret Four is *Feed Your Brain*. If you think you know what a big feeder looks like, think again. Your brain has an outrageous appetite for just about every nutrient known to food science and for about 20 percent of all the oxygen you inhale every day. You might think of your brain as a permanent adolescent: constantly growing, chronically hungry. Skillful use of nutrition, diet, herbs, and supplements can build more brain power.

BRAIN BUILDERS! Secret Five is *Move Your Brain*. While you cannot literally move your brain and exercise it in the same sense that you work out your leg muscles when you go jogging, exercise is still a vital key to better brain power. It gets more oxygen into your brain cells. Learn how to move your brain through exercise, yoga, qigong, breathing exercises, and twirling.

BRAIN BUILDERS! Secret Six is *Sound Your Brain*. Did you know that music, sounds, even electronic frequencies are food for your brain? Your brain emits a spectrum of energies, or frequencies, called brain waves, and these change according to your activity. Feed your brain nourishing sound waves and watch your brain power grow.

BRAIN BUILDERS! Secret Seven is *Exercise Your Brain*. Finally, here is the cart of brain power, now that you have put the "horse" in its rightful place. Brain-building exercises can get much better traction and results when you do them in a prepared environment. Creating this environment is what all the earlier BRAIN BUILDERS! secrets are about; now even a little practice with some of the exercises in this section will give you far better results than if you had tried them first.

So these are the seven BRAIN BUILDERS! Secrets. But there are also 86 brain building secrets that are the substance of this book. Each of the seven major secrets has many examples, techniques, and exercises by which you can gain mastery of each stage. You might think of the 86 brain building secrets as the step-by-step instructions for the recipes by which you will build more brain power.

The 17 foundational BRAIN BUILDERS! Secrets are like the main courses in your meal. There are also 17 extra features in your brain-building meal. Each of these 17 sections talks about an aspect of THE ANATOMY OF BRAIN POWER. You might think of these as the cook's commentary on the recipes. Then to get you right into the brain-building spirit of the day, you'll find 36 BRAIN BUILDERS! Workouts interspered in the early chapters of this book.

This book is meant to be interactive (and fun) to use. For example, you can read all 17 Anatomies at once, as a kind of separate book within a book. Similarly, you can go through all 36 Workouts at once, if you like, even before you read the main text of 86 *Secrets*. I do recommend, however, that you practice the 86 Secrets in order as they are carefully sequenced to give you the maximum benefit, in that order.

Between the 86 Secrets, the 17 Anatomies, and the 36 Workouts —that's 139 easy-to-use and fun BRAIN BUILDERS! techniques in all—you'll finish the book with a very thorough and, I hope, inspiring view of your own brain power potential. Your 139 keys to smartening up and building better brain power start on the next page. And remember: *Use your brain*!

1 BELIEVE YOUR BRAIN

▼▼▼▼▼▼▼▼▼▼▼▼▼▼▼▼▼▼▼▼▼

How to Smarten Up Your Attitude to Gain More Brain Power

Believe your brain. You must start believing that it is possible to gain more brain power. The secret is really your attitude. It sounds paradoxical, but the secret to claiming the power of your mind is to believe you have this power in the first place, even before you see any proof of it. So you need to believe in your brain and in your ability to gain more mastery of it.

There are seven brain-building secrets within this category of *believe your brain*. Here you will learn how to work on your attitude about being smarter, study the smart study habits of top students, and learn that there are many kinds of intelligence. You will see that your brain is very flexible and moldable—"plastic" is how the scientists describe it—if you make the effort.

Here you'll see how to develop the right attitude to make the effort your brain requires. You'll learn how to take charge of how your brain functions and how to make it work for you, and you'll see unexpected ways to make your home environment a better brain power environment.

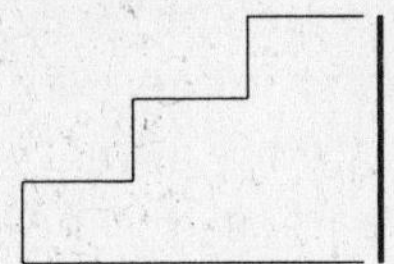

BRAIN-BUILDING SECRET #1 Your Attitude Is the Key to More Brain Power

Do you privately and secretly think you are stupid? Are you convinced that there is no way you could become smarter?

Be honest with yourself. If you answered "yes" to either of these questions, you have just revealed to yourself the power of attitude in shaping brain power. And I am here to assure you that even if you did answer yes, you are mistaken.

The correct answer to both questions is no. To be more precise, it is your attitude alone that is denying you your natural share of brain power.

Your first brain building secret is both the simplest and most important of any you will find in this book: *Believe it's possible to be smarter, wield more brain power, and have a wider, sharper range of mental abilities. Resolve to transform your attitude.*

DON'T DRAW THE WRONG CONCLUSIONS ABOUT YOUR MENTAL ABILITIES

Possibly the most important fact to keep in mind is that nothing about your mental abilities is permanent or incapable of change and improvement. Perhaps you carry, unthinkingly, an attitude from high school that since you did poorly on your college boards or unexceptionally on your IQ tests, that is your lot for life, as far as brain power is concerned. This is a mistaken view.

It is quite easy to form an erroneous view about your mental abilities and about the possibilities for improvement. You may admire others for being exceptionally smart but privately feel that this could never possibly be your lot. Often, at an early age when we are particularly sensitive, we listen too much to the opinions of others.

Let me dip into autobiography for a moment to make the point. My early schooling from about age 12 to 16 fostered the impression that I was of mediocre intellect. I was not in the top classes; I was put in classes with students who were a little dull from my perspective. When I was 13, I had a glimpse at my IQ test and wasn't impressed with the numbers. I did not score particularly high in grades in high school, although I did well in English. I spent many years, including high school, college, and afterwards, living under a mistaken impression about my mental abilities.

In ways common to my generation, I took certain steps to change my life-style at an early age, including conversion to a vegetarian diet, starting up a meditation practice, and practicing hatha yoga. I became more aware of the state of my mind and began to see things shift.

My point is simple and I hope you will see its relevance to your own situation. It took many years and much inner effort to throw off the mistaken views I had uncritically accepted from my peers, parents, teachers, and my own opinion about the situation, to see that I was smarter than I thought and I could be even smarter.

Once my attitude shifted, everything became possible. I was happier with my brain. I thumbed my nose at the teachers who had misread me. The same can be true for you.

7 QUESTIONS TO ASK YOURSELF ABOUT YOUR ATTITUDE

1. What is your own intellectual history?
2. What conclusions do you draw when you examine the personal history of your attitude about your intellect?
3. What is the autobiography of your attitude about your brain power?
4. When did you form the ideas you now have about your mental abilities?
5. Did someone ever tell you that you were a dummy?
6. Did you agree with that person?
7. Can you see what this did to your attitude about brain power?

You may make similarly interesting and liberating discoveries, as I did. You may find that increased brain power is merely an *attitude shift* away. And what shifts attitude is *focused motivation*, which is our focus in this brain-building secret.

GET YOUR MOTIVATION IN GEAR FOR GREATER BRAIN POWER

The life-changing power of motivation is a prime tool for improving the quality of any aspect of how you feel, think, and live, according to the latest discoveries of holistic health and popular psychology. Motivation is another way of saying "will," which means your will power. When it comes to getting smart faster, the skillful use of will, or motivation, requires only one thing: You must believe it is possible to gain more brain power.

Belief is what happens when, through your will, you make motivation a permanent habit of mind. Then it continually energizes you and moves you closer to your goal of more brain power. One way to make this belief a regular habit of mind comes from practicing affirmations. You affirm that it is entirely possible for you to gain brain power; then all the exercises you do have a stronger, deeper effect.

This is a sly way of reprogramming your mind to a new way of thinking. It is a bit like dropping a powerful suggestion into the dark basement of your unconscious mind. You wait a little while; then it throws it back up as a new automatic way of thinking and acting. Some call this approach *Neurolinguistic Programming*, or NLP for short.

TELLING YOUR NEURONS DIFFERENTLY—WHY WORDS MAKE A DIFFERENCE

Neuro refers to neuron, the brain cells within your nervous system that store information and provide reactions (and responses) to all life situations, both inside and outside your body.

Linguistic refers to the way you describe events and situations to yourself, your particular choice of words. The specific words and phrases you use carry innate value judgments and assessments; when you speak them, your brain is listening and acts accordingly. If you say you are *incredibly forgetful* or *not good at numbers* or *a slow reader*, your unconscious mind acts accordingly and keeps you precisely that way.

Programming means you can change it. You have already programmed your mind the first time to have these negative self-attitudes. This program runs on automatic pilot and serves you up preformed attitudes and reactions.

Now you can put a new positive "tape cassette" in the VCR of your self-attitude and generate entirely new, more self-affirming responses. One way to do this is to *reframe* the situation. You see that all the facts and data can actually add up to something entirely different than you thought. You put your picture of reality into a new frame of perception and understanding.

A QUICK REVIEW OF POSSIBLE NEGATIVE PROGRAMMING IN YOUR HEAD

Here are some negative programs that you may recognize and that may be making it difficult for you to learn, to increase your brain power, and to believe that IQ can be improved.

These are inner, secret attitudes you may be carrying around with you as automatic neurolinguistic programs that constantly feed back to you your own faulty and negative input.

12 WAYS YOU MAY BE UNDERMINING YOUR BRAIN POWER

1. I am stupid.
2. I don't want to learn.
3. I had a bad experience with this subject once.
4. My teachers made me feel bad about myself.
5. They won't let me learn this in my own way.
6. They always discouraged me from being original in my thoughts.
7. I got punished for being too clever.
8. I don't feel comfortable being open and curious.
9. I don't have the mental software.
10. My creativity is dead.
11. It's too scary to change now.
12. Frankly, I don't deserve it.

Do you see how things can work?

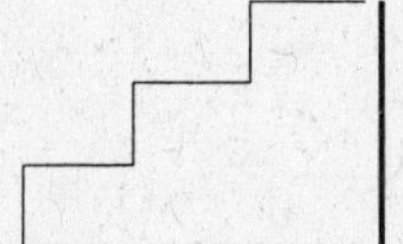

BRAIN-BUILDING SECRET #2
More About How Your Attitude Is the Key to More Brain Power

Do not underestimate the suggestive power of your early schooling. Often this sets the tone for a lifetime, and usually a lifetime of disinterested alienation or lack of confidence in one's ability to be a competent learner. For example, in 1982 a self-esteem researcher reported the results of a study of 100 school children during a typical class day. On average, each child received 460 negative or critical comments from the teacher or peers and only 75 supportive or positive ones.

THE WRONG KIND OF SCHOOLING—AND ATTITUDE—CAN ROB YOU OF YOUR NATURAL BRAIN POWER

This kind of chronic negative feedback can be disastrous to your self-image and confidence as a young learner, and unless you consciously overcome this conditioning, it will remain with you as a strong, unacknowledged influence throughout your adult life.[1]

The result is a very large number of Americans have been schooled to think dumb, to think they are dumb, and to believe that nothing can be done to change this. The result is a learning shutdown and an IQ stalemate. But it needn't stay this way.

Suggestion is a powerful tool. If you developed all your present attitudes from a pattern of negative suggestions, then what is to stop you from turning this all around and developing a new pattern from *positive suggestions*? You need to affirm your untapped brain power every day, and you do this by changing your programming, changing your inner attitude, and refueling your positive motivation.

6 WAYS TO AFFIRM YOUR MOTIVATION EVERY DAY

1. Say to yourself: "I *can be* smarter than I think I *am*. I am smarter than I think. I *can* master the basics of developing a sharp mind."
2. Repeat this sequence three times, saying it with conviction.
3. Repeat these affirmation sequences at least three times daily, preferably as soon as you wake up in the morning, at midday, and just before falling asleep.

4. It is psychologically more effective to say your affirmations out loud in a strong, clear, confident voice. Speaking them actually gives them energy and brings you closer to their realization in your life.
5. Use them like medicine: Every time you doubt your abilities, feel mentally sluggish, stupid or dense, repeat them, preferably out loud, to bolster your confidence.
6. Make this a daily practice: Write out your brain power goals; draft new or different affirmations, and say them out loud daily.

YOUR MIND IS THE KEY TO YOUR BRAIN POWER

Affirmations work because they actively engage your will, helping you to overcome and eventually silence the inner voice that keeps telling you the contrary, that you are no Einstein, that you are stupid. The approach is astonishingly simple, yet it's founded on a profound truth.

The power of the mind and our attitude to shape, influence, and alter reality is enormous— provided we believe it's possible.

Affirming our motivation that greater brain power is easily within our reach puts into practice the famous saying that with an ounce of faith we can move mountains. In this case, the mountain is a 3 $^{1}/_{2}$-pound universe—your brain.

Working with affirmations is like being a slick salesman, except you are also the customer and the goods are worth buying. The whole business is to convince the doubter in us that he or she is wrong. The doubter has that carping voice in the mind that always takes the negative side of any issue; generally we are only subconsciously aware of it, but this doesn't prevent it from being successful in making its case.

Through affirmations we bypass this inner doubter and appeal to a more positive aspect of ourselves. We tell the doubter that we can in fact improve ourselves despite all objections and arguments to the contrary, using the same guile and subtlety that the inner doubter normally uses to make you think you are not particularly smart or mentally agile.

So the key is this: *Pretend that it's possible to actively believe that you can enhance your brain power and resolve that you shall make it happen.*

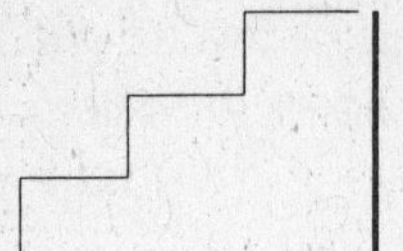

THE ANATOMY OF BRAIN POWER #1
Meet the 4 Players in the Game of Brain Power

In your quest for more brain power, it helps to know what are the elements of stronger brain function. Although we prefer to think of the brain as a whole, integrated, smoothly functioning unity, there are times when one aspect of brain power rather than another comes into the foreground.

If you think of these qualities as "mental muscles," then you must start seriously thinking about getting some *brain exercise* to keep them in working trim. So let's have a quick look at the major players in the game of higher brain power.

1. *Mental Strength*. When you need to concentrate on a difficult, challenging, or novel mental task, you need strength of mind. You have to be able to "lift" the problem and hold it before your attention.

   For example, mental strength comes into play when you are doing math calculations, weighing the factors in a hard decision, balancing your checkbook, preparing your income taxes (here you'll also need patience, detachment, and a sense of humor), or narrowing your focus to a single topic, problem, or factor.
2. *Mental Flexibility*. This quality refers to your ability to shift from one kind of mental task to another, such as writing a sentence to determining spatial relationships, or working up your math calculations to discussing creative marketing ideas on the telephone. It also means you can do mental gymnastics in your mind, turning issues inside out, looking at them sideways, backwards, upside down—in other words, creatively.
3. *Mental Endurance*. Say you have to write a marketing report, term paper, magazine article, or some other written product. You need endurance to sustain your mental focus on the task, to keep your level of inspiration and focus on line, to maintain the linear, logical thread of the presentation, and to generally stay brilliant on the task from start to finish. Endurance means you can shake off distraction, fatigue, and boredom until the task is finished.

4. *Mental Coordination*. This means you can do *three* marketing reports at the same time. When your mind has coordination, it does mean you can juggle several different but equally demanding mental tasks at once or in the same day.

   It also means you can maintain your focus in the foreground of each of their demands as well as to stay in focus regarding all three of them, as a kind of project manager. Mental coordination further means you can learn as you work, acquire new information, and create new solutions.

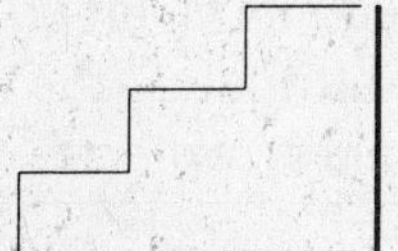

BRAIN BUILDERS! WORKOUT #1
"May I Have Your Attention, Please?" Says Brain Builder to Brain

Paying attention and being in command of your attention are essential tools to brain building. You might think of your attention as a kind of mental "muscle." The more you exercise this muscle, the stronger, more flexible, more dependable it becomes.

After all, if you want to wield your brain in a variety of mental tasks, you need to be able to hold its concentration steady on a given task, subject, object, or thought. Here is the first of many brain-builders exercises to tone up your attention muscle.

WATCHING THE CLOCK

- ▼ You need a large clock with a second hand for this exercise. Sit down comfortably, follow your breathing for a few cycles.
- ▼ Now for the next 2 minutes rivet your attention on the second hand. Do not be distracted by a single thought, sensation, or outer event for this 2 minutes.
- ▼ Give the slow-moving second hand your undivided, absolute attention. If your attention wanders, as soon as you catch it, start over again, and do the 2-minute clock watch again until you can remain undistracted for the full 2 minutes.

- When you have mastered this, increase the time to 5 minutes, then 7, then 10 minutes. Do this once a day for a month.

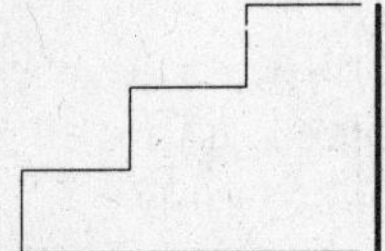

BRAIN-BUILDING SECRET #3
What the Smart Students Know—And How to Copy Them

Where better to look for brain-building secrets than the real professionals at the game of learning—students?[2] If there is a single key word that describes what makes smart students smart it is *attitude*. As you learned in brain-building secret #1, attitude is the key to everything: how you set up your experiences, beliefs, expectations, assumptions—your world view, in short.

Here are some elements that could usefully be part of your new attitude about learning. You might consider all of this a pep talk at the beginning of your new brain power building program. This is the key: *Start by assuming you are a smart student already, no matter what your age or background.*

THE 12-STEP SMART STUDENTS BELIEF SYSTEM

1. You can teach yourself any subject better than any other so-called teacher.
2. You may think you are doing enough when you listen studiously to your instructors and complete your assignments, but you're wrong.
3. Of all the assignments you get for reading and study, they are not all equally important; you need to rank and prioritize them.
4. Don't live your life worrying about grades; they are mostly only subjective opinions dished out by teachers.
5. If you truly want to learn and improve yourself, prepare to make mistakes and even appear foolish on behalf of being smart at the end of the day.
6. The next time you hear a question, remember the point is not to answer so much as it is to be stimulated to think more.

7. The whole point of being in school—or studying anything at any age—is not to simply repeat back what the teachers or books tell you, but to learn how to think for yourself.
8. Even though certain subjects may seem to bore you and lack relevance, the act of being actively engaged in studying them, thinking about the materials, mulling them over, is the key. Think of it as exercising your brain power muscles.
9. When you sit down and really start to learn, you may find this is unexpectedly intimidating and frustrating, yet it is—guaranteed—rewarding and enriching at the end of the day.
10. How well you do in school or in any course of study—whether independently undertaken or as part of a curriculum—depends more on your *attitude and method of study* rather than any particular scholastic ability.
11. Don't be seduced into studying and excelling at intellectual matters for the praise of your fellows or teachers, because this robs you of the true source of your hard-won self-esteem—your own sense of accomplishment.
12. School, learning, education, the life of the mind—they're all a kind of wonderful but important game.

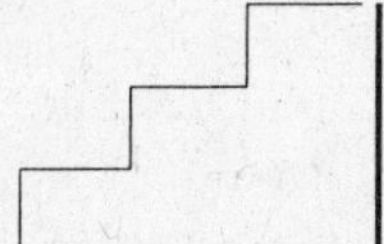

BRAIN-BUILDING SECRET #4
More About What the Smart Students Know—And How to Copy Them

I mentioned "method of study" earlier. Here are 12 tips for how to study.[3] When you sit down to a new course of study, or anything requiring your mental concentration and output, ask yourself these questions. You may find it helps you quickly organize the information and commit it to memory.

12 KEYS TO HIGH BRAIN POWER STUDYING

1. *What is your purpose for reading this*? Before you read even the first sentence, be clear in your mind what your intellectual goal is for this project.

2. *What do you already know about this topic*? Rummage through your mental file cabinets to call to mind what you already know on this subject. You might make some preliminary notes based on your initial recall.
3. *What is the big picture here*? Focus on the forest before you study the individual trees. Determine what the main points are, what the context and background for the subject are, and where it fits into a larger body of knowledge and experience.
4. *What is the author likely to say next*? Here it doesn't hurt to stay one step ahead of the author, if you can. If the material follows a logical, linear presentation, you should be able to anticipate the next stage in the information. This in itself will help you master it and remember it later.
5. *What are the key questions and topics in this field*? Every subject has a certain innate organizing structure to it, complete with jargon, special terminology, and key discussion topics. When you learn these, you have already understood half of the field itself because everything else is detail slotted into this master outline.
6. *What impact does this material have on my own thought processes*? Undoubtedly the material will raise questions, spark discussion, disagreement, or insight in you. Keep track of these reactions; they help to build your knowledge base and sense of familiarity with the subject. Again, these are supports that later will enable you to recall the material easily.
7. *What is the essential information*? You need to evaluate, rank, and prioritize the information as it comes in; not all belongs at the top of your study list; some is worthy only of footnotes. Put it all in order as you go.
8. *Can you see ways to paraphrase and summarize the information*? This is like making an outline in your head as you move through the material. Translate the author's words and jargon into your own working vocabulary; personalizing the information is another learning and memory support.
9. *How can I better organize this information*? After you have completed your first pass through on the study material, see if there is a way you can organize it even more intelligently than the author. The more contact you have with the material you are trying to learn, the easier it gets.

10. Is *there any way you can picture this information*? See if you can translate the material into a compact set of symbols and pictures as an abbreviated outline form.
11. *What is your hook for remembering all this material*? This is a single memory device (or gimmick) such as a story, picture, rhyme, expression, or summary phrase that encapsulates the subject so well that when you see it again it brings the whole field back into active memory for you.
12. *How does the material you're studying integrate with what you already know*? Context and relevance are crucial to any real learning and ability to recall. When information assumes a natural, integral part of your life and concerns, it becomes incredibly easy to remember it.

BRAIN BUILDERS!
WORKOUT #2
A Brain-Builder's Reminder

- ▼ Practice this for an hour during whatever activities you might be engaged in. Keep repeating to yourself, internally, I *am paying attention*!
- ▼ When you notice that you have forgotten to repeat this phrase in your mind, restart your brain-builder's reminder.
- ▼ When you discover you have been seriously distracted and suddenly snap back to your resolve to repeat this phrase, say I *am paying attention*! out loud 5 times; then return to voicing it mentally.

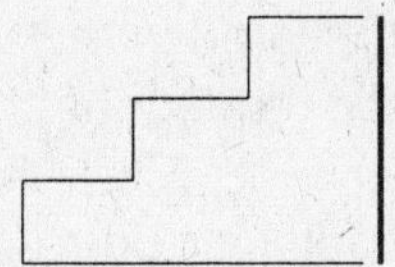

BRAIN-BUILDING SECRET #5
There Is More Than One Way to Be Intelligent —Introducing the 7 Kinds of Brain Power

One of your biggest obstacles to increasing your brain power is your idea of intelligence itself and how much of it you have. Here it is very easy to be misled and misinformed and to form mistaken impressions of the amount and quality of your own natural brain power. That's why the breakthrough insights of psychologist Howard Gardner are so valuable for building the maximum brain.

GET IN TUNE WITH YOUR 7 NATURAL INTELLIGENCES

Over a period of 15 years, Gardner developed a theory that each person has 7 *intelligences*, all different and equally important. These multiple intelligences, says Gardner, are the following:

1. *Linguistic*: the ability to use words skillfully and to express concepts fluently,
2. *Logical-mathematical*: understanding numerical relationships.
3. *Spatial*: the ability to think in pictures and images and to transform the visual-spatial world.
4. *Musical*: the ability to hear and produce rhythms, melodies, and harmonies.
5. *Bodily/kinesthetic*: athletic intelligence to control one's body with dexterity.
6. *Interpersonal*: the ability to understand and interact with other people.
7. *Intrapersonal*: intelligence of the inner self.

In light of this theory, standard IQ tests clearly cannot measure very much of your brain power, perhaps only 2 of the 7 intelligences everyone has.

There might be 7 different and relatively independent brain systems, corresponding to each of these multiple intelligences. For example, scientists believe that linguistic intelligence is seated in the left-brain hemisphere, while the musical, spatial, and interpersonal intelligences may be situated in the right hemisphere.

This means that insult or injury to specific regions of your brain may impair the full functioning of each of these intelligences. The 7 intelligences concept about human IQ is based in biology, in the actual physiology and anatomy of the brain itself.

This means we need to redefine our idea of intelligence based on the best examples of each of the seven kinds.[4]

EXAMPLES OF THE 7 INTELLIGENCES AT WORK

1. A novel like Herman Melville's *Moby Dick* may represent a high example of *linguistic intelligence.*
2. The chess mastery of world champion Bobby Fischer represents a high degree of *logical-mathematical intelligence.*
3. Pablo Picasso's *Guernica* painting may be a top example of *spatial intelligence.*
4. The group work of a leading psychotherapist like Arnold Mindell may represent a state of high *interpersonal intelligence.*
5. The highly sensitive soul-searching poetry of Rainer Maria Rilke might illustrate *intrapersonal intelligence.*
6. The violin virtuosity of Itzhak Perlman may demonstrate extraordinary *musical intelligence.*
7. The Olympic figure skating artistry of Oxana Bayul may stand for the highest in *bodily/kinesthetic intelligence.*

In other words, if you do not excel in either linguistic or logical-mathematical intelligence, there are still five other legitimate categories in which your brain power may in fact surpass those who are only word or number smart.[5]

A CHECKLIST THAT GIVES YOU A NEW VIEW ON YOUR BRAIN POWER

So here is a checklist quiz to reassess your intelligence.[6] You may be sure that it will prove you are smarter than you think because your idea of intelligence itself needs to be expanded to include all "7 kinds of smart." This exercise will show you something new and exciting about your own brain power. The value of this exercise and new way of thinking about intelligence, Armstrong says, is that through this you can get "a full-spectrum video of your total abilities as a learner and not just a black-and-white snapshot that tags you with a meaningless label."

Simply check each question that pertains to you. Then when you're finished, see which categories have the most checks.

WORD INTELLIGENCE: IS YOUR INTELLIGENCE VERBAL/ LINGUISTIC?

___ Are books important to you, more than other ways of gathering information?

___ Do you hear words and sentences in your mind before you talk and does it seem like taking dictation when you write?

___ Do you prefer radio, audiocassettes, or books-on-tape to visual media such as television or movies?

___ Do you excel at word games like Scrabble, Anagrams, or Password?

___ Are you a punster, entertaining friends with wordplays, jokes, puns, and deliberate slips of the tongue?

___ Do you find you are consulted as a walking dictionary, in which friends ask you to explain obscure words or that you use words in your own communication that are foreign to them?

___ In school, were subjects like English, history, social studies, and art history easier and more interesting for you than math and science?

___ When you're speeding along the freeway, do you compulsively read all the billboards and highway signs and ignore the scenery?

___ Do you often refer to things you've recently read or studied when you're in conversation?

NUMBER INTELLIGENCE: IS YOUR INTELLIGENCE LOGICAL/MATHEMATICAL?

___ Can you easily figure numbers and columns in your head?

___ When you were in school, did you prefer and excel in math, science, statistics, and logic?

___ Do you particularly enjoy working brainteasers, puzzles, or games that require logical thinking?

___ Do you have the kind of mind that delights in posing "what if"? scenarios as little experiments to see how things would change if you changed certain factors?

___ Do you habitually look for regularities, rhythms, patterns, and logical order in events, relationships, or activities?

___ Do you follow new developments in science and technology with keen interest?

___ Do you believe that everything can be rationally explained?

___ When thinking, do your concepts sometimes appear without words or images, but as clear abstractions?

___ Without trying, do you identify the logical flaws and inconsistencies in what people tell you or how they go about their work?

___ Are you more at ease after something has been translated into quantities, categories, measurements, and thoroughly analyzed rather than when it remains vague and mysterious?

PICTURE INTELLIGENCE: IS YOUR INTELLIGENCE SPATIAL/ PICTORIAL?

___ When you close your eyes do you often see pictures and clear images?

___ Are you especially sensitive to color and appreciate its nuances, subtleties, and energy?

___ Do you like recording events around you with a camera, sketchbook, or video recorder rather than taking notes?

___ Do you enjoy picture puzzles, crosswords, mazes, and other puzzles that are visual in nature?

___ Are your dreams especially vivid, like watching movies?

___ Can you easily find your way around unfamiliar territories even without a map?

___ Do you enjoy doodling, sketching, or drawing?

___ In school, was geometry easier for you than algebra?

___ Can you easily visualize with your mind's eye what an object would look like if you could see it from different angles or from above?

___ When it comes to books or magazines, do you prefer texts that have lots of pictures, charts, and diagrams?

BODY INTELLIGENCE: IS YOUR INTELLIGENCE BODILY/ KINESTHETIC?

___ Do you practice at least one physical sport, such as tennis, basketball, volleyball, racketball, golf, or surfing on a regular basis?

___ Are you unable to sit still for extended periods of time?

___ Do you especially enjoy, if not prefer, working with your hands in hands-on activities such as sewing, weaving, pottery, sculpting, jewelry making, carving, or carpentry?

___ Do you get your most inspired ideas when you're outside, walking, running, canoeing, hang gliding, or doing some another kind of active motion sport?

___ Do you spend as much of your leisure time outdoors as possible?

___ When you're talking with a friend, do you find you use your hands, arms, head, and torso to emphsize points?

___ Are you the kind of person who has to touch things to be able to know it or learn more about them?

___ Do you consider yourself well coordinated?

___ When it comes to learning about a new skill, do you need to instantly put it into practice rather than watching it or reading about it?

MUSIC INTELLIGENCE: IS YOUR INTELLIGENCE MUSICAL/ RHYTHMIC?

___ Is your voice pleasant and sonorous when singing?

___ When listening to music, can you easily tell when a note is off key?

___ Do you spend a lot of time listening to music, much more so than reading or watching movies?

___ Do you play a musical instrument or do you daydream of doing so?

___ If all the music were removed from your life, even your ability to sing in the shower, would your life be impoverished?

___ Walking down the street or driving your car, do you sometimes break into singing or whistling a familiar jingle, pop song, show tune, cantata, or oratorio, or do these things play in your mind like records?

___ Using a simple percussion instrument or even tapping your fingers, can you keep a rhythm?

___ Do you know the tunes and melodies to a variety of songs and pieces?

___ After hearing a new piece of music only once, can you reproduce it fairly accurately?

___ When you're working or studying, do you often tap your fingers, whistle, hum, or sing little melodies to yourself?

PEOPLE INTELLIGENCE: IS YOUR INTELLIGENCE INTERPERSONAL/INTERACTIVE?

___ Do people at work or in your neighborhood naturally come to you for guidance and consultations?

___ When it comes to games and sports, do you prefer group and team activities such as volleyball and softball rather than swimming or jogging?

___ When a problem arises, do you typically seek out the advice and discussion of friends rather than struggling with it alone?

___ Do you have at least five good friends?

___ When it comes to entertainments, do you prefer social games such as Monopoly or bridge instead of solitaire or video games?

___ When you know how to do something, do you enjoy teaching others?

___ Do you or your friends consider yourself a leader?

___ Are you comfortable and at ease in crowds and among lots of strangers?

___ Do you tend to get involved in community-based activities?

___ Would you rather spend a free evening at a social gathering rather than reading a book alone at home?

INNER INTELLIGENCE: IS YOUR INTELLIGENCE INTRAPERSONAL/INTERIOR?

___ Do you often spend time alone in reflection, contemplation, meditation, or inner work and thought?

___ Have you been to counseling sessions or personal growth workshops?

___ Do you enjoy learning more about yourself?

___ Do your opinions set you apart from the crowd of your contemporaries?

___ Is there a special interest, hobby, or line of study that you enjoy but keep private from others?

___ Do you often stop to assess how you're progressing with respect to your short- and long-term life goals?

___ In your opinion, do you have a sober and realistic idea of your strengths and weaknesses, based on your own reflection and the feedback of others?

___ Would you rather spend a weekend alone in a rustic cabin in Maine than at a bustling casino hotel in Las Vegas?

___ Are you strong-willed, independent, and do you think for yourself?

___ Do you keep a diary or journal to record the important inner events of your life and what they mean to you?

___ Are you self-employed or have you thought favorably about trying it out as a life-style choice?

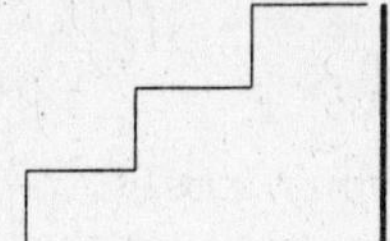

BRAIN BUILDERS! WORKOUT #3
Pay Attention to Your Attention Paying

- This exercise develops two levels of paying attention. Pick up an illustrated magazine, one that you do not normally read, and casually thumb through it, pausing for a few moments at each page. Keep repeating to yourself I *am paying attention*!
- Notice which articles, pictures, words, or illustrations distract you.
- Notice how your mind gets distracted. Notice how it is like a dog on a leash that suddenly darts out, yanking the leash out of your hand.
- Rein your attention back in. Pay attention to the way your attention comes and goes, to how easily it is to be distracted.

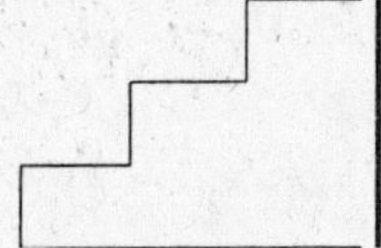

BRAIN-BUILDING SECRET #6
7 Ways to Hone Your Intelligences For Greater Brain Power

Now that you have reassessed the state of your mind and come to the conclusion that you are smarter than you thought and have intelligence in areas you never before thought even counted when it came to intelligence, here are some simple practical exercises to hone your various intelligences into an even sharper edge.[7]

1. Word Intelligence

- Read a complete book each week and write a report describing its contents, theme, plot, whether it was well written and why, whether you liked it and why, and how it might rank with other books of its kind.
- Get a good dictionary and start with the A's. Learn three new words a day, the stranger and more unfamiliar the better. Try them out in sentences. Look for them when you read. Go through the entire dictionary.

- When you come across unfamiliar words while reading, circle them, look up their meanings, and memorize them.
- Listen to audiotapes of writers and poets reading. Listen to books-on-tapes in which actors read famous books out loud. Study how the words and sentences sound. Note dialects and speech intonations. Try to imitate these.
- Select a short story, poem, or brief essay that particularly appeals to you. Memorize it completely, perhaps three lines a day. When you have it committed to memory, practice reciting it out loud.
- Study fine writing and classical literature to see how good writing is done. Consider reading works by Thomas Mann, Marcel Proust, Virginia Woolf, Henry James, and Lawrence Durrell. Note how they put sentences together, how they bend the grammar, how they use unusual adjectives to make a point.

2. Picture Intelligence

- Work on jigsaw puzzles, Rubik's cube, mazes, graphics software programs for your computer, or the game Pictionary.
- Take up photography, video-recording, drawing, sketching, geometry, and the principles of architecture and design.
- Analyze topographical maps, flowcharts, engineering diagrams, architectural floor plans, visual dictionary, or any other kind of visual representations. Walk your way through these illustrations. Try to visualize them in three dimensions.
- Watch the movies of film masters such as Alfred Hitchcock, Stanley Kubrick, and Bernardo Bertolucci, and note how they compose each shot, what colors they use, what perspective, how things move.
- Visit an art museum. Select one painting that especially appeals to you. Find out why you like it. Figure out its design strategy. Commit it in all its detail to memory. Later, recreate the picture in your mind.

- With your eyes closed, visualize these scenes and images: your mother, father, and siblings on the ceiling of your bedroom; your face when you were 6 years old; the exact contents and layout of your garage; a black cross with seven red roses at its central crossing.
- Select an object such as your coffee table or favorite padded chair and while seated close to it, visualize seeing it from every possible angle and perspective. See it from underneath, directly overhead, from the side on, from 360° in 30° segments. Then walk around the actual object and examine it from all the perspectives you have just visualized. Compare the results.
- Take a blank piece of paper and using a pencil, make a sketch of the inside of a washing machine, the inside of your body, the floor plan for your bedroom with all furniture in place, your neighborhood for up to three blocks.

3. Music Intelligence

- While sitting comfortably in a chair, your shoes and glasses off, try bringing to mind these musical sounds, one at a time: the theme song from your favorite television show or movie; the sound of your singing voice; the sound of rain on the roof and windows; the sound of an oboe, clarinet, trumpet, and harp, one at a time; the sound of wind chimes; the sound of church bells.
- Select an instrument that appeals to you, such as a clarinet or oboe. Find music that features it; listen to it until you have memorized the quality of the sound. Consider learning how to play that instrument.
- Listen to new, unfamiliar kinds of music every week.
- Listen for music, melodies, rhythms, and harmonies in exotic unmusical formats, such as the sound of machines, automobiles, traffic, weather, nature, your own bodily sounds.
- Make up your own music and tunes while in the shower, driving, walking. Hum, sing, whistle, scat it.

4. Body Intelligence

- Using a pair of tweezers, transfer 100 grains of rice from one bowl into another, as quickly as possible, without spilling any.
- Bring to mind a physical skill you excel at or which you practice often, such as a golf swing, a swimming stroke, a hatha yoga posture, a gymnastics drill, a figure-skating double axle, a ballet jump, an over-the-head soccer kick. Now, while sitting in a chair and without moving a muscle, *visualize* your body moving through all the steps in any of these actions. Take yourself through this action in all its detail. Sense how your muscles are stretched, the position of your body, your rate of breathing, the symmetry of your torso.
- Study a martial art like karate, akido, judo; learn tai chi chuan, hatha yoga, pantomime, charades, sign language, Eurythmy, mudras, or dance.

5. Number Intelligence

Make your best guess regarding these questions:

- How many dimes would you have to stack to reach the top of the World Trade Center in Manhattan?
- How many times have you inhaled in your life?
- How many words have you spoken in your life?
- How many sentences have you heard spoken in your life, including television, movies, and radio?
- How many people in the world are kissing at this very moment?
- How many full-body prostrations would you have to make if you were to do a prostration pilgrimage from where you are to where you were born?
- How many grains of salt have you consumed in your life, including the salt that was in prepared food products?
- How many bottles of champagne would it take to turn your house into a swimming pool so that the water was up to the ceiling in all rooms?

- How many photographs does your favorite daily newspaper publish in one year?
- How many windows are there in all the houses and buildings in your hometown?
- How many minutes would it take you to write out all the contents of this book in the hand you never use for writing?

6. People Intelligence

- Turn on the television or a movie but keep the sound off. Study the body language of the people before you. Watch their facial, hand, and torso gestures. What are they saying to one another? Can you figure out the plot based on body cues alone?
- Watch a "foreign" movie in its own language without subtitles or dubbing. Or watch a Spanish or French language channel on cable. Make sure it's a language and culture you are unfamiliar with. Can you figure out what's going on based on the body language and the language sounds?
- Spend 10–15 minutes a day actively listening to somebody. Ignore all your own thoughts, emotions, and opinions, Listen. Study their gestures, facial expressions, posture, tone of voice. Be as objective as possible.
- Spend 10–15 minutes sitting on a park bench or a rotunda within a mall, an airport lounge, a restaurant—any place where you can watch people. Pretend you are an anthropologist or an extraterrestrial. Observe everything. What can you learn about the people you are observing?

7. Inner Intelligence

- Find out who you are. Make a picture of yourself. Take a few pages from a newspaper, magazines, plus art materials such as scissors, glue, transparent tape, crayons, pencils, pastels.
- Make a collage of all the different aspects of yourself. Include descriptive words, adjectives, or nouns that pertain to you. You might picture all of your personalities as planets revolving around the central sun that is the real you. Use pictures and words to show it all.

- Read autobiographies of celebrities and literary, historical, and spiritual figures. Notice what they emphasize, how they describe themselves, what they have learned about themselves. Listen to the narrative voice and tone. What does it tell you about the person?
- Pretend you are about to die or go away on a lifelong trip, never to return. Write a personal statement or life testimonial to leave behind for the loved ones left. Tell them who you thought you were, what you tried to accomplish, whether you think you succeeded, what it all meant.
- Spend the next week trying to remember your dreams. Write down the dream stories in as much detail as you can remember. When you have a handful of dreams, choose one.
- Select the one with the most vivid imagery or the most mysterious plot. Spend the next week thinking about it. If the dream had several characters, pretend being each one.
- Try to understand what role the characters play in your dream. Have a dialogue with each of them. Ask them what they have to say to you.

THE ANATOMY OF BRAIN POWER #2

Your Brain Can Change—Why Your Brain Power Should Never Cease Growing

When you were born, your brain had an estimated 100 billion nerve cells, or neurons. Your neurons are concentrated in a 2-millimeter-thick layer on the outer surface of your brain's cortex, the famous "gray matter." During your life, your brain must process 3 billion stimuli every second just for you to stay awake.

Now consider these facts. The average human IQ is 100; genius is 160; yet a typical person uses only about 4 percent of his total potential brain power. Clearly there is a good reason to improve your brain power: 96 percent more brain function awaits you.

THE SECRET LIFE OF YOUR BRAIN— A BIOLOGICAL BIOGRAPHY

The brain grows astonishingly quickly during the prenatal period. The nervous system begins forming itself within 20 days of conception; around day 35, the brain begins to develop. Neuroblasts, which are precursors of neurons, the basic brain cells, are generated at the rate of several thousand a minute. After 12 weeks of growth, the fetus adds new neurons at the rate of 2,000 a second, provided the mother is keeping her nutrition in order. (See Diagram 1-1.)

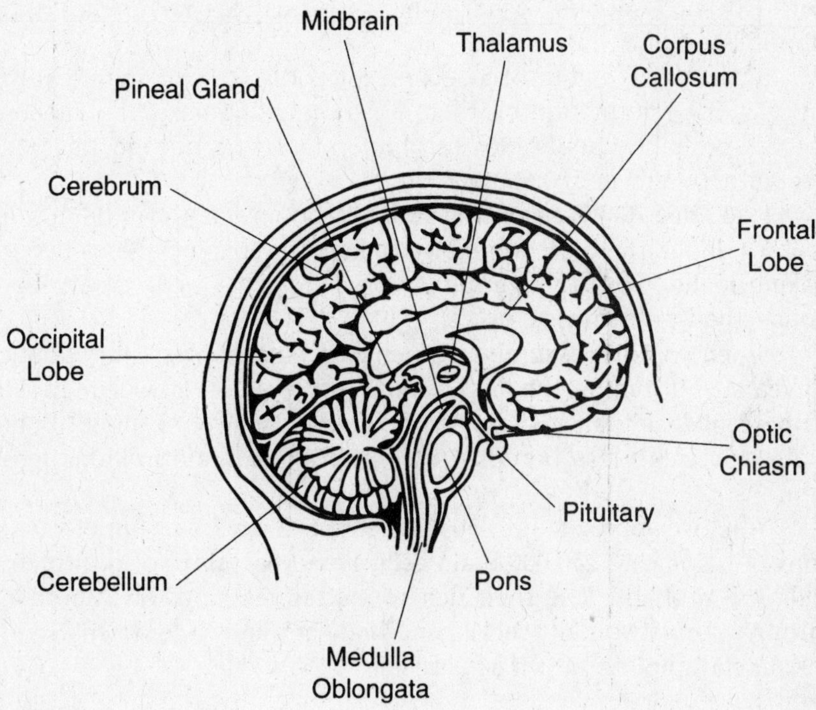

Diagram 1-1

Malnourishment of the mother can lead to children with 50 percent fewer neurons than average, adequately nourished children. Then at 20 weeks after conception, the fetus's entire nervous system is complete, with its 15 billion neurons in place. Although this prodigious network of brain cells comprises only 2 percent of body weight, it will require up to 20 percent of your bodily oxygen supply.

YOU'RE LOSING NEURONS AS YOU COUNT THEM

Incidentally, are there mathematical limits to how much you can perceive in a given moment of time? Perhaps. According to scientific research, most of us can manage seven different bits of information—such as sounds, visual stimuli, or nuances in thought and emotion—at one time.

It takes one eighth of a second (or about 0.00165 minutes) to process one information bit then move on to the next. This means you can probably handle 126 bits of information per second, or 7,560 a minute, or almost 500,000 per hour.

If you live 70 years and stay awake 16 hours a day, your brain will process about 185 billion bits of information. This includes all your waking reality, your thoughts, memories, feelings, actions, perceptions—the whole movie.

When you die, assuming you enjoy a natural lifespan of about 75 years, your brain—the "3 1/2-pound universe"—will weigh about 10 percent less than it did when you were a newborn infant. Your brain will weigh less because it will literally contain millions less neurons.

You lose approximately 50,000 neurons a day from your cerebral cortex, or some 18,250,000 brain cells every year. Many of your brain cells will probably lose their rich connectedness with one another, through the network of tendrils and branches known as *dendrites* and the junction points known as *synapses*. [8]

MENTAL EXERCISE CAN STOP THE BRAIN DRAIN

What is most remarkable about these statistics is that in no way does it mean or guarantee there will be (or should be) the slightest drop in your brain power.

In fact, with "mental exercise," you may not regenerate brain cells, but you will surely stimulate their connectivity, ensuring that you can potentially finish your life in full command of your natural brain power despite the massive brain cell loss every day.

This fact underlies the optimistic conclusion of neuroscientists that the human brain is astonishingly plastic, flexible, and resilient; it can adapt, get by with less, grow more connections between existing cells so that no significant loss of brain power will ever be registered. In fact, it may be virtually insignificant that your brain loses 16 million neurons a year because neuroscientists now think you never needed 100 billion in the first place.[9]

Anyway, the secret is how you use (or sculpt) the neurons that remain. That's why mental exercise, or brain-building techniques described in this book, is the secret to keeping your brain power intact throughout your life. As you learn more, you grow more synapses; as you stimulate your brain more, you grow more dendrites.

GETTING OLD DOESN'T MEAN YOUR BRAIN POWER HAS TO DROP

One brain scientist remarks that after examining the brains of normal elderly people over 90, he finds them "indistinguishable" from the brains of healthy people in their midtwenties. These are "perfect" brains with "absolutely nothing wrong at all," which is why he concludes that there simply isn't enough evidence to say that aging alone negatively affects the function of the brain.[10]

Instead, it seems that even as you age, your brain can change its structure, grow more synapses, sprout more dendrites, and increase its *neuronal connectivity*. If you go about it correctly (which means practice brain-building exercises), your brain cells will continue to form new connections (which means faster, more complex processing abilities) throughout the life of your brain.

A single neuron can have 100,000 synapses that connect it with neighboring brain cells. All told, there are probably *trillions* of interconnections made possible by your dendrites and axons. In fact, if you take the conservative estimate that, on average, each neuron has 1,000 synapses, that gives your brain a total of 100 *trillion* possible connections. That is why it's possible to improve your brain power and why it is possible for you to make instant, far-reaching intuitive connections far faster than a computer.[11]

Challenge your mind daily and you are literally stimulating your dendrites to proliferate their connections with other brain cells. The key is *stimulation*. Keep your brain *stimulated* and you feed your brain cells the "energy" they require to keep active and connected. Keep your mind *enriched* and its synapses will hum.

And the key to brain stimulation are the brain-building secrets outlined in this book.

AN INSPIRING SCIENCE-FICTION STORY ABOUT YOUR BRAIN

If the human brain is indeed this plastic, might it not be genetically improvable? The idea of using genetics to artificially enhance human intelligence is of course an idea that has already occurred to science-fiction writers.

In his recent science fiction novel *Jupiter's Daughter*, Tom Hyman imagines a Nobel Prize-winning geneticist manipulating the human gene pool to gain a 100 percent increase in IQ, so that a child would be born with an IQ of 200.

The scientist's technique was to reactivate about 800 of the thousands of dormant genes in the human DNA, to switch them back into life. In this way, he created a new human being with extraordinary capacities, enhanced intelligence, health, and strength.

This new girl, the first daughter of the Jupiter project, had 804 extra and active genes, but that made all the difference. In addition, a brain scan of the girl's corpus callosum showed a high degree of brain chemical activity. In other words, her two hemispheres were working as virtually a single integrated brain, and she was processing a great deal more information, and faster, than the average brain.

Let's remember that what is the science fiction of tomorrow may well be the inspiration of today. The essential inspiration of *Jupiter's Daughter* and the fact that aging does not spell the end of your mental abilities is that your brain power, like any muscle, can be built, strengthened, flexed, and improved during your lifetime.

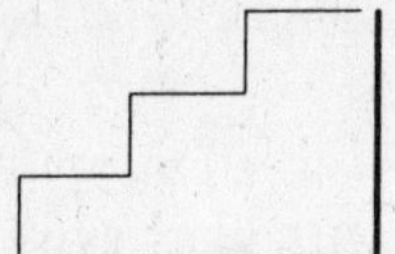

BRAIN BUILDERS! WORKOUT #4
Counting Your Change at the Basketball Game

This exercise trains your attention on several levels simultaneously. First, run through a series of number expansions:

1. Count backward from 100 in 4's.
2. Keep doubling a number for as long as possible, as in 3, 6, 12, 24, 48, 96, 192, . . .
3. Count in 4's, as 4, 8, 12, 16, 20, 24, . . . while visualizing the number sequence 5, 10, 15, 20, 25, . . .
4. Now while practicing one of these number sequences, visualize in as much detail the following scenes, one at a time:

   a. Watching a championship basketball game
   b. Touring an art gallery
   c. Having dinner at a sushi bar
   d. Building a stone wall around your house.

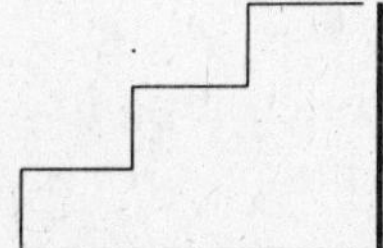

BRAIN-BUILDING SECRET #7
How to Anchor In More Effective Learning and Memory

There is a witty saying attributed to Marilyn Monroe that pertains to our interest in developing better brain power: "I can't memorize the words by themselves. I have to memorize the feelings."

This exercise is called *anchoring*, because it involves a method of linking positive emotional qualities to your learning experience and your body through creating *magic buttons*. The idea is to match an external stimulus with an internal emotional or psychological state as a way of reinforcing the memory.[12]

7 STEPS TO TRULY CHANGING YOUR MIND WHILE YOU WAIT

1. Sit in a comfortable chair in a relaxed way, with your eyes closed and your breathing calm and slow. Establish rapport with yourself, as if you were both teacher and student.
2. Bring to mind a situation or experience in which you felt happiness, acceptance, success, triumph, and joy, and savor it like a good wine. This experience could be a moment when, during study, you understood a subject, had a wonderful insight, received a teacher's praise, or had some kind of enjoyable educational breakthrough.
3. Move your attention fully into this remembered experience. Try to recreate the entire episode, visualizing all its details. Picture how your body was in this earlier time and "step" into it as if you were donning a costume. Note what you are seeing, hearing, and feeling, and enter these sensations in depth. Be sure to cast all your descriptions—whether you say them aloud or in your mind—in the present tense, as if it's all happening now.
4. When you feel you are really here and now in this happy experience, touch your earlobe or wrist and hold the spot for 5 seconds. This creates the "magic button," which is to say, a trigger point on your body where, when you touch it again, you should be able to evoke the same pleasant memory, or at least the sensation of pleasantness.
5. Wait 10 minutes, then touch your magic button again. Do you experience the same sensation as you remembered earlier? The magic button can now work for you as a *positive conditioned response* (as opposed to an unconscious negative conditioned response) which you can deliberately use as a trigger to generate a positive state of mind and emotions suitable for learning.

   You have *anchored* this positive trigger in your body. When you can change your mental state to one that is positive and uplifting, this is an excellent learning environment.

6. As a variation, you can install a series of *linked anchors*, or magic buttons in sequence. Say you have an exam, sales meeting, marketing conference, or television interview, and you wish you weren't so nervous about it. You can set up linked anchors along the lines of anxiety, calmness, and confidence.
7. Following the same procedure just described, anchor a feeling of anxiety about exams on the first knuckle of your right hand. Anchor the feeling of calmness in the face of pressure on the second knuckle. Then using your third knuckle, anchor in the feeling of confidence, ease, and success. Wait 10 minutes; then test the anchoring.

   The next time you are confronted with an exam or conference, you can knuckle your way through to a calm, confident state of mind in seconds by pressing these preset body triggers or "magic buttons."

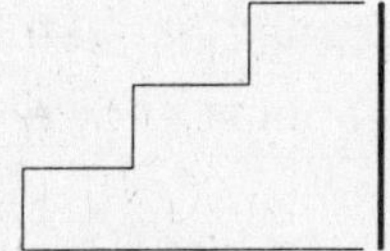

BRAIN-BUILDING SECRET #8
How to Be in Charge of Your Own Brain—At Least the Movie Division

The essence of this new brain-building secret has to do with memory and the emotional quality you attach to its contents. Here is the key: *By changing the emotional quality of your memory of the past, you can build better memory powers in the present.*

Say you had a seriously unpleasant experience in your past, such that you prefer not to recall it or when it comes up you pass over it fleetingly, sparing yourself most of the details. Think of your memories as similar to a television image; your television has controls for adjusting every aspect of the picture, including the brightness, contrast, speed, and duration.

Your mind has far more "controls" over the pictures, or visual memories, it serves up to you, often unbidden, so why not learn how to work the knobs on your brain's picture-generating function?

HOW TO REDIRECT THE MOVIE OF YOUR LIFE—NOW IN PROGRESS

The reason for doing this is that when you can voluntarily—consciously—adjust the brightness or intensity of these remembered images, you can change the way you *feel today* about them.

This means you can defuse the emotional pain or discomfort from past memories by readjusting your memory of them in the present. You can change your emotional response to your memories by changing the form in which you remember them by *reframing* them—changing the way you picture them in your mind.

These are some of the adjustable "controls" on your brain's image-generating function. As you read through this list of 13 changes you can make, bring to mind first a highly pleasant memory and go through all the picture control options; then repeat this exercise making the adjustments on a miserable recollection. As you make each adjustment, note how you now feel about the contents of the memory.

With this exercise, you are retracing the steps consciously that your brain and emotions took long ago unconsciously to put the experience into a *frame* of reference. Maybe it wasn't the best choice in frames.

13 WAYS TO REPROGRAM THE WAY YOU REMEMBER

1. *Color*. Change the intensity of color from bright, vivid colors to a dull black and white.
2. *Distance*. How far away are you as viewer from the scene? Bring it in closer, then push it farther away.
3. *Depth*. See the picture as a flat, two-dimensional image, then deepen and broaden it so it is fully three-dimensional, even a "wrap-around" picture.
4. *Duration*. Pan quickly across the scene, taking it in only superficially, then go over it along with long steady shots, registering the scene in depth.
5. *Clarity*. This is the focus control: Make the image fuzzy and indistinct, now sharpen it so it is perfectly, vividly clear in all its details.

6. *Contrast*. Here you can play with the relative degree of light, dark, and gray in your picture memory.
7. *Scope*. You can switch from focusing on the foreground with only close-up items filling the frame or zoom back to include all of the background that even includes events happening behind your head.
8. *Movement*. Freeze the frame so that it is a still-life photograph, now fast-forward so that it is a living, moving image.
9. *Hue*. Here you can adjust the color balance. Highlight the reds and oranges; then try the blues and greens.
10. *Transparency*. Make the image transparent, like glass, so you can see through it to what's happening behind and beyond it.
11. *Aspect Ratio*. You can reframe the image into a tall, narrow frame, then into a wide, short, squat frame.
12. *Orientation*. Tilt the top of the picture away from you, then toward you; do the same with the bottom half of the image.
13. *Foreground/Background*. You can pull the foreground up close, forgetting about the background, or zoom in on the background entirely so the foreground becomes fuzzy.

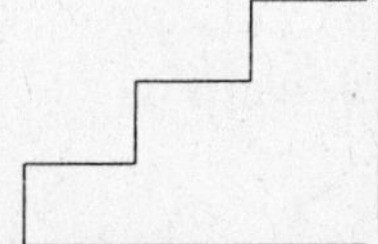

BRAIN-BUILDING SECRET #9
How to Be in Charge of Your Own Brain—The Sequel

So much of how you feel about a situation—and thus your ability to remember it—depends on how you framed the experience in the first place.

Experiences are reframeable—that's the brain-building secret here.

"I think *everything* is unfinished in this sense: You can only maintain any memory, belief, understanding, or other mental process from one day to the next if you continue to do it," psychologist Richard Bandler comments.

Think of unpleasant learning experiences you may have had earlier in your life, in school or at work. You may have developed a math phobia, an initial frustration with arithmetic that developed into an insecurity, then a lifelong aversion to numbers, and to a lifelong lack of self-confidence in having any ability to be good with numbers. Psychologists call these "school phobias."

HANGING A NEW PICTURE FRAME—OF YOUR BRAIN POWER

You might as well call it a "brain power phobia" because it may work as a serious obstacle at the start of your resolve to enhance your intelligence. These events could have framed your inner attitude about learning (and thus brain power) for life and will continue to frame them negatively unless you change it.

In other words, when you combine the attitude-shifting work of Brain-Building Secret #1 with the reframing technique for adjusting memories in this brain-building secret, you get a powerful and effective tool to start your brain-building program. Here is another technique to try in complement with reframing your past.[13]

5 EASY STEPS TO ELIMINATE OLD ANTIBRAIN POWER HABITS

Use this exercise for shifting old, entrenched habits or "automatic pilot" states of mind, such as I *am too dumb to boost my brain power, because that's what my parents, teachers, friends, and associates have always told me*. It might also be a math phobia, a learning phobia, a fear of complex intellectual ideas, nail biting when nervous.

1. *Identify the context*. Select which long-term habit you wish to remove. Think about it, get the matter clear in your mind.You will probably need to close your eyes for this exercise.
2. *Identify the cue picture*. Let's say it's a reluctance to work with numbers, balance your checkbook, figure your taxes. You might picture yourself pushing away a table of numbers such as a bank statement, burying the calculator under some magazines, and telling yourself you're no good with numbers.

Try to summon up the feeling you normally experience when confronted with a task like this; no doubt, it is some degree of unpleasantness, discomfort, irritation, and impatience. When you have the "taste" of this feeling, you have found your cue picture.

3. *Visualize a picture of a better outcome*. Here you create a second image of how you would see yourself differently if you were the master of the thing you are avoiding—something on the order of a math genius, or at least someone able and interested in balancing the checkbook.

   Find an image that is highly complimentary and pleasurable; perhaps you should exaggerate this a little and picture yourself as a certified public accountant, working with 10-digit numbers for a giant corporation. Smile at this image, as if you are proud and satisfied with your accomplishment.

4. *Swish*. Give the cue picture plenty of light, color, and brightness; make it large, vivid, and in full contrast. Remember, this is the picture of yourself as a math incompetent.

   Put the second image of yourself as a math genius as a small, dark image in the lower right corner of the cue picture. Say "swish" out loud, and reverse the pictures.

   Make the math genius picture grow to full size and fill with light and brilliance; make the cue picture of math incompetent shrink down to a postcard stamp in the corner. Do this as fast as possible, in a second or less. Open your eyes and forget about both images for a moment; look around the room. Notice how you feel. Repeat this swishing reversal 5 more times.

5. *The test*. Bring to mind your first cue picture, yourself as a math phobic. Does it feel or look different now? If you swished correctly, the cue picture will tend to fade away and yourself as the glorious math genius will take its place.

   To be really sure, unbury your calculator from under the magazines, fetch the bank statement from the wastebasket, and start balancing your checkbook—you math genius, you.

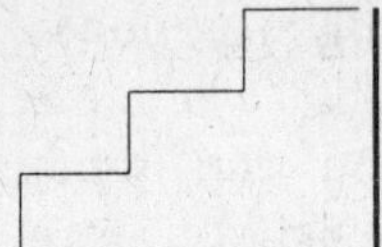

BRAIN BUILDERS! WORKOUT #5 Keeping Your Attention on the Word Family

- Select a word with many meanings and references, such as "imagination" or "medicine." Write the word at the center of a large piece of paper. Draw a circle around it.
- Now start writing down all the ideas and relationships that connect with this single word; draw a circle around each and connect it to the central word with a straight line.
- Keep building up your associations and generating your word family until you have filled the page. Don't allow yourself to be distracted by any thoughts unrelated to the main word theme.

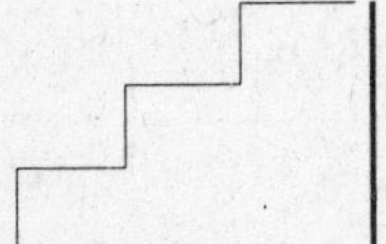

BRAIN-BUILDING SECRET #10 How to Create an Environment Your Brain Would Be Happy to Live In

Your work environment can exert either a supportive or a harmful effect on your use of your own natural brain power. It all depends on how you set it up, so here are some tips.

Step 1. Feed Your Brain with Negative Ions

Take a moment and remember the last time you enjoyed a waterfall, when you were close enough to feel the energy and vitality of the flowing water but perhaps not quite close enough to get drenched. There is a biochemical reason why you felt so astonishingly refreshed, alert, inspired, and generally uplifted after spending time before the waterfall. It's called *negative ions*, and here, for once, the word *negative* means something good for you.

Negatively charged air molecules (or ions), which are common around any falling body of water or immediately following an electrical storm, have proven effects in improving mood, heightening concentration, inciting inspiration and creativity. They are literally the molecules of refreshment.

One connection might be through the neurotransmitter serotonin. Scientists have found that the higher the negative ion level in an environment, the lower the serotonin level in your brain; remember, serotonin is what puts you to sleep. So fresh, unpolluted air, rich in negative ions, can produce a lift in spirits and a gain in mental output.

Consider these environments for their negative ion content and ratio of positive to negative ions:

- Clean mountain air: 2,500 positive ions (PI), 2,000 negative ions (NI); ratio 1.25:1
- Rural air: 1,800 PI, 1,500 NI; ratio 1.2:1
- Urban air: 600 PI, 500 NI; ratio 1.2:1
- Prestorm air: 3,000 PI, 800 NI; ratio 3.75:1
- Poststorm air: 800 PI, 2,500 NI; ratio 0.32:1
- Light industrial plant air: 400 PI, 250 NI; ratio 1.6:1
- Office or typical apartment air: 200 PI, 150 NI; ratio 1.33:1
- Office without windows air: 80 PI, 20 NI; ratio 4:1
- Closed moving vehicle, car, bus, plane, train air: 80 PI, 20 NI; ratio 4:1

PUT A WATERFALL IN YOUR OFFICE AND SKIP THE COFFEE

You can see clearly from the preceding list why you probably feel sleepy on an airplane and energized at a waterfall. The trouble is that in your typical modern office building and recently built home, the place is generally so tightly sealed and then fortified with heating and air-conditioning systems, that the negative ions do not stand a chance.

As a result, your streamlined, fax-equipped office may not be a place conducive to brain power tasks. Your office may be filled with dead, brain power–defeating air.

On the other hand, if you want to stay perky and on focus in your windowless office (or office in which the windows do not open), you need to get negative ions back into the work environment to relieve the doldrums and keep you alert.

Negative ion generators (sometimes marketed as air purifiers) are available to fulfill this precise task, usually for around $100. See if you can install windows that open, put fans near the windows; you might even invest in a miniature waterfall to generate a small measure of brain power–boosting negative ions.

Step 2. Put Your Brain in a Room with a View

Why do writers, at least according to popular myth, prefer a quiet, rural environment for their work with words? Because the view inspires and the countryside continually refreshes—especially if you can see both from your desk, out a large picture window. The visual content of your work environment can have a measurable effect on the quality of your brain waves and thus on your output.

A study actually proved that people who can view natural settings that include water and vegetation while they work have higher levels of alpha brain waves than when they confront a dull, lifeless urban environment. Alpha waves are associated with relaxation and creativity.

In other words, views in which nature predominate are provably better for brain power work in a wakeful, relaxed state than blank walls or vistas of urban blight. If you can't rearrange your desk or office to include an inspiring view, why not hang one on the wall in lieu of a sylvan vista.

Step 3. Keep Your Brain Well Lit

While you're redecorating, why not install full-spectrum lights. Studies show that you get higher productivity under natural light than under artificial, incomplete-spectrum fluorescent lighting.

Light is a nutrient required by your entire system, which means if you work indoors, you will flourish if you can absorb full-spectrum light during the day. It will keep you energized and alert. This is especially true in the winter months when there is far less natural sunlight available outdoors.

Many who live in the Northeast become susceptible to a condition called seasonal affective disorder, or SAD, which is a kind of nutrient deficiency, in this case, natural light. Productivity drops, the need for more sleep and food increases, and often mild depression ensues.

What happens is that as the amount of light diminishes, your body thinks it's nighttime already and secretes more melatonin, the brain chemical that puts you to sleep. The thing you most want to do in these circumstances is hibernate until April—hardly appropriate if your livelihood depends on your brain power.

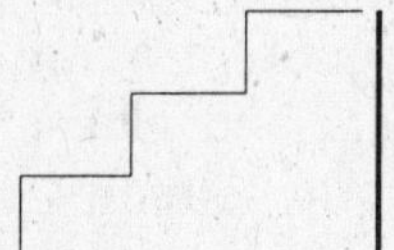

BRAIN-BUILDING SECRET #11
Keep Your IQ Intact—How to Make Your House Brain Fogproof

As long as we're outfitting your house to be a better brain power environment, here are additional suggestions to consider.

In earlier brain-building secrets you learned that many aspects of your life-style, diet, attitude, and other personal factors may act as prime obstacles to having more brain power. You will see in Brain-Building Secrets #24, 25, 26, and 27 the effect of allergenic foods on the state of your mind. Now we need to add another important factor to the picture: your living environment itself.

Owing to the ultratechnological state of the typical American home or work environment, a great many components of your taken-for-granted environment may not only be generally toxic to your health but decidedly bad news for all aspects of your natural brain power.

Here is a guide to the possible brain power poisons in your typical home or work environment that can interfere with your intelligence and create a condition some experts call *brain fog*.

THE BRAIN POWER FRIENDLY HOUSE—YOU CAN LIVE THERE

First, these are conditions to be wary of because they can drain your brain power:

▼ *Kitchen*. Chlorine in tap water, inadequate ventilation with buildup of gases, oven fumes and cleaners, refrigerator gases.

- *Dining and livingroom*. House dust mites in carpet, possible formaldehye and other contaminants in carpet, wall insulation, new carpets that sometimes do not fully outgas for 20 years, pesticides in wood treatments, particle board subflooring.
- *Bedroom*. Outgassing from all synthetic materials; carpets; blankets; lacquers and laminates on nightstands, dressers, tables, headboards of bed; all glued joints in furniture; foam mattress; polyester draperies; vinyl wallpapers and glues; fake wood panelings; scented detergents; fabric softeners, dry-cleaned clothes; shoe polish.
- *Bathroom*. Synthetic shower curtains, synthetic antiseptics, perfumes, deodorants, bleach, formaldehyde from plastics, solvents, paints, and glues.

Second, here are some steps to take to make your house a brain power–friendly environment:

- *House construction*. Avoid UFFI walls, as the formaldehyde continues to outgas into the indoor breathable air for years. Avoid spraying materials with antifungals; avoid products that are destined to be permanent fixtures in your environment if they are known to release formaldehyde—such as wood, boards, plastics, glues, paints.[14]
- *Furnishings, decorations, fixtures*. Remove and replace as many synthetic materials as possible, including fabrics, carpets, foams, curtains, plywood floors, plastics.[15]
- *Ventilation*. Take measures to double the natural ventilation of your living space; make sure all windows can be opened; install wall fans in the kitchen and bathroom if necessary. Airtight may save you money in heating bills now, but it will cost you more money in doctor's bills later.
- *Personal clothing*. Consider wearing fewer polyester or synthetic materials; use natural fibers, cottons, wools with natural dyes; avoid clothes treated with pesticides for moth control. Eliminate dry cleaning as a mode of cleaning clothes.

- *Bedroom*. Do not use an electric blanket, as this wraps your body in an unhealthy low-potency electromagnetic field. Do not situate the head of your bed near an electrical outlet, for the same reason. If your bedroom is situated near an electric power line pole or wire crossings, relocate your sleeping arrangements elsewhere in the house, for the same reason.

This completes all the exercises in your first major Brain Builders Secret. By now you are probably seeing how important your attitude is for the success of the goal of gaining more brain power. By now, I trust you are beginning to *believe your brain*. With this new positive, upbeat attitude about the possibility of building your brain power, you are now ready to move on to the next 6 major Brain Builders Secrets. In the next chapter, you will learn ways to *free your brain* from obstacles that keep your natural IQ tied down. Just by making moderate changes in how you live and eat can gain you IQ points, even before you begin any brain-building exercises.

2 FREE YOUR BRAIN

▼▼▼▼▼▼▼▼▼▼▼▼▼▼▼▼▼▼▼▼▼▼

How Your Diet, Emotions, and Life-Style May Be Draining Off Your Natural Brain Power

Free your brain. There are many factors in the way you live that directly interfere with the full expression of your natural brain power. In other words, you may be far smarter than you are capable of acting because of certain obstacles that drain your brain yet can be removed. These include stress, depression, alcohol use, dietary style, inadequate nutrition, chronic constipation, and brain allergies. When you correct these factors, you free your brain to start developing itself.

In the last chapter, you saw how important your initial *attitude* about developing brain power can be. Once your attitude is engaged, you need to start removing obstacles in your body and life that keep your natural brain power suppressed. That's what this second chapter is all about: how to gain IQ points simply by removing obstacles to the full flowering of your intelligence.

This brain-building secret has techniques based on the idea that you need to free your brain from all the obstacles your life-style has put in its way. This may be the first time you've heard this, but many things you take for granted in your life, such as meat, alcohol, prescription drugs, stress, your eyes, constipation, and others, can all work against your brain power. But they can all be corrected and adjusted by following the brain-building secrets in this chapter.

It's not so much a matter of elimination but management. Certainly you do want to eliminate the serious brain power damaging effects of stress, depression, and constipation. You might want to consider making adjustments in what you eat and drink on behalf of your greater IQ. And there may be a few facts in this chapter that surprise you altogether. Those moments of fuzziness and fog that come over your brain may be due to undiagnosed allergies to foods and substances; they are correctable. This chapter also gives you some tips on how to start a brain-boosting program of detoxification to help free your brain.

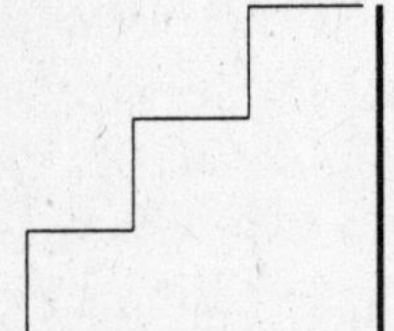

BRAIN-BUILDING SECRET #12 Chill Out and Put Your Brain on Ice Because Stress Destroys Your Brain Power

High blood pressure, chronic stress, and hypertension all work against your natural brain power. They can also lead to stroke, which can really put a clamp on your neuronal fitness. Stress, whether it's to do with pleasure or danger, triggers a kind of biochemical alarm reaction in your body that produces up to 1,000 different chemical reactions or physical changes.

Numerous hormones and neurotransmitters are released during a moment of stress, and under normal healthy conditions, they are reabsorbed into your system with no harmful effects. But if you are stressed often, or chronically, this means you may have too much of certain hormones and too few of others, and your health may start to suffer in terms of increased blood pressure and other factors.

Our brain-building secret regarding stress is this: *Examine your life-style, your moods, thoughts, and ways of reacting to demanding situations to see if you are under more stress than is healthy for your brain, then take steps to reduce or "absorb" the unhealthy stress.*

TOO MUCH STRESS CAN AGE YOUR BRAIN

Chronic stress and high levels of stress hormones may start to age your brain prematurely and lead to a decline in your usable brain power. In fact, stress can actually kill brain cells.[1] This tells us that *how you cope with stress* will directly affect how much and how fast your brain ages.

Stress and untreated hypertension can eat away at your vital brain power during your adult years. In general terms, chronic stress is regarded as a major contributing factor to a great variety of serious illnesses, in as much as 80 percent of cases. It contributes strongly to insomnia and sleep disturbances, which in turn interfere with brain power. Obviously, stress and hypertension are also major risk factors in coronary artery disease and stroke.[2]

Scientists believe that chronic high blood pressure (which involves a thickening of the cerebral arteries) cuts down the normal flow of oxygen into your brain. What should be a flexible hose—your arteries and capillaries—have become an inflexible pipe. Continue this pattern for 10 years and small lesions and microscopic tissue damage will form in your brain; these, too, can slow down blood circulation and oxygen flow to your brain cells.

The negative effect on mental abilities seems to build slowly with age. The longer you have high blood pressure, the worse the decline; you start seeing its effects after 10 years of prolonged high blood pressure, and after 15 years, there are marked drops in memory function.[3]

YOU MAY BE LOSING VALUABLE NEURONS TO STRESS AS WE SPEAK

With this in mind, note that studies show that people with diastolic readings of 90 and higher start showing significant declines in general memory, mental tasks involving short-term memory, and the fluidity (or flexibility) of intelligence. In fact, for each rise of only 20 millimeters of mercury in the diastolic blood pressure reading, continued, untreated, over a 10-year period, there is a drop of one quarter of a standard deviation on memory tests.

That translates out as 2 to 3 points on an IQ scale of 100. That's a 2 to 3 percent drop in IQ from high blood pressure and stress alone. When you consider all the other factors that interfere with your natural brain power, you begin to see that you are "leaking neurons" all over the place with every breath you take.

Now let's have a look at some practical steps to take for stress and high blood pressure. Technically speaking, if you have high blood pressure, you should consult a qualified natural health practitioner (such as a naturopath or acupuncturist), nutritionist, or a conventional physician for professional advice. Still, there are safe, simple steps you can take immediately to help things along.

HIGH BLOOD PRESSURE: 7 BRAIN POWER-PRESERVING STEPS

1. Lose weight, eat more fiber, reduce saturated fat in your diet, drink less alcohol, use less table salt, and consider a semi-vegetarian to fully vegetarian diet.
2. Increase your intake of *calcium* to 1 gram daily for two months.
3. *Magnesium* deficiency is directly related to high blood pressure, particularly as you need magnesium to dilate your blood vessels to allow more blood flow. Increase your daily intake to 400 mg for two months.
4. The amino acid *taurine* is related to lower incidence of high blood pressure. Try a dosage of 2 grams, three times daily for one week.
5. The amino acid *tryptophan* has been shown to reduce high blood pressure when consumed in sufficient amounts. Take 1 gram three times daily for a three-week trial period.
6. *Garlic* has a blood pressure-lowering effect. Ingest three fresh garlic gloves (9 grams) daily or a garlic extract (according to product instructions) for four weeks.
7. Regular aerobic *exercise*, such as walking, running, swimming, and other motion activities, can reduce blood pressure. Start with only moderate exertion so as not to overtax your system.

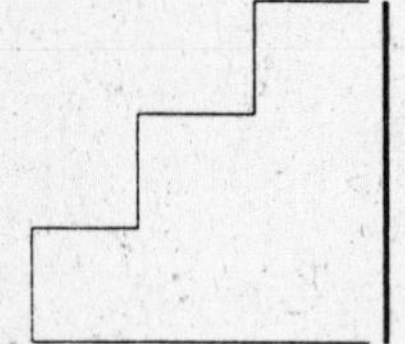

BRAIN BUILDING SECRET #13
8 Exercises for Chilling Out and Removing Your Brain Power Drain from Stress

Now let's look at the 8 steps you can take to start reducing the effect stress has on your brain power.

1. **Get truly relaxed**. Learn what *true, deep relaxation* actually feels like. This may sound obvious, but most people do not know what it feels like to be completely relaxed. *There are various ways to achieve this*:

- Treat yourself to a luxurious day at a professional spa, complete with sauna, full-body massage, whirlpool, herbal teas, aromatherapy, and cleansers.
- Spend an hour without distraction listening to music specifically composed and engineered to promote relaxation. Consult Chapter 6, Brain-Building Secret #67 (page 283), for more detail on music and brain power.
- Spend one day absolutely pampering and indulging yourself.

2. **Collect yourself**. Stay calm in the midst of agitation. Part of the damage that stress exacts on your nervous system and brain power is that you don't see the hit coming. When you start to feel stressed out, anxious, nervous, impatient, rushed, and pressured, stop everything; note the sensations, thoughts, attitudes, and your general mood objectively, as if you are compassionately observing the inner workings of somebody else.

- Take a mental inventory; assess your situation; breathe with attention.
- Take 5 minutes to sit down, close your eyes, put your attention on your inhaling and exhaling.
- You might even say to yourself: *In this moment I am aware of my stress and agitation and am releasing it with each breath*.
- Let your worries take a breather. When you give yourself this moment of detachment, it acts as a wedge, prying open your stress to allow a little beam of calm clarity to enter.

3. **Breathe with attention**. You can even do this standing up, in the midst of problems, right on the subway.

- Put all your attention on your inhale.

- As you inhale, count from 1 to 5.
- As you exhale count from 6 to 10.
- Do this without losing count for 5 minutes. *Don't do this while driving a car; do it only if you're the passenger.*

4. **Alternate your nostrils**. If you can take 10 minutes off every time you feel the stress building, do this breathing exercise from the hatha yoga tradition. It will calm your nervous system, rebalance your brain hemispheres, and actually restore a clear sharp edge to your mental abilities for the next several hours.

- Sit down in a chair with your back straight but comfortable.
- Close your eyes. Take your right index finger and gently block your right nostril.
- Inhale slowly and steadily through your left nostril to the count of 5 or 6, without straining.
- Remove your right index finger from your right nostril. Use it to block your left nostril.
- Exhale slowly through your right nostril to the count of 10 or 12.
- Now inhale through your right nostril.
- Unblock your left nostril and block your right nostril. Exhale through your left nostril.
- Then inhale through your left nostril, and so forth.
- Make your exhale twice as long as your inhale. If you can inhale to the count of 6, 8, or 10, this is even better; then exhale to the count of 12, 16, or 20.
- Repeat this cycle of inhaling through one nostril, exhaling through the other for 5–10 minutes.
- Consult Brain-Building Secrets #62 and #63 for more exercises involving breathing.

5. **Take flower essences**. There are a number of useful flower essences that can help you chill out quite effectively. Take

- *Lavender*, to soothe and calm an overwhelmed nervous system

- *Cherry Plum*, if you fear that too much stress will lead to a loss of control and breakdown
- *Five Flower Formula* for temporary relief from trying circumstances
- *Indian Pink*, if you need to stay calm and centered in the midst of intense activity
- *Impatiens*, if you're trying to go too fast and are feeling seriously irritated
- *Chamomile*, to deeply relax and mellow out after intense emotional experiences or concentrated stress

Consult Brain-Building Secrets #14 and #34 for more detail on flower essences.

6. **Take a bubble bath**. This can be remarkably restorative at the end of a stressful day. Use pure lavender oil or a prepared lavender bubble bath mixture or a combination of these with a neutral high-bubble-content preparation.

- Pour a half-dozen drops or a teaspoonful of the lavender liquid into an empty quart yogurt container.
- Fill this with hot water from the tap in the bathtub.
- As the bath water flows out of the tap into the tub, let this mixture dribble into the water flow. This will create the maximum amount of bubbles and distribute the essential oil uniformly in the bath water.
- Remain in the tub soaking and relaxing for at least 20 minutes.
- On other occasions try rose oil, chamomile, jasmine, or melissa.

7. **Become a corpse**. Essentially the first and last pose in many series of hatha yoga positions is a relaxation posture called *Savasana*. It is loosely translated from the Hindu texts as corpse pose because you lie on your back and gain such a state of relaxation you might possibly be mistaken for having passed on.

- Put on loose-fitting clothes like a sweat suit or pajamas.
- Remove shoes, jewelry, watches, glasses.
- Lie down on a carpet or floor mat, on your back.
- Spread your legs about 18 inches.
- Extend your arms about 12 inches out from your side.
- Have your chin in alignment with your groin; do not tilt your head to either side.
- Rotate your legs in and out, then let them flop to the side. Do the same with your arms.
- Gently, slowly turn your head to the far right then to the far left, then return it to the center.
- Stretch yourself out fully as if someone were pulling gently at your head, feet, and arms, elongating you.
- Feel as if someone were pulling your shoulders down away from your neck, your legs away from your pelvis.
- Feel the pull of gravity across the underside of your body. Feel it wrap around you like a blanket.
- Breathe deeply from your abdomen. Feel your belly rise and fall with each breath.
- As you exhale, let the outgoing breath meet the "gravity blanket" and disperse like a cushion of air around you.
- Now as you inhale, focus your attention on your body, starting with the ankles.
- First, tense your ankles then release.
- Then as you breathe in, direct your attention to and imagine your breath is entering and bathing your ankles with light.
- As you exhale, blow all the stress and toxins out of your ankles.
- Next, do this same attentive breathing, slowly, and one by one, for your calves, then knees, thighs, groin, abdomen, chest, fingers, forearms, upper arms, shoulders, neck, ears, chin, nose, face muscles, eyes, scalp, and skull.

- Remember to first tense this individual body area, then release it before inhaling and exhaling in that area.
- You might also say this to yourself as you work with each body part: I *relax the calves. My calves are relaxing. My calves are relaxed now.*
- When you have finished flushing your body with fresh, light air and attention, let go of this focus and simply lie there following your breathing.
- Try to stay awake in a relaxed alertness; if you fall asleep, that's okay.
- As an additional boost, you might do this exercise while listening to relaxing music.

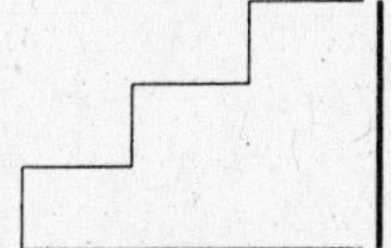

BRAIN BUILDERS! WORKOUT #6

How to Remember Your Sneakers

- Find a pair of shoes, preferably sneakers, preferably yours. Study them in detail for 5 minutes, as if you've never seen shoes like this before. Bear in mind that you are creating memories as you file away the visual details of your shoes—so pay close attention.
- After 5 minutes, put the shoes away and recall everything you have just seen. How much have you already forgotten? Take a break.
- After 15 minutes have passed, recall your last recollection of the shoes. How much have you forgotten since your last memory visit with your sneakers?
- As you try to remember your last remembering, bear in mind that you will be trying to remember this act in 15 minutes from now. Take a break.
- After 15 minutes have passed, recall your last recollection of the shoes. How much have you forgotten since your last memory visit with your sneakers?

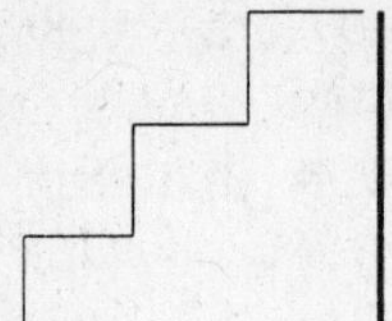

BRAIN-BUILDING SECRET #14
Get Undepressed: Use Flowers to Clear Up Your Emotions and Regain Your Natural Brain Power

You may think you're growing stupid, but in fact you may be depressed with all your brain power on reserve. As many as 10 million Americans suffer at least one bout of depression during their lives, psychologists estimate. Most of us are subject to periodic bouts or short-lived moments of low spirits or depression. This is especially so with the elderly; in many cases physicians mistake depression for Alzheimer's.

THE BEST TRANQUILIZER COMES NATURALLY FROM FLOWERS

The increasing popularity of tranquilizers and prescription anti-depressants further shows that depression is a problem for many people. Depression, whether short term or chronic, detracts from your brain power.

That's because depression is the most common cause of *reversible* memory loss and intellectual deterioration. A lifetime of depression or chronically low spirits can actually drain off your brain power. That means, in practical terms, your emotions exact a toll on your *usable* brain power.

Certainly you experience daily, weekly, and monthly swings in your feelings. If you could see this pattern from a distance and over time, it would be like a rollercoaster; you ride the highs and lows, the peaks and flatlands of joy, elation, indifference, boredom, sadness, grief, resentment, anger, and happiness. Some of these emotions affect your ability to process information, to remember, compute, organize, learn, and generally go about your mental life with efficiency.

These have a short-term effect on your brain power. Of far greater importance to you should be the chronic, or long-standing, emotions, feelings you have had for as long as you can remember. Depression is probably the most common cause of *reversible* vital memory loss and the loss of brain power.

When you're depressed, your brain power suffers. You can't remember well; you're easily distracted; you have too much already on your mind; your attention span is short; you can't easily take in new information; and, generally speaking, you don't want to. You forget things quickly and more frequently; it becomes harder to summon up recent memories.

That's why as part of your brain power building program you need to take a few simple measures to get *undepressed* by clearing up your emotional pain, confusion, sorrow, and other states.

A QUIZ TO SEE IF YOU NEED TO GET UNDEPRESSED

Here is a quick quiz to give yourself, a friend, or family member to see if you are depressed rather than losing your brain power:

Is your mood one of dejection, sadness, the blues, shame, worry, humiliation, uselessness, hopeless, or feeling miserable?

Do you have negative feelings toward yourself and feel worthless?

Do you get less gratification from your favorite foods, pastimes, objects, pets, work, friends, parties, vacations, and feel bored more often than not?

Are your emotional attachments to your spouse, family members, friends, relatives, even yourself slipping away with respect to your appearance?

Do you have untypical crying spells, when you have tears for no particular reason or at almost the drop of a hat?

Have you lost your sense of humor and no longer respond well to jokes, kidding, and teasing?

Has your self-esteem plummeted? Has your outlook on life become gloomy and pessimistic?

Are you unable to make decisions quickly or at all anymore?

Is your body image distorted, which means, is your idea or perception of what your body looks like suddenly strange, weird, out of focus, even inaccurate?

Have you lost all your drive and motivation to accomplish things?

Do you experience self-destructive, even suicidal thoughts running through your mind?

Have your appetite for food, your sexual interest, and your ability to sleep undisturbed through the night all disappeared?

REVIEWING THE QUIZ RESULTS—HAVE SOME MUSTARD

If you answered yes to at least 5 of these questions, quite likely you have some degree of depression; if all 12 questions perfectly describe your state of mind, then you definitely have depression.

However, a diagnosis of depression is not a death sentence; it's purely descriptive and should help you understand why you are not wielding your natural brain power with as much spunk as you once did. And depression is easily reversible and, with it, a return of your natural brain power.

Now let me show you how a drop of mustard can improve your brain power and how to let the flowers melt your heavy emotions.[4]

It may surprise you that in this project of getting undepressed, flowers may be your chief ally. Somehow infusions of flower blossoms, when taken orally as drops, actually clear up heavy emotions like depression, anxiety, fear, worry, grief, and others. Dr. Bach devised a series of 38 Flower Remedies, which are water-based preparations made from the plants; they are widely available as over-the-counter remedies at natural foods and health outlets throughout the country and directly through mail order (see Resources).

PRESCRIBING FLOWER ESSENCES FOR YOURSELF—AND YOUR BRAIN

Here are some examples of Flower Remedy applications of interest to our project of getting undepressed. The remedies listed here are ready-to-use preparations made from common flowers:

- *Gentian*. Are you someone who is easily discouraged, melancholic, disheartened, and lacking the faith to continue after setbacks? Take gentian.
- *Gorse*. For despair, great hopelessnes, resignation, darkness, loss of will, and chronic depression, take gorse.

- *Borage*. Do you feel heavy-hearted, empty of confidence and courage in the face of difficult circumstances, and are you burdened with grief, sadness, and general disheartenment? Borage is the flower essence for you.
- *Mustard*. For intense, sudden, periodic depression and gloom without obvious cause; for melancholy, gloom, despair, and generalized unspecific depression; for manic-depressive mood swings or the feeling that a "black cloud" is sitting over your head, take mustard.
- *Hornbeam*. For fatigue, weariness, for when your everyday responsibilities are too big a burden and seem monotonous and uninteresting, take hornbeam.
- *Milkweed*. For a deeply depressed state; an inability to deal with everyday affairs; a desire to wipe out your consciousness with drugs, alcohol, overeating, or sleep and your own self-awareness; and for a sense of extreme dependency and emotional regression, take milkweed.
- *Sagebrush*. Do you feel personally devastated, that you've hit rock bottom, that you cannot accept the emptiness and loss that seems to surround you, then sagebrush will help you.
- *Wild oat*. For a sense of chronic dissatisfaction with your work and life; for despair, confusion, or indecision in the face of your life's direction; for lack of focus and committment, wild Oat is the flower essence to help you.

HOW TO PUT FLOWERS TO WORK FOR YOUR BRAIN POWER

Here are some general instructions for how to use flower essences to get undepressed.

- Generally, use one remedy at a time at a rate of perhaps three to six times daily, one dropperful each time, until the bottle is used up; usually a bottle will last about two weeks. As you start to feel better, gradually reduce the number of times you take the essence so that after a couple of weeks you are taking it perhaps only once or twice a day.

- During this time, keep a daily journal of your emotions, thoughts, and state of mind; when you finish the remedy, review all your notes and look for changes and shifts in attitude.
- Notice dramatic shifts in tone, effect, and attitude as you moved through the remedy experience.
- Wait another week at least before starting another remedy. The effects are subtle but cumulative, and generally require a few weeks to become apparent. Flower essences have positively no side effects, are absolutely safe, inexpensive, easy to use, and produce remarkable results, often very quickly.[5]

So consider the flower remedy as a friendly ally in your quest for more brain power through clearing any negative emotions that weigh down your natural intelligence.

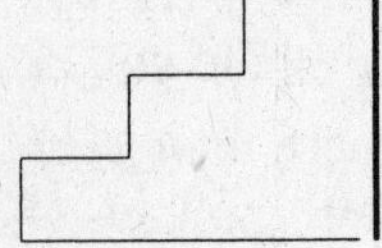

BRAIN BUILDERS! WORKOUT #7 Keep Your Eye on the Star

- In this exercise you train your attention on an imagined image inside your body. For the next 60 minutes, try to keep your attention, without distraction, on the following inner image: 2 *inches above your belly button and* 2 *inches inside there is a single brilliant pinprick of light, like a tiny blazing star inside your body*.
- No matter what you do in the next 60 minutes, keep as much of your attention as possible on this pinpoint of absolutely brilliant light.
- Whether you're washing dishes, reading the newspaper, talking to your children, don't let the star out of your sight.

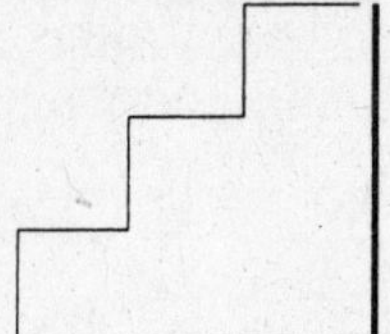

BRAIN-BUILDING SECRET #15
Get Even More Undepressed: Making the Food-Mood Connection Work for Your Brain Power

While taking flower essences will certainly work miracles in your emotional life and thus free up brain power, you might need to make changes in other aspects of your life at the same time.

Certain aspects of your diet may be draining off your natural brain power; you may be taking in too much of one substance and too little of another—in either case, your brain power is paying the bill for the dietary mistake.

Eliminate all caffeine, from coffee, teas, nonprescription drugs, chocolates, and sodas; sugars of all kinds; and all processed foods from your diet for a week. At the same time, eat a high-protein, low-carbohydrate diet for a week.

Nutritionists have observed that by making this simple but dramatic dietary intervention, depression in many individuals can lift as quickly as within 4 days or in 3 to 4 weeks. In many people excess caffeine (4–5 cups daily) and processed sugars upset the body's metabolism and through the digestive system lead to imbalance; often the result is a cluster of symptoms that either resemble hypoglycemia (chronic low blood sugar) or imitate it. The result can often be a condition similar if not identical to depression.[6]

MAYBE YOU'RE NOT DEPRESSED BUT LOW IN BLOOD SUGAR

These are the typical symptoms of low blood sugar, also known as pseudohypoglycemia and actual hypoglycemia, which can *mimic* depression.

- depression
- suicidal thoughts
- detached feelings
- apathy
- exhaustion
- fatigue
- blurred vision
- dizziness
- disorientation
- weakness
- excessive worry
- poor memory
- negativity
- poor judgment
- irritability
- crying easily
- speech difficulties
- poor vision
- forgetfulness
- mental confusion
- moodiness
- nervousness
- loss of appetite and sexual interest
- headaches
- an inability to tolerate stress

A QUIZ TO SEE IF YOU ARE ACTUALLY DEPRESSED

Here are some questions to ask yourself as to whether you should consider trying this change in diet to lift your depression.[7]

- Do you feel low, "down in the dumps," and depressed but cannot figure out why? Or are you having a good time when suddenly a wave of depression breaks over you and swallows up your good spirits?

- When you think about it, are you unusually moody?
- Do you find yourself tired and worn out most of the time? Even when you sleep 8 hours at night, do you wake up unrefreshed and still tired?
- Do you feel as if all your energy drains out of you as from a leaky drum?
- Do you frequently have headaches, especially dull aches?

Consider this case of a person strongly affected by sugar and caffeine in her daily diet. A 21-year-old woman had mood disturbances, psychological distress, depression, anxiety, and nervousness. When she started a diet high in protein, low in carbohydrate, free of sugar, caffeine, and alcohol and followed it for two weeks, virtually all her psychological symptoms had disappeared.

When as an experiment she reintroduced sweets and caffeine into her diet, her emotional distress started to return. After three weeks on this modified diet with sugar and caffeine, she again felt anxious, nervous, and depressed. You can see how reversible was her so-called depression.

6 DIETARY FACTORS THAT CAN DEPRESS YOU AND DRAIN YOUR BRAIN POWER

Here are some additional dietary factors—vitamin deficiencies—that can contribute to depression and thus to a loss of your natural brain power.

1. *Folic Acid Deficiency*. The average American adult gets only 60 percent of total required folic acid (folate). Low levels of folic acid are commonly associated with depression; in fact, the more depressed you are, the more likely you are deficient in folic acid.

   A folic acid deficiency can mimic the symptoms of senility and central nervous system disorders; it might even represent a distinct state of depression itself, known as *folic acid deficiency depression*.

   Researchers have found that typical signs of the onset of senility may actually be caused by a folate shortage in the body that begins to short-circuit normal nervous system operation. *Recommended healing dosage*: 800 micrograms (mcg) daily, dropping down to a maintenance dose of 400 mcg daily.

2. *Riboflavin (vitamin* B2) *deficiency*. A shortage of this vitamin can contribute to a depressive state. In one study one fourth of the 172 people in a psychiatric hospital were found to be deficient in riboflavin; this same one fourth had already been diagnosed with mood disorder. *Recommended dosage*: 40 milligrams (mcg) daily.
3. *Thiamine (vitamin* B1) *deficiency*. Even psychologically stable individuals can start showing signs of depression, irritabilty, and fearfulness if their thiamine levels start to drop. In cases where mental illness is so pronounced that it requires hospital treatment, thiamine deficiency is commonly found in as many as 30 percent of admissions. *Recommended dosage*: 40 mg daily.
4. *Pyridoxine (vitamin* B6) *deficiency*. This vitamin helps to convert the amino acid L-tryptophan into the neurotransmitter serotonin. Decreased levels of vitamin B6 are linked with depression, especially the kind due to factors originating within the person rather than the environment, because less serotonin is produced, which leads to depression. *Recommended dosage*: 40 mg daily.
5. *Vitamin* B12 *deficiency*. A medical study showed that 5 percent of patients admitted to a psychiatric hospital were deficient and 10 percent had subnormal levels of this vitamin. A vitamin B12 deficiency can show up as a mood disorder or chronic tiredness, and it can be mistaken for early senility. *Recommended dosage*: 1,000 mcg, by intramuscular injection, once weekly, by your physician.
6. *Vitamin* C *deficiency*. People dangerously low on this common vitamin may manifest mild symptoms of scurvy, including chronic depression, irritability, tiredness, and a vague feeling of mental ill health.[8] *Recommended dosage*: 2 gm daily, in 1 gm installments spaced 8 hours apart.

THE AUTOBIOGRAPHY OF MY BREAKFAST, LUNCH, AND DINNER

Here is an additional brain-building secret approach that will help you see the relationship between what you eat and how you feel in yourself.

- For the next week, keep a food-mood journal.
- Take seven blank pieces of paper. Label each for one day of the week.
- Mark off three vertical columns on the right half of each page.
- Label these Breakfast, Lunch, Dinner, or Meal 1, 2, 3.
- Divide each of these into two more vertical columns, labeling them Before/After.
- Down the left margin, enter these words, making another vertical column: Alert, Vigorous, Sharp, Motivated, Relaxed, Calm, Focused, Patient, Irritable, Grouchy, Tense, Agitated, Sluggish, Apathetic, Slow, Sleepy, Sad, Blue, Despairing, Unable to cope.
- Say it's breakfast time. Note how you feel *before* eating anything.
- Check off which words listed best describe your state of mind.
- Eat breakfast. Now note which words describe your condition after eating.
- If your mood has shifted from *alert* to *sluggish*, have a careful look at what you ate.
- Try to determine which food item or groups of foods produced these effects.
- If they make you sluggish, you might want to reduce your intake or eliminate them or perhaps eat them at a different time of day.
- If you go from *focused* to *despairing*, you better act fast to change your diet.

- Study your results at the end of the week and make appropriate changes in your diet.

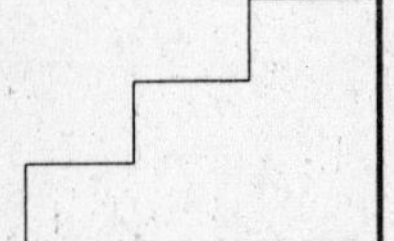

BRAIN BUILDERS! WORKOUT #8 Newspaper Word Scan

- You need a light-colored felt-tip marker or highlighting pen and a kitchen timer.
- Pick up the daily newspaper. Randomly select a word of at least three syllables, such as *instrument*, *Pacific*, *factory*, *prevalent*, *President*, *redundant*, and *argument*.
- Set the timer for 5 minutes. Scan the newspaper, column by column, for repetitions of this same word you have selected. When you see it, underline it with the felt-tip marker. Continue until the timer rings.
- Do this twice a day for a week. The goal is to train your mind to process verbal information both quickly and accurately.

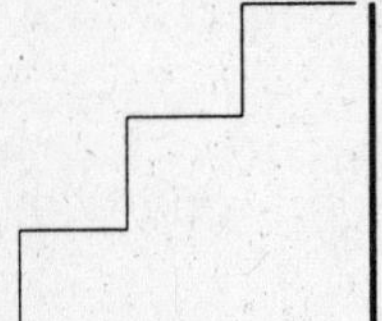

BRAIN-BUILDING SECRET #16 Seeing Correctly Makes Learning Possible— Are Your Eyes Draining Off Your Brain Power?

It's well known that learning disabilities, dyslexia, attention deficit disorder, and other clinically labeled conditions afflict several million American schoolchildren. It's equally obvious that unless these conditions are corrected, the children grow into adulthood bringing with them the same difficulties in learning and the same shortcomings in their brain power.

What is not nearly as well known is that in many cases these conditions are correctable by a most unexpected route: the eyes. According to the burgeoning field called behavioral optometry, visual defects may lie at the root of many learning disability problems.[9]

Our brain building secret is this: *If you have otherwise unaccountable difficulties in learning, reading, or comprehension with visually acquired information, consider having your eyes and your entire vision system examined by a behavioral optometrist.*

You may need special corrective lenses that a conventional optometrist would not know how to prescribe for you.

THE WRONG GLASSES—OR NO GLASSES—CAN DRAIN AWAY BRAIN POWER

The essential idea in behavioral optometry is that imbalances in your visual-perceptual system (the full combination of muscles and nerves among your eyes and brain) can lead to faulty processing of visual information. This can then trigger numerous problems in behavior, learning, work, and health. The trick here is that the connection is often overlooked by conventional optometry.[10]

It may surprise you to learn that behavioral optometrists have definitely correlated faulty, uncorrected vision with such seemingly unrelated problems as travel sickness, bed-wetting, migraines, sensitivity to light, tension, depression, alcoholism, and schizophrenia.

These are correctable problems in the vision system, yet they can significantly impair the use of your intelligence. It is essential that your eyes and brain are working smoothly together, as a visual-perceptual team. This partnership between your eyes and the rest of our body and mind matures as you actively experience and use your vision.

The eyes are so interrelated with the mind that you may have lived many years seeing incorrectly, probably from undiagnosed visual stress as a child. Vision therapy, or behavioral optometry, is about restoring full, healthy perception so that you see everything. When you remove all the obstacles to your vision system, your natural brain power is set free from the heavy weight of faulty perception it has carried most likely for years.

A CHECKLIST FOR SYMPTOMS OF IQ-DRAINING VISION PROBLEMS

There are many factors involved in vision-related learning disabilites, say the behavioral optometrists. Here is a sampling by which you might evaluate your own vision system or that of your child.

The key point to remember is this: *These are not a reflection of brain power but are vision-based obstacles to the successful use of your* IQ.

- *Eye appearance and complaints.* Closing one eye; one eye turning in or out; excessive blinking; sties, red eyes; squinting in mild light; squinting or frowning when concentrating; swollen lids; frequent tears; eyes hurt or headaches after use; eyes burn, itch after use; objects appear double, blurred, moving; dizziness, sensation of a film over eyes.
- *Problems paying attention.* Inability to remain with a visual task for long; tendency to daydream or to become fatigued during visual tasks; difficulty in eye tracking; moving head during reading; losing place during reading; using a finger to mark the spot; omits small words; difficulty in following the sequence of printed instructions.
- *Difficulties with eye-hand coordination.* Difficulties in writing on printed lines; prints slowly; not easy to connect *t's* or dot *i's*; hard to mark the correct space in tests; avoids eye-hand activities such as tying shoelaces, playing catch, sharpening pencils.
- *Problems with eye-teaming abilities.* Hard to judge where objects are in space; double vision; closes or squints a single eye; misaligns numbers in a column; misaligns head or body while working at a desk; easily distracted from visual tasks.
- *Problems with form and perception.* Mistakes similar geometric shapes or letters; confuses words with the same beginnings; hard to use a dictionary or file cards; misreads similar numbers.
- *Difficulties with spatial and perceptual abilities.* Mixes up left and right; hard to understand spatial words, such as above, below, outside; writes crookedly; transposes letters; confused with maps; problems with reading directions; takes wrong turns even when traveling to familiar places.

A CASE STUDY THAT DRAMATICALLY MAKES THE POINT

A child named Kevin, an average but shy student in the third grade, had been classified as learning disabled on the basis of some educational tests. But as his IQ was 127, there must be something to account for the discrepancy between ability and performance.

He had difficulties in the area of visual and hearing perception and memory; he was unable to keep up with his school work, and his handwriting and composition skills were below the norm for his age. Beth Bazin, O.D., a behavioral optometrist, made a 21-point evaluation of Kevin's vision system and started to get to the core of the problem. Kevin reported that words often blurred and floated, he saw images double, and he lost his place while reading.

Dr. Bazin's diagnosis was that Kevin's eyes had difficulty in changing focus from far to near objects, making it hard to see clearly at different distances; also his eyes did not work well together as a visual team. For Dr. Bazin, this explained why an otherwise bright young boy was performing poorly in his school work. She started Kevin in a special program of vision training that would correct these perception problems; she also prescribed a special pair of lenses to use for reading.

A year later his vision system had improved greatly in the key areas Dr. Bazin had been working on. His eyes worked together as a team; no longer did words blur or float. In effect, his learning disabilities had vanished. As Dr. Bazin saw it, the behavioral optometry intervention in Kevin's problem *removed the obstacles* that made it hard for him to learn and to use his otherwise impressive brain power.

The annals of behavioral optometry are rich with case studies like this. Often behavioral optometry can be useful even when there are no outstanding symptoms, such as with Kevin. People who read little may actually read poorly because of undiagnosed vision problems; since they read infrequently, it never comes to their attention.

The paradox is if they could read better, meaning with greater visual ease, they might read more often. That in itself would help them "grow" their brain power.

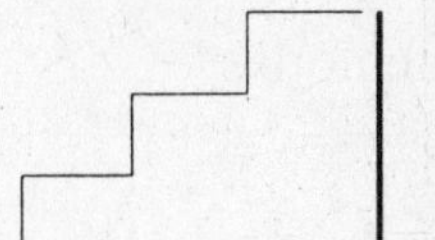

THE ANATOMY OF BRAIN POWER #3
Alzheimer's Disease: Does It Have to Be the Nightmare of Brain Power?

In the 1990s, known as the decade of the brain, Alzheimer's disease is regarded as the nightmare at the end of your brain power. In fact, an entire generation, now in their seventies and eighties, has come to look upon Alzheimer's as almost the inevitable price of old age—the gruesome state that happens when your mind loses its muscle in your declining years.

It all started back in 1906 in Germany when a 55-year-old patient of Dr. Alois Alzheimer died. For nearly 5 years this woman had shown strange mental symptoms. She lost her memory, she couldn't reason, and her overall mental abilities declined seriously. After she died, Dr. Alzheimer did an autopsy on his patient's brain and found evidence of strange formations. Within a few years, what had been called *presenile dementia* was now named after its discoverer and called *Alzheimer's disease*.

It refers to a person's unusual but rapid mental decline, loss of memory and the ability to reason, personality change, confusion, lethargy, disorientation regarding time and space, and the shutting down of nearly all conscious brain functions. Alzheimer's is the end of all brain power as we know it, and if the doctors are right, the end of the individual's brain itself.[11]

Scientists estimate that of the 3 to 5 million Americans over 65 years old who develop symptoms of senility, 10 percent suffer from brain tumor, Parkinson's syndrome, psychiatric illness, or other rare brain diseases; 17 percent have symptoms produced by hardening of the brain's arteries related to hypertension, arteriosclerosis, or heart disease; and 7 percent have conditions that are unclear in origin; but for 66 percent of "demented older patients," the cause is Alzheimer's.

If the "cause" of this much elderly senility is Alzheimer's, what exactly is this disease? In terms of what you can tell about a person from the outside, most doctors agree that these are the telltale signs of Alzheimer's:

- progressive loss of memory
- a decline in vocabulary and word understanding
- repeating the same questions
- failure to remember short- and long-term memories
- difficulties with numbers
- taking metaphors and proverbs literally
- problems with orientation in space and time
- forgetting simple words and familiar names

▼ severe impairment in speaking fluently

Two *anatomical* changes happen during the onset of Alzheimer's. Neuron fibers in the brain appear to twist around one another like pretzels, and clusters of these twistings (called neurofibrillary tangles) combine with other abnormal tissues to form a brain lesion called neuritic plaques. These two events take place in the brain's hippocampus and cerebral cortex, two key brain regions associated with memory and the activities of the intellect.

But even this finding is not definitive, because the brains of numerous alert elderly men and women, on autopsy, revealed numerous lesions; similarly, the clearly demented often have brains with no signs of plaques or lesions. A medical study showed that about 99 percent of people older than 80 have some brain lesions but are not necessarily senile.[12]

Aluminum concentrations in the brain may have a lot to do with the formation of the lesions, because when doctors studied the brains of Alzheimer's patients they found 10 to 30 times the normal level of aluminum.

Another theory regarding the possible cause of Alzheimer's suggests that people with this form of dementia may be lacking a brain enzyme needed to make the neurotransmitter acetylcholine. This brain chemical is believed to be involved in thinking and memory. The doctors determined that as the brain levels of acetylcholine dropped, the amount of brain lesions increased.

What makes a healthy but aging brain fall apart into Alzheimer's is still a mystery to physicians. Brain experts do know that as you age, your brain becomes measurably smaller, lighter, and more loosely packed. They also know that as the years pass, you lose literally billions of brain cells (neurons), not to be replaced; and they understand that many of the remaining brain cells lose their ability to connect with other cells through the dendrites.

Infants start with an estimated 15 billion neurons; what's most interesting is that you actually lose the greatest amount of brain cells ("neuronal death") between birth and age 30. From age 30 into old age, you lose neurons at a slower pace.

Nor do you lose brain cells in every region of your brain; some areas lose none, others may lose up to 80 percent of their dendrite connections and 40 percent of their cells by age 80.

Dendrites are like the leaves on your brain tree; as you age, the "leaves" fall off. This means there are fewer of the tiny, hairlike filaments that connect the brain cells with one another and through which nerve impulses and nutrients are transmitted. Strangely, scientists have discovered that when you age, you lose dendrites and grow new ones at the same time. In other words, advancing age is not entirely a death sentence for your brain cell's dendrites.

Further, debris collects in the spaces between cells and even inside them, including a yellowish age pigment. This substance, called "old age pigment" or "liver spots," can appear on the backs of your hands and in the cell body of your brain's neurons. It's basically a form of cellular rubbish from old insoluble fats and broken-down cellular membranes, and in ways not well understood, it seems to interfere with the normal activity of your brain cells.

KEEP YOUR BRAIN LITHE AND AGILE DESPITE YOUR AGE

As the brain ages, the amount of key neurotransmitters—called "the ferrymen of the brain's communication system"— also declines so that, if you are elderly, your brain probably has much lower amounts of acetylcholine, dopamine, epinephrine, norepinephrine, and gamma-aminobutyric acid (GABA).

Even so, all these major changes do not always add up to Alzheimer's; for the majority of the elderly, old age means slower brain processing and response time and a more sluggish memory but not senility.

The famous anthropologist and writer Margaret Mead, who lived to be 78, never lost any of her considerable brain power. Her advice was simple: "Change all your doctors, opticians, and dentists when you reach fifty." What she meant was that when you are in your twenties to forties, most likely your physicians are older than you; when you're 50, most of these doctors will be 65 or older.

When you get to this point, Mead suggested, start all over and get yourself a roster of younger doctors. "Then as you grow older, you'll have people who are still alive and active taking care of you. You won't be desolate because every one of your doctors is dead."

What Dr. Mead is saying is this: *Fortify your attitude against the depression of seeing all your doctors die on you by getting new, healthier ones as you age. Then their upbeat attitude will inspire you to stay cheerful as well.*

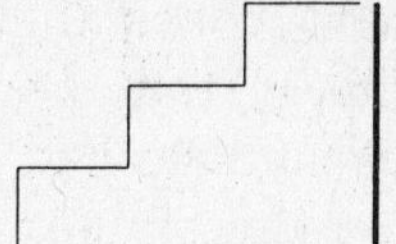

BRAIN-BUILDING SECRET #17
Eliminating Brain Poisons: Alcohol and Memory Loss

Despite the popular image of the writer downing a glass of wine to get inspired for intellectual work, alcohol is actually an enemy of your brain power. You need only think of the image of the "lost weekend," made real by the movies, to realize that ultimately alcohol makes you sleepy, even unconscious, and entirely forgetful. Memory impairment is built right into the substance.

People drink alcohol to relax their social inhibitions, to forget in part who they are; eventually you forget everything you did while you were drinking to forget yourself. In other words, in excess, alcohol is bad for your memory; in fact, it directly contributes to memory loss and dysfunction. That's why many doctors, especially those concerned with maximizing brain function, regard it as a potent brain poison.

Our brain-building secret regarding alcohol is simple: *If you want maximum brain power and fully working memory, reduce your alcohol consumption to a minimum.*

TOO MUCH ALCOHOL PICKLED HIS BRAIN

This dictum depends on your body weight and the way your system absorbs and detoxifies alcohol and how fast it reaches your brain, but most experts on the subject recommend no more than one glass of beer or wine a month. According to medical studies, even as few as two alcoholic drinks a day will diminish your ability to remember. People over 40 are especially susceptible to this alcohol-induced memory impairment even if they are drinking only moderately.

Here is a dramatic case of how alcohol severely damaged a man's brain and its function:

A 27-year-old man was admitted to Boston City Hospital neurology ward with uncontrolled epilepsy. Prior to his admission, he had been drinking a cheap wine steadily for nearly three weeks. He ran out of money, then abstained for a week, and got epileptic seizures as a kind of nightmare form of the DTs. The doctors attending him determined that he had no previous personal or family history of epilepsy, and that it must have started with his drinking bouts.

Apparently the fact that he stopped the high alcohol consumption brought on his seizures. CAT scans of his brain showed that the tissues in the center of his brain had shrunk while the ventricles had expanded, filled with fluid. In addition, his cerebellum had shrunk. The alcohol had actually produced a measurable loss in his brain substance.

This, of course, is an extreme example of the damaging effect alcohol has on the human brain; actually, even very small amounts can trigger the same serious reactions in different people, as the following example shows.

Ten people were given a pint of whiskey over a period of a few hours. Then they were tested for recall from a movie they had just watched. Of the ten inebriated subjects, only five could remember the objects from the film after 30 minutes; of these five, after 24 hours they could remember only 60 percent of what they had recalled after 30 minutes. The other five subjects couldn't recognize the movie objects after only 30 minutes. They had blacked out and never committed the material to short-term memory in the first place.

HOW TOO MUCH ALCOHOL CAN PICKLE YOUR BRAIN POWER

Let's look at this in more detail. The key point is that, physiologically, alcohol is a brain poison. Neuroscientists talk of a *blood-brain barrier*. This is a membrane around your brain's capillaries that normally keeps out harmful substances from the brain; it also keeps brain chemicals and ions (such as calcium) in their appropriate concentrations for proper brain function. A number of factors can break down this blood-brain barrier, including tumors, infection, injury, excessive bleeding, and alcohol.

Large amounts can break through and contaminate the entire brain, while smaller amounts break down the barrier in the limbic brain, a section believed to be associated with emotions. As a result, the limbic brain, which includes the hippocampus and amydala, which are the inner parts of the temporal lobes, and the thalamus and hypothalamus, is poisoned. In addition, alcohol destroys the dendrites that link neurons.

YOU CAN'T DRINK AND THINK (TOO WELL) AT THE SAME TIME

Light or moderate drinking can impair your ability to form concepts, do abstract reasoning, learn, adapt, and perform other sophisticated mental tasks. Alcohol also interferes with your ability to process new information and to store it as memory. It is worth repeating that alcohol is a *brain depressant*: It depresses or turns down most of the important brain functions. This is the long-term permanent effect.

Alcohol can produce both short-term forgetfulness and long-term chronic memory loss because it affects the limbic area of the brain, which scientists believe is the seat of memory function. It becomes harder to gain and store new information; when you remember things, the memories are shallow and incomplete, and you easily forget recently learned items.

Add to this the fact that alcohol robs your body of vital nutrients, especially the B vitamin complex (especially B1, or thiamine) which are essential for brain function. Serious thiamine deficiency can produce Korsakoff's psychosis, in which memory loss is severe.[13]

TOO MUCH ALCOHOL CAN SHRINK YOUR BRAIN

Long-term alcohol consumption (and abuse) actually changes the physical structure of your brain permanently.

The brains of chronic alcoholics are actually softer to the touch than the brains of nondrinkers. Animal studies have shown that after five months of alcohol consumption, there were pathological changes in their brains and in the way their nerve cells conducted impulses.

One medical study showed that the brains of chronic alcoholics and heavy drinkers tended to *weigh less* than the brains of nondrinkers, even though they were otherwise similar in height and weight. Scientists conducting this study determined that the brains (frontal lobes, specifically) of alcoholics actually had *smaller and fewer* neurons, which are the basic stuff of brain power.

Not only that, but the reason long-term alcohol abuse may lead to serious, even permanent, memory loss is because it makes the liver toxic. It's well known that alcoholics sometimes die from cirrhosis of the liver, but those who don't succumb in this way may suffer with Korsakoff's syndrome. This is a state of extreme liver toxicity named after its Russian discoverer, Sergei Sergeivich Korsakoff, who died in 1900.[14]

Speaking frankly, if you have a history of heavy alcohol use, you would be wise to consider a program of liver detoxification, ideally using herbs and acupuncture to restore this essential organ to health and, with it, your potential for excellent, full-ranging memory.

Self-help herbs to use in the meantime are dandelion root, burdock, yellow dock, and celandine, alone or in combinations, as concentrated tinctures or as strong herb teas taken twice daily.

BRAIN BUILDERS! WORKOUT #9
Reading Upside Down

- Take a magazine that has a lot of text, such as *Time*, *The New Yorker*, or *Scientific American*.
- Hold it upside down. Set the timer for 10 minutes. Start reading it upside down.
- When the timer rings, count how many lines you were able to decipher.
- Do this twice a day for a week. See how many more lines you are reading at the end of 14 sessions.

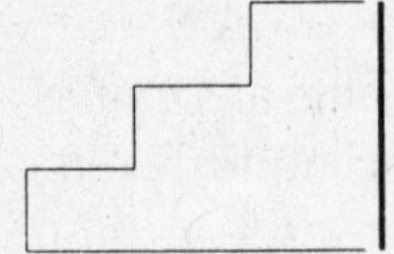

BRAIN BUILDING SECRET #18
9 Brain Poisons Worth Reducing or Eliminating from Your Life

There is another class of powerful brain poisons that include recreational drugs, hallucinogens, prescription drugs, opiates, sedatives, depressants, and stimulants, all of which are known to suppress brain power. As with alcohol, they primarily affect the limbic brain and can generate hallucinations, false euphoria, and a veil between your mind and the acual world.

Not only do these substances have negative effects on how your brain works, but they contribute to the overall load of toxic materials in your body. Further, the negative effect of these substances increases with your age. That's because as you age, your brain cells, of which there is a fixed number at birth, continually decrease in number, which means your brain becomes more vulnerable to the toxic effect of all the brain poisons.

▼ Our brain-building secret regarding these substances is simple: *If you want to safeguard your natural brain power and create the conditions in which you can increase it, avoid as many of these products as possible; if you need to use any for medical reasons, keep your use at an absolute minimum.*

1. *Cocaine*. An estimate in the late 1980s suggested that 15 million Americans had tried cocaine and that about 3 million Americans were using it regularly. In some cases, cocaine abuse can lead to seizures and epileptic convulsions, which are obvious signs that the brain is being negatively affected if not permanently damaged. It appears to impair every aspect of memory, concentration, and the ability to process, learn, and store new information.

   In the case of one cocaine addict, not only did his habit lead to epilepsy, but it warped his personality, making him paranoid, and lessened his ability to concentrate and avoid distractions. In certain sensitive individuals, even a small amount (a single dose) of cocaine can lead to a stroke or brain hemorrhage.

   Not only does this substance generate electrical seizures, abnormal electrical activity in the brain, and a general state of anxiety and hyperactivity, but it increases the level of another brain chemical called dopamine, which seems to affect the personality in strange ways.

2. *Amphetamines*. This is a class of stimulant, including various substances called "speed," STP (methyl amphetamine) or "angel dust," MDA (methylene amphetamine), certain diet pills, and other "designer drugs" that are all dangerous brain poisons.

Chronic use of these addictive substances can lead to a loss of mental abilities, memory capacity, and changes in personality, including paranoia and aggression.

As with alcohol at small preliminary dosages, there is an initial, short-lived increase in your ability to focus with greater concentration on mental work and to retain information. However, there is also the tendency to forget the new information after a few days.

You may experience a temporary elevation in mood, which in turn helps your concentration, but as you increase your dependence on these substances, suddenly things turn around. Your ability to acquire, store, and retrieve information begin to fall apart, and your overall performance in terms of learning declines.

The more you take, the more your brain power collapses. Your powers of concentration worsen; you become agitated, hyperactive, and easily distracted; and you cannot marshall enough attention to learn the new material. Conditions may even deteriorate into states of confusion and disorientation, even hallucinations. Obviously, you won't be learning much or setting records as a mental prodigy in this state of mind.

3. *Barbiturates*. This is a class of prescription and over-the-counter sedatives that depress brain function, decrease your mental abilities, and impair memory. This class of products includes tranquilizers, sleeping pills, and various brand-name drugs such as Valium, Ativan, Librium, Serax, Xanax, and Atarax.

   Originally, barbiturates and sedatives were developed to subdue epileptics and to prevent further seizures. That is why, years ago, people suffering with this condition and on barbiturates gave the impression of being "walking zombies," hardly awake and aware of their environment.

   To some extent, this remains indicative of the effect these substances have on the healthy mind: They depress mental function and, particularly, memory. Tests have shown that a substantial drop in memory function happens within the first day of taking these products. Studies also show that of the millions of Americans who use these drugs, nearly all have a measurable decline in their ability to recall information.

As a general rule, if a drug can alter your normal brain function, it will most likely also produce some negative effect or impairment on your memory, depending on how much you take over how long a time period.

4. *Tranquilizers*. Such drugs as Thorazine, Prolixin, Compazine, Mellaril, and Stelazine, commonly prescribed by psychiatrists, can produce severe problems in brain function and a high degree of memory loss. Normally, these powerful psychoactive drugs are used for people suffering from extreme degrees of agitation, hallucinations, and delusions.

5. *Antidepressants*. Such drugs as Elavil and Prozac, which are powerful mood-altering substances, have been used by psychiatrists to treat people with extreme states of depression. A 57-year-old female advertising copywriter started experiencing memory loss while she was taking Elavil for her depression. The drug helped her mood but interfered with her mental abilities.

   Technically, it obstructs the network for the brain chemical acetylcholine, believed to be crucial to memory function. Prozac, another now very popular antidepressant, tends to impair intellectual ability and memory capacity to a lesser degree, so her doctor changed her prescription, and within a short time, her brain power was restored.

6. *Antihypertensives*. This class of precription medications includes beta-blockers such as Atenolol and Propanalol, which are designed to calm people down, and pain relievers such as digitalis. Unfortunately, these drugs can also interfere with your ability to remember and commit things to memory.

   Drugs that suppress the blood levels of glucose, eyedrops taken for glaucoma, and some drugs for the stomach (Cimetidine) are known to block memory and interfere with other mental abilities.

7. *Multiple Drugs in Combinations*. Physicians call this polypharmacy, that is, the somewhat unpredictable effects of taking several powerful drugs at once.

   One patient taking many prescribed medications, including ones for his heart, high blood pressure, and asthma, showed definite signs of decline in his memory and general intellectual abilities. As he was gradually eased off some of the medications and the dosage on others reduced, his brain function returned to normal.

A 68-year-old man took antihistamines every spring for his allergies. Only one spring he complained of accelerated memory loss, constant forgetfulness, and long periods of confusion. When his doctor reduced his antihistamine dosage, his confusion disappeared and all aspects of his brain function returned to normal.

A 72-year-old woman showed symptoms that her doctors called agitated depression. She was put on several psychiatric drugs, but soon after she became confused, more agitated, delusional, and drowsy and had periods of stupor. Was she on the fast track to senile dementia and Alzheimer's? No, her brain was poisoned and toxic from a bad combination of drugs. As these medications were discontinued, all her mental powers came back.

A 62-year-old woman was put in a nursing home with suspected Alzheimer's disease for 17 months. Her doctor discovered she was taking 27 different psychiatric medications at the same time. In his judgment, the combined effect of this drug cocktail was the progressive decline in her mental ability and the steady increase in her mental problems.

In short, her brain was severely poisoned by too many powerful drugs. It took him nearly 7 weeks to ease her off these damaging drugs, after which her symptoms of Alzheimer's disease completely disappeared. She was the victim of brain poisoning.

8. *Partial List of Brain Poison Drugs to Avoid or Limit in Use*. Psychiatric drugs that interfere with memory or brain function include barbiturates, bromides, benzodiazepams, phenothiazines, Haloperidol, Lithium, antidepressants.

   General prescription drugs used by physicians that interfere with memory or brain function include

- antihistamines
- antidiabetic medicines
- analgesics

- antihypertensives
- Cimetidine
- Inderal
- Reserpine
- Darvon
- Symmetrel
- seasickness pills (containing scopolamine)
- glaucoma eye drops
- digitalis
- Methyldopyl
- antiasthma drugs (aminophylline)

9. *Other Brain Toxins to Avoid*. There are additional substances that are known to irritate, poison, or damage brain cells:

- mycotoxins
- aflatoxins, which are produced by mold and found in agricultural products (wheat, peanuts), shellfish, and industrial pollutants
- chemical additives such as aspartame (a sweetener)
- erythrosine
- Red Dye No. 3
- polyacrylimide, a food packaging material that leeches into food

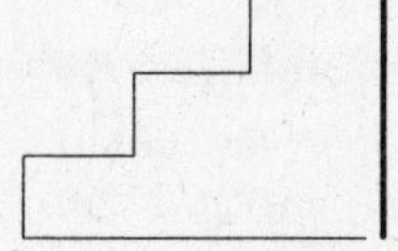

BRAIN-BUILDING SECRET #19
2 Brain Poisons Worth Cutting Back On in Your Life

1. *Caffeine*. The brain stimulant called caffeine is most commonly found in coffee, although it is also present in tea leaves, kola nuts, cacao seeds, ilex leaves, soft drinks, and numerous over-the-counter and prescription drugs. It may surprise you, but Coca-Cola was marketed originally as an "intellectual beverage" and "brain tonic" because of its known effect on the nervous system and brain.

Caffeine is absorbed even faster than alcohol and, at low doses, has an immediate stimulating effect on your brain, removing drowsiness and fatigue and enhancing alertness and focus. It can also produce irritability and nervousness in those not accustomed to it, but fatigue and headaches in those who overuse it.

The paradox of coffee is that while it certainly is a brain power stimulant, coffee can also produce the opposite effects. It may arouse your brain, but it does not actually increase the blood flow in this direction.

In fact, one or two cups of coffee actually *significantly decreases* blood flow to your brain. That's why caffeinated coffee is used to treat migraine headaches—it helps to contract the distended blood vessels in the brain. Also, and equally strange, coffee will calm down especially hyperactive children.[15]

In practical terms, it is probably best to use coffee *sparingly*, one to two cups daily maximum, as an extra booster for your brain power but not as your brain's primary power pack. Nor is it prudent, physiologically, to *rely* on coffee to get you started in the morning, as a substitute for what should be your body's natural vitality.

Remember, too much caffeine in your system and a chronic dependence on this stimulant for getting through the day adds to the toxic overload your body is probably carrying.

2. *Nicotine*. This stimulant, most commonly found in cigarettes, is another problematical substance when it comes to brain power. When you inhale nicotine through a cigarette, it reaches your brain in about 8 seconds; there it stimulates the release of brain chemicals (acetylcholine and vasopressin) associated with memory function and neurohormones that make you feel very good.

   You feel more alert and relaxed and you probably will be able to perform mental work even better, with greater speed and accuracy—for about the next 30 minutes. Then you need a new infusion of nicotine to keep the brain power cooking at the same level.[16]

   Nicotine gives you a temporary boost in usable IQ that carries a potentially deadly price tag: lung cancer. Don't forget that nicotine is also a poison commonly used in rat poisons and insecticides. For the few degrees of increased brain power you gain and for its short-lived presence, the nicotine route to higher mental abilities is not worth the cost.

Researchers have shown that smokers who switch from nicotine to aerobic exercise can experience the same kind of brain high and state of *relaxed alertness* resulting from the release of beta-endorphin, acetylcholine, and adrenaline.

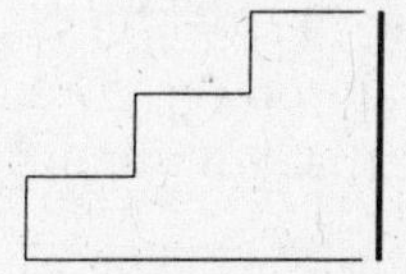

BRAIN BUILDERS! WORKOUT #10
Put Your Reading Eyes In Backwards

- Read each of these statements correctly, in which each of the words is written in reverse.
- A gnirettams fo gnihtyreve, dna a egdelwonk fo gnihton.—selrahC snekciD
- elihW morf a duorp rewot ni eht nwot/htaeD skool yllacit-nagig nwod.—ragdE nellA eoP
- teL su ereht etamina dna egaruocne hcae rehto, dna wohs eht elohw dlrow taht a nameerF, gnidnetnoc rof ytrebil no sih dnuorg, si roirepus ot yna hsivals yranecrem no htrae.—egroeG notgnihsaW

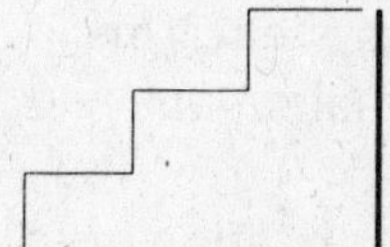

BRAIN-BUILDING SECRET #20
Unclog the Brain Drain—The Intestines and Your Mind

This may strike you as a topic you'd rather not consider, but the vitality of your intestines and general digestive process are crucial to enhancing brain power.

In fact, this brain-building secret, and the related ones dealing with bodily detoxification, are among the most important and crucial of everything recommended in this book.

The health, or stagnation, of your colon underlies every aspect of your mind/body, whether it be well-being or ill health. You must remember that brain power and the flexibility and competence of your mind is entirely dependent on the general state of your organism.

A CLOGGED INTESTINE MEANS A CLOGGED BRAIN

Problems in the large intestine can create toxic conditions within your body that can help generate a host of serious health problems, such as disturbances in your pancreas, liver enlargement, heart and stomach trouble, imbalances in menstruation, and bladder function. If the colon is one of the prime keys to your brain power, constipation and long-term colonic stagnation guarantee that your brain will not function at its highest level.[17]

A clogged intestine directly interferes with your brain power. The more constipated (or intestinally sluggish) you are, the less brain power you have available. That's because there is a direct link—not so much in terms of anatomy and function but in terms of energy—between the mind and the digestive process, particularly the intestines. This means that for many of us, the digestion and assimilation of food and, most important, the elimination of waste may be sluggish, incomplete, and possibly unhealthy.

Natural health experts and specialists in the field of "colonics" claim that most of us are chronically constipated, even if we move our bowels every day. Even with one bowel movement daily you may still be using your large intestines for long-term storage space for undigested food. Worse than chronic constipation is a condition called *autointoxication*, as when your body carries so much old, putrified fecal matter that it begins literally to poison your system. This in turn compromises the healthy action of all your internal organs and physiologic systems.

Here are some of the typical symptoms of autointoxication from a stagnant bowel. See if any of them apply to you:

- lack of energy
- tiredness
- irritability
- restlessness

- intolerance
- a tendency to quarrel
- fatigue
- lack of endurance
- frequent illnesses

PRACTICAL STRATEGIES TO CONSIDER TO UNCLOG THE DRAIN

Before I go any farther with this explanation, let me make some practical suggestions on how you can convert your intestinal storage space into brain power production. Here are a few strategies to consider:

- *Colonics, irrigation, and enemas*. These produce immediate results (within a few hours) but may not appeal to everyone; they also do not affect the entire bulk of the intestines.
- *Short-term fasting* (2–4 *days*). You consume only liquids (fruit or vegetable juices) to give the intestines a chance to unclog themselves.
- *Herbal bowel cleanser*. This is slower, cheaper, easy to self-administer, and more thorough, requiring 10–12 days.

Laxatives and bowel cathartics are not a good idea. They are short-term palliative measures that do not address the problem, nor do they clean out your intestines. They are simply a boost to the sluggish process of peristalsis, the rhythmic contracting movement of your intestines that pushes fecal matter along the track. Laxatives irritate the colon, tire it out, and are no better than constantly jump-starting your car's battery when you really need a new one.

11 STEPS TO UNCLOG YOUR BRAIN IN 2 WEEKS

Prepared herbal colon cleansers and special herb formulations are available in the marketplace and easily obtained at natural foods and health outlets and through direct mail See the Resources for addresses. Here is a sample approach:

1. Take V.E. Vit-Ra-Tox No. 19 Intestinal Cleanser two times daily, per directions on the package, usually once first thing in the morning, once before bed. This preparation is made from powdered plantago and psyllium seed husks, both of which have a high fiber content necessary for unclogging the colon. A jar should last you 10–14 days.
2. On rising, on an empty stomach, mix a heaping teaspoon of the dry mixture with water or a fruit juice, *immediately* shake vigorously, then drink immediately because otherwise the solution congeals into sludge. Repeat before going to bed; make sure it's been at least 3 hours since eating dinner. Do this twice daily for about 10–14 days.
3. Depending on the initial state of your intestines, it may take 3–6 days to start the elimination process. It is working from the moment you take your first dose, but remember that to start moving the matter takes time.

   When it does start working, you may find yourself doing 4–6 bowel motions a day for several days. You may also find these to be of an unusual character, appearance, and odor. Don't worry; this is *very old* matter indeed being purged from all the "nooks and crannies" of your intestines.
4. If you start getting cramps or diarrhea, stop the treatment. Your body is telling you it's had enough. Wait a few days and resume. On the second or third day of the program, you may experience some temporary bloating; you may also experience a fair amount of churning, bubbling, and rumbling in your intestinal tract. These are normal occurrences. It means the product is doing its job and your intestines are responding with a major house cleaning.
5. Try to avoid eating any foods that will cause bloating, such as beans. Eat light foods that are high in fiber, such as whole grains. Go easy on the fats and sugars; these will interfere with the bowel clean-out. Drink more than your usual amount of pure water. Try to avoid "junk foods" during this period.
6. As a complement, to stimulate the detoxifying action of the liver and intestines, take Yerba Prima Kalenite Herbal Formula, in pill form, after every dose of the bowel cleanser.

7. For an even more thorough detoxification program, you might consider the Purifying Program, made by Eden's Secrets, which includes 8–25 different cleansing herbs, depending on the formula.
8. Be prepared for some possible psychological and emotion repercussions. You are literally stirring things up in your mind-body system. Depending on your temperament, you may experience 1–2 days of mental turbulence, in the form of strange thoughts, too many thoughts, or memories from the distant past.

   You may also experience surges of unaccountable anger or depression. Don't worry about these and don't give them too much mind. They are transient events literally generated by the cleaning out of your intestines.
9. Flower essences can help you through this important brain power-enhancing process.

- ▼ Take *crab apple* four times daily during the entire period of time you are on the bowel clean-out. This will help your emotions deal with the cleansing activity.
- ▼ If you feel unusually irritable, take *beech*.
- ▼ If your thoughts keep churning and repeating themselves, take *white chestnut*.
- ▼ If you feel a lot of anger, take *holly*.

10. Consider taking *acidophilus pills* every day while you're on the clean-out. Each pill has 50-million live lactobacillus organisms that are of great benefit to your intestine. They are part of the normal healthy intestinal flora that live in your colon and are crucial to the normal activities of detoxification in your colon. There are in fact some 400 different species of intestinal microorganisms, weighing 3–5 pounds in total, active in your colon.
11. Consider repeating this program in 3 months; then again in 6 months; then make it an annual affair as a kind of internal spring cleaning on behalf of improving your brain power.

ADDITIONAL GUIDELINES FOR DOING THE BRAIN BUILDERS! BOWEL CLEAN-OUT

- Generally, it takes about 2–4 days for the mixture to start producing results, but they will be remarkable.
- You may find yourself regarding your intestines with awe when you experience the amount of matter that has been stored within them, unknown to you.
- You may find your waistline slims down, your posture improves, your walking gait lightens up, and your clothes fit better.
- You may find that certain long-standing emotions, grudges, peeves, complaints, and attitudes shift or even disappear.
- Your overall disposition may grow sunnier, more optimistic, more confident.
- On the other hand, it's important to see that your mind also conditions your colon. Mental tension, stress, worry, and emotional pains can irritate your intestines, producing inflammation, contractions, or constipation.
- If you are attentive, you may also directly experience the working connection or energy link between the intestines and the mind.
- For one day or perhaps two, you may feel riled, agitated, stirred up, spaced out, and unfocused as the bowel-cleansing process moves into full gear. The negative impact on your mind passes in a couple of days, so do not take any of these transient experiences seriously.
- But when the bowel clean-out program is finished, you will feel unexpectedly light and mentally agile, as if a great load has been taken off your mind in exchange for millions of liberated neurons now ready to enhance your brain power.

A PERSONAL PEP TALK ON IMPROVING THE CONNECTION BETWEEN YOUR MIND AND YOUR INTESTINES

Here are some personal reflections on this most astonishing process of intestinal house cleaning. I learned the connection between thinking and the intestines quite directly.

As a writer, mental clarity—the ability to focus, remember, connect, organize, and explain—is more central to my profession than the working status of my computer and typewriter. And a clogged colon makes me work harder to get the same mental clarity and to keep up the same mental performances than I ought to.

According to naturopath and health educator Dr. Bernard Jensen, you can have 3–4 bowel movements a day and still have a chronically constipated colon. Dr. Jensen also estimates that most people are at least 10 meals behind in their eliminations.

Consider the statistics: the small intestine is 20 feet long; the large intestine about 5 feet long but twice as wide and full of little pockets and convolutions. That is a lot of *storage* space. The trouble is that when fecal matter gets stored in the 25 feet of our intestines, it starts polluting us from the inside, making our system toxic. A clogged intestine can produce headaches, mental dullness, drain our energy, and leave us fatigued or irritable. And those are the milder symptoms.

What clogs the intestine? A meat-centered diet—typically a standard American diet that is high in animal protein and saturated fats, low in vegetables and fiber—will clog the intestines quicker and more thoroughly than a vegetarian or semivegetarian diet, which is high in vegetable fiber and grains, low in fats, and only moderately high in nonmeat proteins. However, even a vegetarian's colon most likely is clogged and carrying extra baggage from the past.

AN ASTONISHING AMOUNT OF STORAGE SPACE ROBS YOUR BRAIN POWER

Here is an astounding fact: if you were to stop eating today and not eat for a week (and go on the bowel clean-out program), and if you had never done anything to purge your intestines, you would surely have at least 25–30 bowel movements during this 7-day period. That is no exaggeration. It is awesome to experience how much old matter we carry about in the 25 feet of our intestines.[18]

There are various reasons that account for this. Meat—animal products—and saturated fats are complex foods that require a lot of energy and time to digest; they have a tendency to putrefy in the intestines. Vegetables, grains, fruits, and nuts are less complex and digest faster, usually more thoroughly, and move through the system more quickly. However, stress, tension, lack of exercise, inadequate water intake, illness, overwork, and other factors can make the intestines of even a long-standing vegetarian sluggish if not overfull.

Even vegetarians do not have completely empty, highly efficient colons, as I discovered. Lack of regular physical exercise, dehydration, overeating, and chronic stress can also contribute to sluggish intestines. This condition shaves off IQ points from our intelligence. Fortunately, there are strategies you might undertake to immediately unclog the brain drain in your intestines.

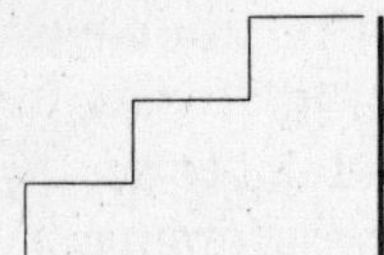

BRAIN BUILDERS! WORKOUT #11
Put Your Reading Eyes In Backwards—Again

Read each of these statements correctly, in which each of the words is written in reverse.

- fltit'nseodeviguoyaehcadaeh, tilliwekamuoytnaillirb. hcaEdrowniesehtdecapsnusecnetnessidellepssdrawkcab. daeRmehttuoyltcerroc.
- llAehts'dlrowaegats.dnAllaehtnemdnanemowyleremsreyalp: yehtevahriehtstixednariehtsecnartne;dnaenonamnisihemit-syalpynamstrap.—mailliWeraepsekahS
- ehTsomiksedahytfifowtsemanrofwonsesuacebtisawtnatrop-mi:erehtthguootebsaynamrofevol.—teragraMdoowtA

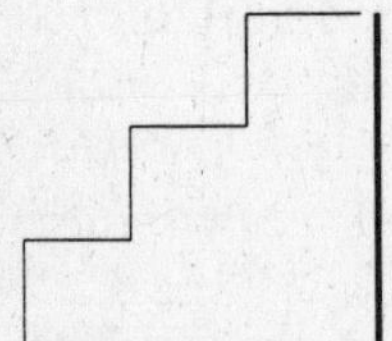

BRAIN-BUILDING SECRET #21
Get the Meat Out of Your Brain—5 Reasons Why Beef May Drain Your Brain Power

Aside from the matter of high cholesterol and saturated fat, if your diet is high in meat (beef, pork, lamb), you may pay a price for this one day in a loss of brain power. Not only does the standard American high-beef-consumption diet raise the average risk of cardiovascular disease, but it can also heighten your susceptibility to a mental decline in your elderly years.

Scientists studied data on diet and disease for 34,000 vegetarians that the Seventh Day Adventists had compiled since 1976. They compared the health status of 136 Seventh Day Adventist vegetarians with people of the same gender and age who were meat-eaters and found that only 3 vegetarians developed dementia compared to 10 meat-eaters.

Further, none of the vegetarians suffered from dementia produced by stroke while 5 of the meat-eaters did. One scientist involved with this study declared that if people stopped eating meat today, in 10 years they would have 50 percent less risk of dementia compared to the average heavy meat-eater.

Our brain-building secret here is straightforward: *Consider reducing your red, fatty meat consumption by half, or even entirely, to preserve your brain power when you are older.*

There are five reasons why it might be prudent to consider reducing your meat intake—both in terms of your general well-being and with respect to your neuronal health.

1. *Atherosclerosis*. Excessive meat consumption is linked to atherosclerosis, or hardening of the arteries, and this in turn is directly related to mental decline. Here's how it works.

   Most American males, for example, eat a diet that is very high in fats and animal protein and low in fiber; in many cases, 50 percent of calories derive from meats alone. The result is thickened, hardened arteries, which eventually stiffens its way into the clinical condition called atherosclerosis.

   Of the estimated 1.5 million Americans who have been diagnosed with severe dementia, nutrition experts suggest that most of the people involved probably had lifelong unhealthy diets. In other words, to a certain extent you can lay the "blame" for so-called age-related brain power decline to ill advised diets.

   Atherosclerosis is directly linked to diminished brain function for a simple reason. Your arteries simply cannot deliver the required oxygen and nutrients to your brain in sufficient quantities because there is so little "pumping" space left in them. They are so clogged that the supplies can't get through.

Remember, your brain not only uses 20 percent of your body's oxygen supplies, but it requires amounts of nearly every known nutrient, vitamin, and mineral to keep itself in thinking trim. There you are trying to think more, use your brain more, pump ions, whatever, yet your circulatory system cannot meet the demand for the needed brain nutrients because your arteries are so clogged.[19]

Expand this scenario over a period of several decades and you have dwindling brain power and eventually, for some people, dementia and Alzheimer's disease. Diminished blood flow to the brain—cerebral vascular deficiency—is extremely common in the United States. The chief reason for this is atherosclerosis, the blocked flow of blood and brain nutrients, largely created by a diet too dependent on meats.

2. *Food poisons*. Most meats and poultry are laced with hidden poisons in the form of hormones, antibiotics, tranquilizers, additives, preservatives, pesticides, and other toxins fed to the animals to fatten them, speed up their growth, or to keep them from getting sick in our modern factory-farming approach to "animal husbandry." If these harmful chemicals are in the meat, when you eat the meat, they're in you, too.

3. *Contaminated meats*. Infected, contaminated meat may have a role in producing dementia. News reports in the 1990s tell us increasingly of incidents of contaminated meats and chickens and of meat-packing and -processing plants that are inadequately inspected and poorly sanitized.

   People get serious food poisonings from prominent fast-food burger franchises as undercooked hamburgers transmit generous supplies of E. *coli* bacteria to unsuspecting consumers.

4. *Free radicals*. More important, a diet based largely on meats may keep you from eating enough fresh fruits, vegetables, and legumes that contain a wealth of valuable micronutrients such as flavonoids and carotenoids, which help protect your body from cardiovascular disease, stroke, and oxidation by free radicals. (See Brain Building Secret #52)

This is an important but not widely understood phenomenon. A free radical is a toxic, highly reactive form of oxygen circulating in the body. A molecule of oxygen becomes "free" in the sense that it is unstable and not yet bonded with other molecules, because they are unbonded, or "free," to need to bond with available electrons to complete themselves. This is where the problem arises.

A free radical robs an electron from other molecules and in the process damages these cells. Many experts on aging believe that free radicals contribute heavily to aging and the decline of mental abilities; free radicals are believed to damage brain cells, interfere with memory, and even cause the brain to shrink in size. In fact, scientists have proven that tissue damage in all parts of the body and all forms of degenerative disease are caused in part by free radicals.

In fact, so prevalent are these damaging free radicals—from pollutants, processed foods, even computers,—that many scientists suggest that they may be robbing youthful and middle-aged brains of their vital brain power. When the free radicals rob electrons, this is called *oxidation*.[20] Free radicals may be involved in mental deterioration, the aging and damaging of neurons, and the early stages of Alzheimer's.

5. H*omocysteine*. Another possible link betwen meat eating and loss of brain power may involve a chemical compound called *homocysteine*.

   For some decades, this chemical has been considered a risk factor in heart disease, but now scientists believe it may be involved in strokes as well. It's produced as a by-product of the amino acid methionine and normally your body converts homocysteine to a harmless form called cystathionine.

   The trouble is, if you eat a lot of meat, your body may produce large quantities of homocysteine but not convert it to its harmless form. Researchers now have evidence suggesting that if your system is high in this chemical, it can lead to a decline in your mental abilities, specifically, to lower scores on standard cognitive tests.

   Also, it seems that people with higher levels of this chemical in their bodies tend to have a much higher risk of cerebrovascular disease, even higher than from smoking, high cholesterol, or high blood pressure.

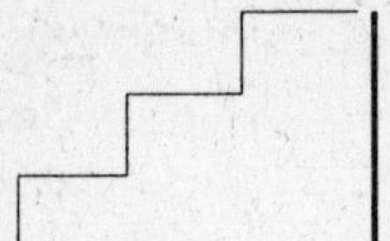

BRAIN BUILDERS! WORKOUT #12 Getting It All Backwards, on Purpose

Rewrite these sentences with the letters in each word reversed. Try to do this first in your mind, pronouncing or seeing the reversed words in the entire sentence; then write it out on paper.

- Land is immortal, for it harbors the mysteries of creation.—Anwar al-Sadat
- Once more, in the great systole and diastole of history, an age of freedom ended and an age of discipline began.—Will Durant
- Facts are stubborn things; and whatever may be our wishes, our inclinations, or the dictates of our passions, they cannot alter the state of facts and evidence.— John Adams

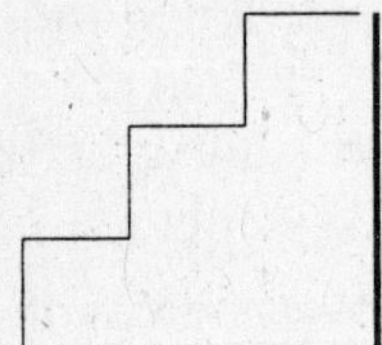

BRAIN-BUILDING SECRET #22 Your Memory Loss May Be Due to Faulty Nutrition—and How to Reverse It

Let's consider the possibility that the main source of your declining brain power is *malnutrition*. Your brain is not getting the nutrition it requires to operate in top form. Here are some suggestions for shoring up the basic nutritional status of an elderly man or woman with signs of brain power loss.[21]

The discussion here is about the negative effects on your brain power due to serious shortages of essential nutrients. For example, it's worth noting that

- The elderly tend to be deficient in many nutrients and often have poor nutrition.
- In one study of elderly people who had recently entered the hospital, 53 percent of the men and 61 percent of the women were diagnosed as undernourished, compared to elderly of the same age living at home.

▼ The hospitalized elderly typically consume less than two thirds of the adult RDAs for many important nutrients.

The emphasis in this discussion is on the numerous ways in which factors in your life-style, diet, and environment may be obstacles to the full expression of the IQ that is naturally yours. Later in the book, you will see many ways to enhance and expand your natural brain power through nutrition.

Folic acid deficiency. If your body is short of this nutrient (also called folate), you may experience apathy, disorientation, gaps in your memory, and an inability to concentrate. A 75-year-old woman had severe dementia and major brain damage that affected all her limbs. After she took folate, her mental abilities gradually improved, according to measurements of her brain waves, the disorders in her neurons improved, and her arm and leg reflexes returned to normal.

Recommended dosage (with medical supervision): 10–20 mg folic acid every day for 7 days; then reduce to 2.5–10 mg daily.

Vitamin B3, *niacin*. If you are seriously short of this vitamin, you may have pellagra, one of whose three chief signs is dementia. In some cases, supplementation with niacin has reversed this condition within weeks.

Recommended dosage: 300 mg every day for one week, then 100 mg daily.

Vitamin B1 (*thiamine*). There are several important brain enzymes whose activity is dependent on good supplies of thiamine. If you are seriously short on thiamine, your memory is probably suffering; taking ample amounts of vitamin B1 may not necessarily reverse damage to a thiamine-starved memory, but it will prevent any further loss of memory power.[22]

Recommended dosage (with medical supervision): 1 gm thiamine 3 times every day for one week, then 100 mg once a day.

Vitamin B12. It's likely that if you are elderly you are not absorbing all the B12 that may be in your diet; changes brought on by aging may be preventing your intestines from *absorbing* all the available B12.

A deficiency in this vitamin is linked to memory loss, confusion, apathy, irritability, emotional disturbances, pernicious anemia, muscle spasticity, general slowness in mental abilities, depression, and actual brain damage.

A medical center evaluating its elderly patients for B12 deficiencies found that 29 of 152 randomly selected men and women didn't have enough of this vitamin in their systems. Other medical studies suggest that 30 percent of elderly patients in general are deficient in B12. Looking at things from the reverse perspective, giving 13 senile patients B12 supplements led to a complete recovery of brain power for 8 of them, which is more than 50 percent.

Over a period of several months, a 73-year-old woman became forgetful and confused, had joint pains, and experienced tingling in her hands. All the medical tests showed that she was technically normal, even down to having enough B12 in her blood. Still, her physician started her on a program of B12 injections, and within a few days she was much improved, and after 3 months, all her symptoms had disappeared and her brain power was restored.[23]

Recommended dosage (with medical supervision): 100 mcg of vitamin B12 by intramuscular injection for 1 week; then a maintenance dosage of 1,000 mcg per month.

Choline. Choline is an essential ingredient in the makeup of the neurotransmitter called acetylcholine, which scientists believe is crucial to the function of memory. It's part of a network of brain cells in your brain's physiology that scientists call the *cholinergic system*. People who have been diagnosed with Alzheimer's disease and even with simple age-related memory loss are known to have much lower levels of acetylcholine and a slower-acting cholinergic system.

Recommended dosage: Take 10–20 g of 95 percent pure phosphatidyl choline, every day for a 6-month trial period.

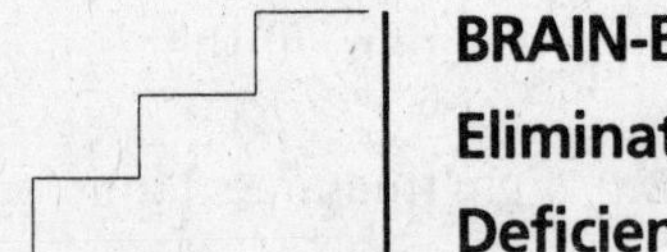

BRAIN-BUILDING SECRET #23
Eliminating Brain Poisons: Magnesium Deficiency Robs Your Brain Power

Here the problem is not that you have yet another brain poison, but rather the fact that your body may be dangerously low in a vital nutrient. If your body is low in magnesium, for example, you may be experiencing unpleasant symptoms of brain fog and the toxic brain. A significant magnesium deficiency can on its own produce nearly all the negative effects on your brain power as being allergic to foods and chemical substances.

Magnesium is an essential mineral that helps your muscles relax; it helps synthesize and break down important brain chemicals; it's also Nature's tranquilizer and a calcium channel blocker—essential to your mind and body's well-being. In fact, magnesium is necessary for the proper function of over 300 enzymes in your body; it keeps your heart healthy and your blood pressure at normal, healthy levels. Magnesium, in short, is essential for nearly every magor biological process in your body to run smoothly.

HOW YOU CAN TELL IF YOU'RE SHORT ON MAGNESIUM

The most common symptoms of a magnesium shortage are

- chronic back and neck pain with occasional muscle spasms and tremors in the same areas
- anxiety
- panic attacks
- nervousness
- cold white-tipped fingers
- irregular heart beat
- fatigue
- spastic muscle symptoms
- asthma
- migraine
- colitis
- angina
- hypertension
- cystitis
- eye twitches
- brain fog
- feeling of being dizzy, dopey, spaced-out
- confusion, depression
- inability to think clearly
- irritability

- feelings of aggressiveness
- sinus misery (sneezing, coughing, watering eyes)

FACTORS THAT ROB YOUR SYSTEM OF BRAIN POWER MAGNESIUM

You must remember that a magnesium deficiency weakens your entire system, especially your body's ability to detoxify itself. Here are additional factors that rob your system (and brain) of magnesium:

- The effect of other brain poisons, such as foods and chemicals that you are allergic to
- The general nutrient-starved state of our food, the standard (fast-food) American diet, and the use of foods grown under modern chemical-based agricultural practices
- The negative influence of stress, chronic illness, and the use of certain medications, such as diuretics for blood pressure or retaining fluids
- Overcooking of foods containing magnesium, which leeches out this valuable mineral
- High doses of vitamin C, high-fat diets, diets high in calcium (as from dairy products) or phosphates
- Poor absorption of magnesium from the diet because of food allergies, chronic constipation, inflamed bowels from candida infection
- Drinking fluoridated water
- Aging

When any of these factors are at play in your life, you can readily see how your brain power may take a nose dive into dumbness.

Magnesium, next to potassium, is the most abundantly found mineral in cells of the healthy human being. Approximately 70 percent of this magnesium is found in bone, while 30 percent is in soft tissue and body fluids. Given the factors of modern life-style, diet, a poisonous environment, your body is probably low if not deficient in magnesium.[24]

HOW TO STOCK UP ON MAGNESIUM

Fortunately, all this is reversible. You can reclaim your natural state of brain power by eliminating the various brain poisons that may be part of your life-style. The RDA for magnesium is 300 mg for women and 350 mg for men, although some nutritionists argue that adults of either gender need a range of 200–450 mg daily.

▼ If you think a magnesium deficiency is your condition, consult a clinical ecologist or physician who practices environmental medicine, or consult a laboratory that can check nutrient levels based on a test of your blood or urine. You might need to have a complete nutrition program prescribed for you to match your unique condition and to restore your magnesium levels.

▼ Consider increasing your magnesium intake by adding these foods to your diet:

- tofu (1/4 cup) for 126 mg
- buckwheat flour (1/4 cup), 112 mg
- raw wheat germ (1/4 cup) 97 mg
- almonds (1/4 cup) 96 mg
- cashews (1/4 cup) 94 mg
- kidney beans, dried (1/4 cup) 75 mg
- whole wheat flour (1/2 cup) 68 mg
- raw beet greens (1 cup) 58 mg
- banana (medium) 58 mg
- avocado (1/2) 56 mg
- blackstrap molasses (1 tablespoon) 52 mg
- potato (medium) 51 mg
- oatmeal (1 cup) 50 mg
- raw spinach (1 cup) 48 mg
- salmon (4 ounces) 43 mg
- raw Swiss chard (1 cup) 36 mg

- Try a nutritional supplement or multivitamin-mineral pill. Make sure the pill contains about twice as much calcium as magnesium, as this is their ideal working relationship. Take according to product instructions.
- Dolomite is a natural dietary supplement high in absorbable magnesium as well as calcium and other essential trace minerals.

BRAIN BUILDERS! WORKOUT #13 Improbable Mind Benders— Limber Up!

Here are quick and fun ways to stretch your brain power in unusual ways, by considering (or wrapping your mind around) the improbable:

a) What would your life be like if time ran backwards for 2 hours every day? Would you have different opinions about events.?

b) What if you could maintain your attention span, unbroken, for 4 hours running? What would you do? How would it feel?

c) What would it be like to be a single brain cell?

d) What would it be like to be a great hurricane in full spin?

e) What would it be like to be pure open space, miles and miles wide?

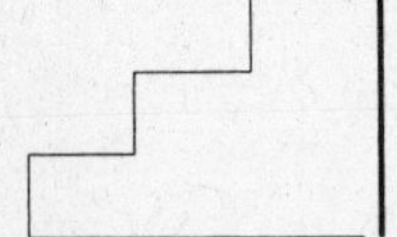

BRAIN-BUILDING SECRET #24 Understanding Mickey Finns, Brain Fog, and the Toxic Mind

Perhaps you remember from the old black-and-white gangster movies where the dissembling moll puts something in a guy's drink to knock him out for half a day. In fact, the same thing happens with Robert Redford in *The Natural* and with Gene Hackman in *The Firm*. Somebody slips them a "Mickey Finn" to put them unconscious.

Technically, the active compound in these Mickey Finns is chloral hydrate, but the surprising, alarming fact is that when your body becomes toxic and can no longer rid itself of a range of harmful toxins that accumulate in the course of living, it slips your brain a Mickey Finn and the next thing you know you are staggering around in a brain fog.

In other words, when your body becomes toxic and essentially poisoned from an inability to rid itself of harmful materials and substances, your brain, too, is toxic, and therefore unable to work at its best. Let's spend a few minutes getting to understand this new concept of bodily *toxicity*.

A LONG LIST OF POLLUTANTS CREATE A TOXIC BODY AND A STRESSED BRAIN

Nobody in Western industrialized societies lives in a pure, chemical-free, pollutionless environment. It doesn't matter if you live in a cabin in Alaska or a 1,000-acre ranch in Montana, your environment is not clean, nor is the food you eat as pure as what your grandparents enjoyed.

The nuclear accident at Chernobyl in the 1980s showed that pollution does not respect national boundaries. Although the accident happened in the USSR, the toxic fumes were blown all across Europe, contaminating agricultural and dairy products everywhere.

The list of environmental and foodborne "insults" to the body is quite enormous and the subject of increasing attention by the media. Simply consider the numerous sources of contaminants that most Americans subject their bodies to:

- ▼ medical drugs and chemicals
- ▼ antibiotics
- ▼ vaccinations
- ▼ pain killers
- ▼ birth control pills
- ▼ hormone-replacement substances
- ▼ recreational drugs
- ▼ alcohol

- processed foods with artificial sweeteners
- colors
- additives
- preservatives
- fruits and vegetables grown with chemical fertilizers, herbicides, pesticides, hormones
- food irradiation
- contaminated water supplies with heavy metals
- chlorine, mercury, lead, and other occasional poisons
- polluted air from car exhaust
- industrial fumes
- radiation and X-rays
- cigarettes
- electropollution
- household pollution
- radon gas
- formaldehyde from building materials, synthetic materials and paints

YOU AND YOUR IQ MAY BE SUFFERING FROM A TOXIC BRAIN

If your body is unable to detoxify itself of all the contaminants your life-style undoubtedly presents it with, your brain power will suffer. In short, with most people today, there are too many "foreign chemicals" in the body. Things have become so severe that even a healthy person who exercises, eats well, avoids drugs, and drinks pure water may still have a toxic body.

Your means of elimination and detoxification—skin, breathing, urine, feces, perspiration, even vomiting—may be unable to cope with the burden of contaminants. Further, heavy metals, often found in car and industrial exhausts, in pesticides, and in some food additives, cause permanent neurological damage—they destroy your brain's irreplaceable neurons.

All this toxicity goes straight to your brain, the precious "3 1/2-pound universe" you bear on your shoulders. If you are among the growing number of people who are *chemically sensitive*, you may find yourself in a chronic *brain fog*. Your mental life may feel like a nonstop Mickey Finn because the main target organ for all these toxins is your brain.[25]

The problem is this: When your normal detoxification pathways are clogged from too many toxins and a chronic nutritional deficiency, your body actually produces chloral hydrate and sends it to your brain.

These are the results:

- You get spacey, dizzy, dopey, and feel unreal.
- You're unable to think clearly or concentrate.
- You're unacountably depressed or exhausted.
- Your memory is faulty.
- You may have attention deficit disorder, learning disabilities, or hyperactivity.
- Your moods swing from manic to lows.
- You may have a tingling or numbness in parts of your body.
- You have headaches.

A QUIZ TO SEE IF YOUR BRAIN IS CARRYING A TOXIC LOAD

Here are some sample questions to ask yourself to see if you are chemically sensitive:

- Do you get foggy-headed when you use a copying machine?
- Are you happy one day and dopey, spacey, and unfocused the next?
- Does your nose register smells much better than most people?
- Does your system have a hard time tolerating alcohol?
- Are you bothered by perfumes and strong cleansers?
- Do you feel worse upon entering certain department stores?

- ▼ Are there common drugs and medications that you cannot tolerate?
- ▼ Do vitamins sometimes make you feel worse?
- ▼ Do you find that your reaction time is slower in city traffic than out in the country?
- ▼ Do you find yourself at times suddenly dumb and as if somebody stole your brain?
- ▼ Do you often feel as if you've had too many alcoholic drinks—and feel dopey, spacey, dizzy, unable to concentrate—when you've not had any?

If you answer yes to most of these, chances are your body is toxic, chemically sensitive, probably low in vital nutrients, and unable to detoxify itself. Chances are, too, that you have some of the symptoms of brain fog described earlier.

In practical terms, this means that if you want more brain power, and the use of even the natural brain power you already have, you must remove this major bottleneck in your mind-body system. Only then will the dozens of brain-building secrets presented later in this book have good results for you.

A QUICK GUIDE TO THE POSSIBLE DRAINS ON YOUR IQ

Here are some alarming facts about toxicity and the brain:

- ▼ *Formaldehyde.* Exposure to a single powerful pollutant such as urea foam formaldehyde insulation, commonly found in homes and offices built in the 1970s, can produce the following brain fog symptoms:
    - ▼ depression
    - ▼ fatigue
    - ▼ poor memory
    - ▼ inability to concentrate
    - ▼ headache
    - ▼ inability to think straight
    - ▼ rashes

- coughs
- arthritis

- *Trichloroethylene.* If you are exposed to trichloroethylene, a chemical found in machine solvents and oils, dry-cleaning fluids, carpet shampoos, floor polish, copy machines, furniture glues, typewriter "white-out," you may develop these symptoms:
  - poor concentration and coordination
  - fatigue
  - drowsiness
  - slow reaction time
  - confusion
  - headache
  - poor decision-making ability
  - confusion
  - limited attention span

- *Pesticides.* In 1989, 2.06 *billion pounds* of pesticides were used in the United States on crops, wood products, and lawns. The common symptoms of pesticide poisoning include
  - confusion
  - fatigue
  - faulty concentration and memory
  - irritability
  - slowness to your thinking process
  - schizophrenic and depressive states
  - severe memory impairment
  - difficulty in concentration
  - poor concentration
  - sluggish thought processes and computations
  - memory lapses

- speech difficulties
- anxiety
- irritability

Exposure to common chemical solvents found in the home and office can produce symptoms that include poor memory, an inability to concentrate, confusion, depression, dizziness, panic reactions, numbness and tingling, nervousness, and exhaustion.

ADD STRESS TO THIS MIXTURE AND YOU LOSE EVEN MORE IQ POINTS

Incidentally, if you're also under stress most of the time, this only makes the situation worse. The toxins in your body plus your nutrient deficiencies plus emotional and physical stress pull the plug on your brain power and it starts to drain out. Your natural IQ goes down the drain and you go down with "toxic brain syndrome."

That's because when your body is toxic and can't detoxify itself anymore, the common primary target organ is the brain, and the brain is the first to be affected. There is now lots of evidence that the cumulative effect of pesticides, chemicals, food allergies, nutrient deficiencies, and abnormal bowel flora together can produce the symptoms of chronic tiredness and the toxic brain.

The longer this condition of toxicity continues, the faster you become *chemically sensitive*. This means an increasing number of common household products will set you off into a range of symptoms while draining off your valuable brain power.

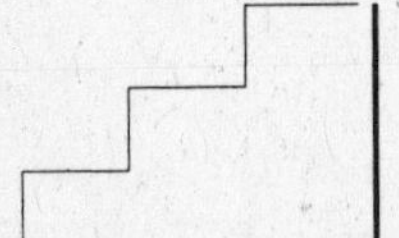

BRAIN BUILDERS! WORKOUT #14
Unscramble and Evict

- The following 8 lines represent 8 words with their letters scrambled. Set your kitchen timer for 3 minutes.
- Do this exercise in your head, without writing anything down on paper.

- Figure out the hidden words in each line. Seven of them belong to the same category, but one belongs to a different category. Find this one and evict it from the list.
- Keep practicing this until you can do it within 3 minutes. (The answers are in the Resources).

C L L I O N N

D I L C A L C A

A J G R A U

T A N A S E P H

E L Y R L O C O S R

E D S C R E M E

X E S U L

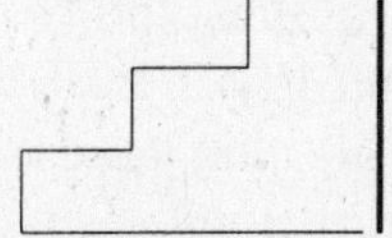

BRAIN BUILDERS! WORKOUT #15 The Zen of Brain Building

Hopefully you've never had the disquieting experience of sitting almost nose to nose with a Zen Buddhist Master who poses a truly baffling question to you, expecting an immediate answer. Zen masters use these nearly unanswerable trick questions, called *koans* (pronounced KOH-ahns), as part of their training of students. The goal is to stretch the mind as far as it will go; for our purposes here, a few *koans* might limber up our brain cells in a useful way.

1. There were two Zen students standing in the monastery courtyard watching a flag rippling in the wind. One student said, "It's the flag that is moving." The other student disagreed, saying, "No, it's the wind that's moving." The Zen master walked up behind them and surprised them with "No, you're both wrong. It is your mind that is moving." *What did he mean*?

2. A Zen master was walking through a village carrying a modest sack on his shoulder. Two young Zen students approached him, drawn by his simplicity and knowing he was a famous teacher. One student, hoping for enlightenment, asked him, "What is the significance of Zen?" The master placed his sack on the ground and stood looking at them, not saying a word. The other student then asked him, "Then what is the attainment of Zen?" The master picked up his sack, threw it over his shoulder, and walked away. *Why did he do this? How was it an answer to the students' questions?*

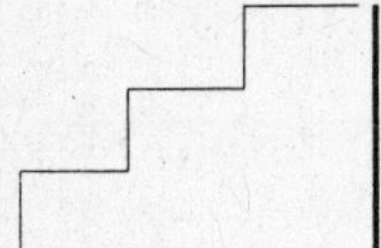

BRAIN-BUILDING SECRET #25

9 Ways to Stop the Brain Drain: You Don't Have to Be "Learning Disabled"

This brain-building secret is particularly important if you have a child who has been labeled learning disabled or dyslexic or who has "minimum brain dysfunction" and is generally having troubles learning in school. This may have nothing to do with your child's intellect, but rather his or her diet, nutritional deficiencies, and possible brain toxicity caused by exposure to heavy metals.

A child who is constantly tired and sluggish or unusually restless and hyperactive has an impaired ability to concentrate and thus to learn in school. But these conditions may be caused by nutritional factors and not be the result of your child's IQ or lack of motivation.

This is the key point: *Malnutrition, even in a mild degree, or any kind of dietary imbalance, can make it harder for a child (and adult) to learn and express their full brain power.*

1. *Junk and sugar foods.* Foods and candies high in sugars can negatively affect your child's ability to learn. For one thing, the excess sugar increases the blood levels of adrenaline, which can then make the child restless and hyperactive. Too much adrenaline in the system of a schoolchild can also increase anxiety, make the child anxious, and reduce his or her ability to concentrate, so that learning suffers.[26]

2. *Caffeine.* caffeine, found in sodas, teas, and coffee, makes learning more difficult. One study of college students revealed that those who were heavy coffee drinkers actually fared worse in terms of grades.

   When nutritional supplements were given to a supposedly "dyslexic" schoolboy, his schoolwork improved dramatically. Although IQ tests proved that this sixth-grade boy was smarter than average, he had difficulty reading and understanding printed words. A nutritional analysis of his body revealed that the levels of his essential fatty acids were out of balance and he was quite low in vitamin B6, iron, and zinc.

   The doctors put him on a diet that reduced his saturated fats but increased the amounts of polyunsaturated fats; in addition, he took vitamin and mineral supplements. He was taken off milk and all dairy products. Almost immediately his physical symptoms improved; his skin and hair looked much better; and within a year after starting this new diet, he had caught up with his classmates in all his studies and was flourishing in school. If he had ever truly been "dyslexic," it had been due entirely to these problems in his diet and nutrition and not at all to anything deep set in his brain power.

3. *Food allergies.* Unrecognized food sensitivities can directly interfere with a smart child's ability to learn. Food sensitivities that interfere with learning can start literally at the moment of birth.

   Two days after a male child was born it showed a severe rash; this soon became chronic eczema. In early childhood this child had trouble pronouncing words; spoke in garbled, unfinished sentences; forgot almost everything; and was confused. He couldn't sit quietly in his classroom and was not learning at the rate normal for his age.

   By the time he was in the second grade, the school authorities had diagnosed him as have a "learning disorder with developmental dyslexia." His behavior was unpredictable; he was moody, easily distracted, and hyperactive.

   At age 9, his parents understood he might be sensitive to foods, so they took him off dairy products and eventually discovered a long list of foods and substances he was allergic to, all of which were blocking his natural IQ. His health improved at once, as did his behavior, penmanship, and school performance.

The crucial point here is that all the professional labels the doctors and teachers put on the boy were not a true indication of his mental abilities. Many factors in his life-style were directly blocking his brain power. All of this was reversible once his parents understood what was really making him "learning disabled."

4. *Vitamin* C. Children who are low in vitamin C are highly likely to increase their IQ (or their ability to use their natural brain power) by taking extra amounts of this vitamin.[27] In other words, if you are low in vitamin C and start taking vitamin C supplements (500 mg/day), your IQ is more likely to climb than if you already were receiving an adequate vitamin C intake.

5. *Iodine*. Iodine deficiency in children has been linked with problems in the thinking processes. The RDA for iodine is 150 mcg, which you can find in sea vegetables (kelp), fish, and most shellfish—including shrimp, clams, oysters, lobsters—and iodized salt. Specifically,

    - kelp powder (1 teaspoon), 3,400 mcg
    - haddock (4 ounces), 454 mcg
    - cod (4 ounces), 209 mcg
    - shrimp (4 ounces), 186 mcg
    - halibut (4 ounces), 74 mcg

6. *Iron*. You don't have to be anemic to have difficulties concentrating that are linked to low levels of iron. Studies have implicated low levels of iron with difficulties in learning, and emotional and social problems in infants, children, adolescents, and adults.

   Infants who are deficient in iron will be irritable and indifferent to their surroundings. Infants who were anemic (severely iron deficient, which means there is less hemoglobin in the blood to carry oxygen to the brain) were more tense, less responsive, more fearful, and more emotionally reactive than were infants who enjoyed normal iron levels;

these same iron-short infants improved measurably when they were given iron supplements. Other symptoms include dizziness, headaches, irritability, constipation, heartburn, loss of appetite, and overall itching.

The RDA for iron varies with age: for infants and children up to age 10, the RDA is 6–10 mg; for men, 10–12 mg, decreasing with age; for women, 10–15 mg, decreasing with age; for pregnant women, 30 mg; for lactating women, 15 mg.

One way to increase your iron absorption is to cut back on how much black tea you drink. The tannic acid found in black tea leaves can reduce your iron absorption by 50 percent; on the other hand, if you drink a glass of orange juice with foods that are high in iron, this more than doubles your iron intake.

Here are some of the high sources of dietary iron:

- ▼ beef liver (4 ounces), 10 mg
- ▼ lean ground beef (4 ounces), 4.0 mg
- ▼ blackstrap molasses (1 tablespoon), 3.2 mg
- ▼ lima beans, dried, cooked (1/2 cup), 2.9 mg
- ▼ sunflower seeds (1/4 cup), 2.6 mg
- ▼ soybeans (1/2 cup), 2.5 mg
- ▼ dried apricots (1/4 cup), 1.8 mg
- ▼ raw broccoli (1 stalk), 1.7 mg
- ▼ cooked beet greens (1/2 cup), 1.4 mg
- ▼ raisins (1/4 cup), 1.3 mg

7. *Zinc*. Children who are chronically low in zinc may be irritable, sullen, prone to crying, and thus poor learners. When you add zinc deficiency to excess sugar intake in a child, you have two of the major factors involved in learning disabilities, as this example shows.

   A 13-year-old girl was diagnosed as having minimal brain dysfunction. She had trouble learning, she was uncooperative and antagonistic in school, and she had frequent temper outbursts. Then her diet was changed to remove all sugars, while increasing her intake of protein, vitamin C, niacinamide, and pyridoxine.

Her doctors also noted that she would be exceptionally alert and cooperative immediately after eating oysters, which they knew are high in zinc. Within one day of starting her on high doses of zinc, her overall behavior and mental abilities improved dramatically.

The RDA for zinc is 15 mg for men, 12 mg for women, 10 mg for children, 3 mg for infants, 15 mg for pregnant women, and 16–19 mg for lactating women. Nutritionists recommend a daily zinc supplement of 15–30 mg for adults and 10 mg for children; they further recommend combining zinc supplementation with copper and selenium, which work together. If you take 15–30 mg daily of zinc, take this with 1.5–3 mg of copper and 50–200 mcg of selenium for best results.

You will find high sources of zinc in these foods:

- lean beef (4 ounces), 7.0 mg
- beef liver (4 ounces), 5.8 mg
- turkey, dark meat (4 ounces), 5 mg
- soybeans (1/2 cup), 3.2 mg
- pumpkin seeds (1/4 cup), 2.6 mg
- sunflower seeds (1/4 cup), 2.0 mg
- Brazil nuts (1/4 cup), 1.8 mg
- wheat berries (1/4 cup), 1.7 mg
- cashews (1/4 cup), 1.5 mg
- tuna fish (4 ounces), 1.2 mg
- roasted peanuts (1/4 cup), 1.2 mg

8. *Aluminum*. Too much aluminum in the body is bad business for your brain power. Aluminum toxicity seems to be linked with Alzheimer's disease.[28]

   Some of the common products that contain aluminum include

- aluminum foil (that may be absorbed by foods)
- aluminum pots and pans
- buffered aspirin
- cake and pancake mixes

- antacids
- drinking water
- pickles
- processed cheese
- products to combat diarrhea
- self-rising flours
- antiperspirant sprays
- douches
- roll-on antiperspirants
- products for hemorrhoids

9. *Cadmium and lead.* A study of 26 dyslexic children from age 6 to 14 showed they had higher lead and cadmium levels in their perspiration and hair than did nondyslexic children. Another study of 150 randomly selected school-age children showed a direct relationship between higher levels of lead and cadmium in their hair and lower scores on standard IQ tests.

   Cadmium is an airborne pollutant found with lead in paint, auto exhaust, and cigarette smoke. Scientists estimate that the average American takes in 70 mcg of cadmium every day.

   The lead goes straight to the brains of the schoolchildren, with disastrous results for their brain power. It produces mild symptoms (depending on exposure) that include irritability, sleep disturbances, behavioral changes, fatigue, loss of appetite, and in higher doses abdominal pain, poor coordination, clumsiness, weakness, vomiting, even brain damage.[29]

   If the lead remains in the system, the children usually develop learning disabilities with emotional problems. The trouble with lead is that it gets right inside the nerve cells, where it disrupts the release of neurotransmitters, the brain chemicals essential to the healthy brain.

   Not only can a low exposure to lead impair your child's brain power, but if your child is already low in calcium, iron, zinc, or copper, this increases the absorption of lead from dietary and environmental sources and only makes the brain power problems worse. On the other hand, increasing your child's intake of these nutrients, combined with higher doses of vitamin C and thiamine, reduces the effects of lead exposure or low-level poisoning.

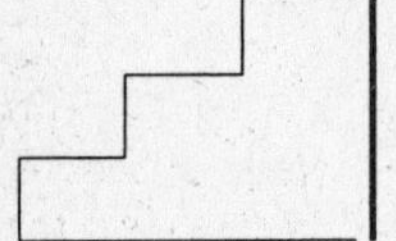

BRAIN BUILDERS! WORKOUT #16
Short-Term Memory Calisthenics

- Study these scrambled letters for 15 seconds; then close the book and look away.
- Set the kitchen timer for 60 seconds and see if you can reconstruct the original word these letters form.
- Keep practicing this until you can get it under 60 seconds. The answer is in the Resources.

---

t m
r n
r n t
a o e
r u t
i e s

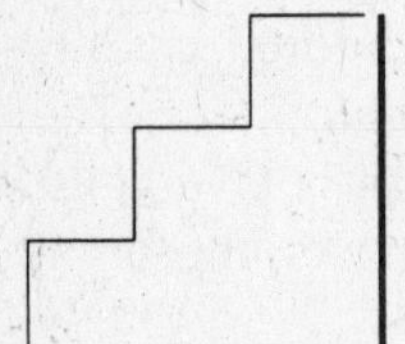

BRAIN-BUILDING SECRET #26
7 More Ways to Stop the Brain Drain: You Don't Have to Be "Learning Disabled"

Here are some more precautions to take against lead toxicity if you suspect it's a factor in your child's (or your own) learning disabilities. Follow these guidelines to build a nutritional "blockade" against pollution. [30]

1. *Eat regular meals* Remarkably, food neutralizes the effects of lead exposure. If there is lead in the foods you eat, little of it will be absorbed in your body; but if you are exposed to lead between meals, somehow 70 percent of it will get into your bloodstream.

2. *Reduce the amount of fat in your diet.* Fats absorb lead faster and more thoroughly than other foods, so cut back on your intake of rich, dairy-based snacks, desserts, and high-fat meats.

3. *Increase your dietary calcium.* Calcium, working with iron, phosphorus, and vitamin D, helps to block lead absorption into the body; if there is already lead in your system, this combination will help pull it out of your bones or fatty tissues before it gets into your organs.

4. *Take more vitamin C and zinc.* These work together to protect you against lead poisoning. According to a medical study, 22 workers exposed to high levels of airborne lead experienced a 26 percent reduction of lead in their blood after 24 weeks when they took 2,000 mg of vitamin C and 60 mg of zinc every day.

   Zinc specifically helps reduce cadmium concentrations in the blood. If you are seriously deficient in zinc, this can lead to a condition known as dementia because it directly causes a loss of brain cells (neurons) and a rise in brain levels of aluminum.

5. *Take more iron.* A deficiency of iron makes you more susceptible to lead toxicity; you may absorb as much as 24 percent of the lead in your foods, compared to only 10 percent if your iron reserves are optimal. Iron also shields your system against toxicity from cadmium.

6. *Add selenium and vitamin E to your diet.* If you have enough selenium, an important trace mineral found in fish and seafoods, in your system, this will block cadmium from entering your tissues. A laboratory study of animals showed that animals with the lowest amounts of vitamin E in their blood had the highest levels of lead after being exposed to it in their food.

7. *Review your level of manganese.* With this mineral, you will have brain power problems with either too much or too little. Studies of children considered learning disabled showed that they typically have higher levels of manganese than did schoolchildren who perform adequately in school. Too much manganese can be toxic and can block the absorption of iron, making you iron deficient; when this happens, it leads to the learning problems associated with a low iron level.

   On the other hand, manganese is needed for certain enzymes in your body to do their necessary detoxification work; it is also necessary to make an important brain enzyme needed to produce two neurotransmitters, one of which produces a natural calming effect.

   The RDA for manganese is placed at 2.5–5 mg, although you may safely take up to 10 mg a day. Proper levels of manganese are necessary for normal brain functioning and for the treatment of certain nervous system disorders, even schizophrenia. Generally, nuts and whole grain cereals are your best bet for high manganese levels.

   Dietary sources of manganese include the following:

   - oatmeal (1 cup), 11,868 mcg
   - whole wheat flour (1/2 cup), 2,580 mcg
   - dried, cooked peas (1/2 cup), 1,990 mcg
   - raw brown rice (1/4 cup), 1,850 mcg
   - banana (medium), 1,120 mcg
   - cooked spinach (1/2 cup), 745 mcg
   - lettuce (1 cup), 682 mcg
   - sweet potato (1 medium), 594 mcg
   - corn (1/2 cup), 561 mcg

   Here are a few precautions regarding manganese:

   - Antacids, laxatives containing magnesium, bran fiber, phytates in vegetables, tannins in tea, and oxalic acid in spinach may cut back the amount of manganese in your system.

- If you take high levels of magnesium, calcium, iron, or phosphate supplements, these, too, may reduce your absorption of manganese.
- If you are going to increase your manganese intake, take it as part of a well-balanced supplement that includes a range of vitamins and minerals.

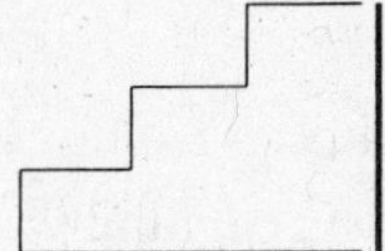

BRAIN BUILDERS! WORKOUT #17
Why Zeno's Paradox Can Build Brain Power

Zeno was a Greek philosopher who posed questions that were tremedously interesting and baffling. The following mind bender is known as Zeno's Paradox.

Suppose you are shooting an arrow from point A to point B. This distance is 50 yards. Before the arrow can travel the full 50 yards, it must travel half this distance. In other words, the arrow must first travel an ever increasing smaller distance before it can cross the full 50 yards, yet this ever increasing smaller distance can be continued indefinitely, into infinity, because you can always divide a number in half and get a smaller number. *So how can the arrow ever arrive at its target 50 yards away?*

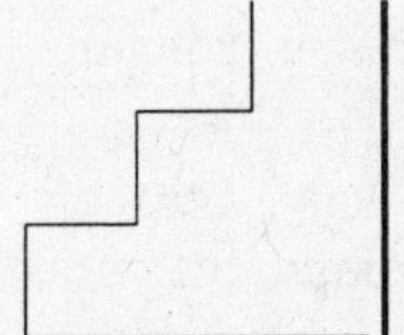

BRAIN-BUILDING SECRET #27
How to Detoxify Your Brain: Start Your Detoxification Program Today and Regain Brain Power

Now that you are aware that factors in your diet and environment may be draining your natural brain power, it's important to take steps to change things in your brain's favor. In this chapter, we're focusing on how to *eliminate* factors in your life-style that *interfere* with your brain power. In later chapters, I'll show you ways to *add* to your brain power by making additional changes in your diet and environment.

For the present, here are some immediate changes you can make in your diet. The goal is to rid your body of its load of toxins, accumulated over the years from foods, air pollution, environmental chemicals—even the way you think and feel.

These suggestions are not meant to be your permanent new diet; rather, they are strong measures to take now and for the next few weeks to help your body rid itself of its many toxins.[31]

Stage One, 1 Week

- Omit all alcohol and products containing alcohol.
- Omit all sweets. This means all prepared products containing sugars, natural and artificial, including maple syrup, honey, brown sugar, fruit drinks, and other imitation sweeteners.
- Reduce your salt consumption. Try to cut your salt intake in half.

Stage Two, 1–2 Weeks

Continue with the omissions in Stage One and add these new ones:

- Omit all foods containing molds or that are made by fermentation. This means such foods as cheeses; breads made with yeast; all processed foods in general from cans, boxes, or bottles; as well as coffee, black teas, vinegar, ketchup, mayonnaise, mustard, and commercial salad dressings.
- Substitute fresh whole vegetables such as kale, brussels sprouts, cauliflower, cabbage, onions, squash, carrots, turnips, and parsnips.
- Omit all dairy products and margarines and all wheat and white flour products, including breads, muffins, crackers, pastas—with or without yeast and all products containing gluten, which is the primary protein in wheat.
- Substitute whole grains such as brown rice, whole unprocessed oats, rye, buckwheat, quinoa, millet, barley, as well as raw, unroasted, unsalted seeds and nuts.

Stage Three, 2–3 Weeks, or Longer

Continue with the omissions in stages one and two and add these new ones:

- Omit red meats and eggs, including beef, pork, and lamb. Substitute poultry and fish; lentils; chickpeas; navy, pinto, and aduki beans; tofu; and split peas.
- Omit all products from the nightshade vegetable family such as potatoes, tomatoes, peppers, chili, eggplant, and tobacco.
- During the early phases of the detoxification diet, you may experience withdrawal symptoms from certain foods that you didn't know you were allergic or addicted to. These symptoms might include headache, depression, mood swings, and other forms of *discharge*.
- You may lose some weight as your pH becomes more balanced.
- You may *temporarily* reexperience some of the symptoms that you started with, such as allergic reactions, mental sluggishness, lack of focus.

LIFE AFTER THE DETOX—7 STEPS TO KEEP YOURSELF HEALTHY

All adverse symptoms are your body's way of telling you it is purifying itself of unwanted food substances and the unhealthy craving to consume them. This stage is temporary, and within a few weeks, you will feel better than ever before as the toxins have been removed from your internal organs, removed from the bloodstream, and eliminated from your body.

How do you know when you are completely detoxified? You will be able to gradually phase back into your diet many of the products you have removed through the detoxification diet.

Following completion of your detoxification program, you might consider making major, permanent changes in your diet. Adopting a healthy life-style will help you avoid atherosclerosis (hardening of the arteries) later in life and, hence, the conditions that impair all aspects of mental ability.

These are the steps:

1. *Adopt a healthy lifestyle.* Eliminate or seriously reduce alcohol, cigarette, and drug consumption. Maintain a positive attitude about life; eat healthy, nutritious foods; keep your body weight in line; learn how to handle stress.
2. *Become more physically active with regular exercise.* According to the research, every hour you exercise adds two hours to your life. Try to exercise in any of a list of activities (bicycling, swimming, golfing, treadmill, stationary bike, aerobics, dancing, jogging, tennis, walking, stairclimbing) for at least 20 minutes daily.
3. *Take a megavitamin supplement regularly.* No matter how well you eat, given the American diet, you will probably still come up nutritionally short with many nutrients.
4. *Take antioxidant nutrients.* See Brain-Building Secrets #52–54 for details about antioxidants and free radicals. These include vitamin C (minimum of 1,000 mg daily) and vitamin E (800–1,200 IU daily).
5. *Supplement your diet with magnesium and potassium.* Both are essential to all aspects of health and both, studies show, are typically low in most Americans.
6. *Take an oil supplement.* Your body needs a regular supply of two polyunsaturated fats, namely, linoleic (omega-6) and alpha-linoleic acid (omega-3). Good sources for omega-3 are fish and flaxseed oils; for omega-6, evening primrose oil, borage oil, black currant seed oil.
7. *Convert your diet to one that is low in fat, high in complex carbohydrates.* This means less animal protein and more fresh vegetables and fruits, whole grains, nuts, seeds, and beans; far less processed, prepared, and fortified foods; less fatty foods in general; higher fiber intake; and reduced sugars and refined carbohydrates.

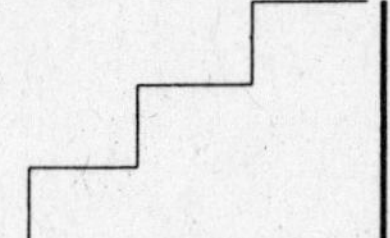

BRAIN BUILDERS! WORKOUT #18
Brain Power
Word Making

- Spend the next 60 seconds studying these four sets of scrambled letters. Each set spells a word when put in the right order.
- For the first two groups, give yourself 45 seconds to reconstruct the original words.
- For the second two groups, close the book and give yourself 45 seconds, without looking at the words, to find the original words in them. The answer is in the Resources.

r d e h n o p n i
e s z r h l i a m e

---

p d e m o n a i
y s e p a s n

3 GET IN RHYTHM WITH YOUR BRAIN

▼▼▼▼▼▼▼▼▼▼▼▼▼▼▼▼▼▼▼▼▼▼▼▼▼

How to Use Your Own Mind and Body Rhythms for More Brain Power

Get in rhythm with your brain. Your brain has its own natural rhythms of activity and rest, as does your body. You can use these to your advantage in this brain-building program. Here you will learn techniques and exercises to develop attention and focus, to prime your memory muscles, and to know the best times for brain activity.

In this chapter you will learn brain-building secrets for using the natural rhythms of your mind and body as a foundation for gaining more brain power. Did you know that every day you have natural highs and lows of brain function and that these come in cycles of 90–120 minutes? Did you know that your nose can tell you which brain power cycle you're in?

You'll learn intriguing techniques in which you use subtle preparations from herbs and flowers to fine-tune your brain power. And you'll learn how to keep your mind in focus acting on your behalf, rather than acting on its own—through mastering the technique called *mindfulness*.

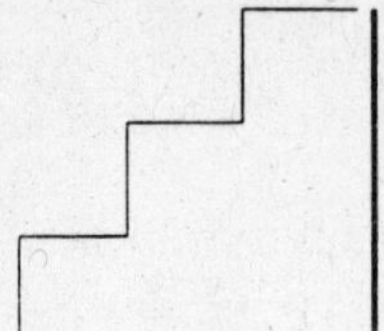

BRAIN-BUILDING SECRET #28
How an Aromatherapy Bath Can Change Your State of Mind and Improve Your Brain Power

You can use many essential oils from the field of aromatherapy as the basis for healing baths that will treat different states of mind. In aromatherapy, essential oils, made from herbs, can dissolve negative states of mind—such as depression, irritability, or panic—as well as enhance the more positive mental expressions, such as sharpening focus and clarity. The essentials oils themselves are widely available at natural foods stores and shops that sell bath products.

Remember, the variety of mind states listed in the paragraphs that follow all drain away your natural brain power. When you learn to change your state of mind and general energy level, using techniques such as aromatherapy baths, you make more of your brain power available to you during the day.

WHAT YOUR NOSE SMELLS CAN HELP YOUR BRAIN THINK

Simply consider how close your nose and its olfactory nerves are to your brain: barely 3 inches. The nerve fibers from your nose and its aroma detectors run directly to your brain's limbic area, which is associated with emotional response. You might even see your two nostrils as a visible protruding part of your brain, sensing—smelling—the outer environment.

One aromatherapist calls the nostrils "brain cells outside the brain." Add to this description the fact that scents and aromas pass directly from your nose across the blood-brain barrier without any interference. This is why smells and aromas can so instantly affect your mind and feelings, triggering joy or disgust or deep memory.[1]

All of this helps to explain why when you inhale the bouquet of an essential oil, its effect goes straight and quickly to your brain. Technically, the aroma molecules never enter your brain, but they are translated into a nerve message that does.

CHOOSING YOUR BRAIN-BUILDING AROMATHERAPY BLEND

Here is a quick review of some of your self-help possibilities. Choose one and try this first, then experiment with the others in the same category.

- *Anger*. Chamomile, melissa, rose, ylang-ylang.
- *Apathy*. Jasmine, juniper, patchouli, rosemary.
- *Confusion, indecision*. Basil, cypress, frankincense, peppermint, patchouli.
- *Depression, melancholy*. Basil, bergamot, chamomile, frankincense, geranium, jasmine, lavender, neroli, patchouli, peppermint, rose, sandalwood, ylang-ylang. Use fresh marjoram and thyme, which are energizers, in salads. Drink herbal teas made of marjoram, mint, verbena, and/or thyme. Burn marjoram or thyme essential oils in a special burner in your room. Rub a few drops of basil, marjoram, neroli, or thyme oil (mixed with grapeseed oil) onto the backs of your hands, stomach, and solar plexus.
- *Disorganization, sense of being in pieces, scattered*. Rosemary.
- *Excitability, overly excited, stirred up*. Lemon, sage, thyme, chamomile, cypress, hyssop, juniper, lavender, marjoram, neroli, rose.
- *Fatigue, from emotional stress*. Lemon, neroli, orange, petitgrain.
- *Fatigue, from physical exertion*. Basil, lavender, neroli, or petitgrain (3 drops in all) with 2 teaspoons soy oil and 2 drops wheatgerm oil; massage around your temples, neck, and chest.
- *Fear, paranoia*. Basil, clary, jasmine, juniper.
- *Grief*. Hyssop, marjoram, rose.
- *Hypersensitivity*. Chamomile, jasmine, melissa.
- *Insomnia*. Basil, chamomile, camphor, juniper, lavender, marjoram, neroli, rose, sandalwood.
- *Impatience, irritability*. Chamomile, camphor, cypress, lavender, marjoram, frankincense.

- *Mental fatigue, poor concentration, weak memory*. Basil, cardamon, peppermint, rosemary.
- *Muscle relaxant for tension held in muscles*. Clary sage.
- *Nervous tension, anxiety*. Benzoin, bergamot, chamomile, camphor, cypress, geranium, jasmine, lavender, marjoram, melissa, neroli, patchouli, rose, sandalwood, ylang-ylang.
- *Overly focused on past unpleasant events*. Benzoin, frankincense.
- *Panic, hysteria*. Chamomile, clary, jasmine, lavender, marjoram, melissa, neroli, ylang-ylang.
- *Shock*. Camphor, melissa, neroli.
- *Sluggishness, fatigue, out of focus*. Pine, eucalyptus, rosemary, black pepper, basil.
- *Stress*. Basil, lavender, mandarin, marjoram, melissa, neroli, orange, petitgrain, clary sage, ylang-ylang. Follow this with a calming tea, such as melissa, orange blossom, mint.
- *Tense, strung-out, overly excited, worried*. Lavender.
- *Tiredness with low spirits*. Thyme (5 drops) with marjoram (3 drops) in a warm bath. After bath, rub your solar plexus and sacrum areas with almond oil (1 tablespoon), wheatgerm oil (2 drops), thyme (7 drops), marjoram (2 drops), rose oil (3 drops).

MORE AROMATHERAPY BRAIN-BUILDING TIPS

- To keep your mind alert and clearheaded, put 2 drops of rosemary oil in a special essential oil burner on your desk. You will inhale the gentle but mind-stimulating fumes as you work, much as you would inhale a pleasant incense.
- If you need to stay alert while driving or in motion, dab a little rosemary on each wrist; as your hands move, you will catch whiffs of the clarifying aroma.

HOW TO USE AROMATHERAPY OILS

Aromatherapy oils are for *external use only*; do not take them orally. While they may seem similar in concept to flower essences and may in fact involve some of the same flowers and herbs, aromatherapy essential oils are far more gross in nature. This means they are direct, concentrated extracts from the plants, whereas flower essences are many times diluted mixtures made from plant blossoms.

- You may add a few drops of a flower essence to your aromatherapy bath mixture. Place 6–8 drops of your essential oil in an empty plastic yogurt container; add a little bubble bath mixture for foam.
- Fill the container halfway with bath water from the tap; now dribble the contents slowly into the stream of flowing bath water as it comes out of the tap. This will disperse the mixture uniformly into your bath water.

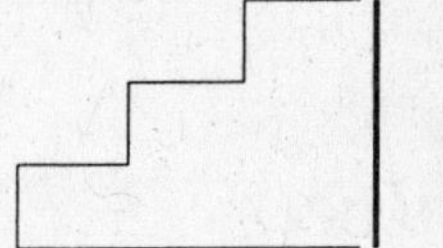

BRAIN BUILDERS!
WORKOUT #19
Number Play

- Examine these numbers for 15 seconds.
- Seven of these 3-digit numbers have something in common, but one does not.
- Find out what that common property is and identify the number unit that does not fit in.
- Set your timer for 30 seconds after you have examined the numbers. The answer is in the Resources.

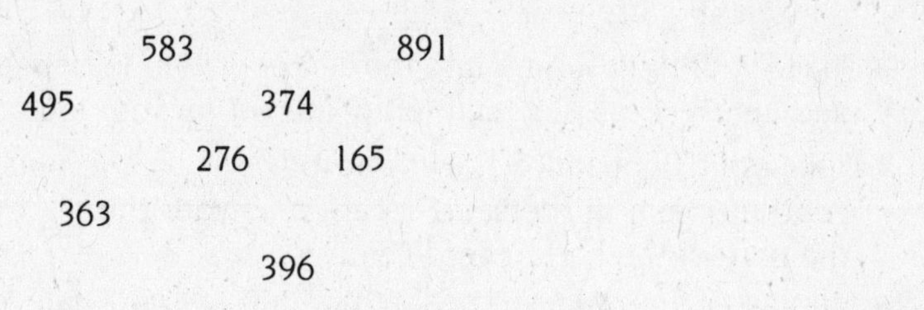

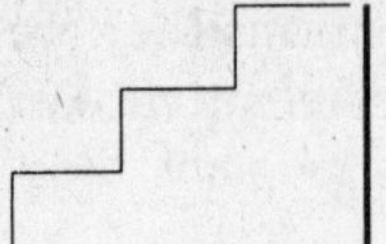

BRAIN-BUILDING SECRET #29 Overcome Stress by Practicing the One-Inch Gate Brain Power Meditation

This is an exercise taken from the Taoist tradition of ancient China. Taoist masters developed numerous ways to build body energy, increase longevity, sharpen all mental abilities, and create mind-body harmony and health. There is a spot one-inch behind the bridge of your nose and between your eyes and one-inch square in size that the Taoist masters called "Heaven's Gate."

According to their models of mind-body energy, which were the basis for acupuncture, energies from the cosmos and planet meet with your own body's energies at this special one-inch square spot above your nose. The goal of this exercise is to reduce and dissolve bodily and mental stress while building your concentration and inner calm.[2]

HOW TO DO THE STRESS-REDUCING MEDITATION

Remember, anything that eliminates stress or fatigue or other mind-body obstacles to your natural brain power in itself *increases* your brain power and your ability to put it to maximum use.

- Sit comfortably in a chair with your back straight, both feet on the floor. Take off your shoes and glasses.
- Breathe calmly and slowly; pay attention to your breathing, watching it rise and fall; inhale and exhale until you feel relaxed and attentive.
- Place your right thumb into the center of your left open palm and gently press. Let your left palm rest on your lap.
- Take your right index finger and place it on the outside of your left palm in the same location as your thumb, only on the back of the hand; press gently.
- While maintaining this position, press your left thumb against the tip of your left index finger and keep this position during the exercise.

- Next, if you are right-handed, cross your left foot over your right foot; if you are left-handed, cross your right foot over your left.
- Now, close your mouth and place your tongue up against the inside roof of your mouth. Don't strain or push it, but keep your tongue in this position during the exercise.[3]
- With your eyes closed, bring your attention to the one-inch square spot between your eyes and at the top of your nose. Don't strain. Think of this spot as a window, or a nest, or a notch.

HANGING OUT IN THE ONE-INCH SQUARE KEY TO BRAIN POWER

- Keep your inner attention focused on this spot, but do not strain or force anything. Remember to keep breathing slowly and calmly, and leave a little of your attention to follow each breath.
- Thoughts may pass through your mind; they may stampede, flood, gallop, or demand your attention. Let them pass like fast-moving clouds against a clear blue sky; pay them no mind.
- There you are, eyes closed, breathing calmly with attention, your inner focus on the one-inch square spot between your eyes. Pretend you are able to see with your eyes closed and that you are calmly surveying this fascinating one-inch window, looking through it, into your brain.
- Smile a little to help your mind and body relax even more.
- Practice this exercise for 5–10 minutes. If you need to look at a clock, squint but don't open your eyes wide open yet.
- When the exercise is finished, *slowly, gradually* open your eyes.
- Note how you feel. Are you relaxed, calmer than when you started, more at ease, more in focus, more confident in your ability to wield your natural brain power? For maximum brain power benefit, do this exercise at least once every day while you're on the brain-building program.

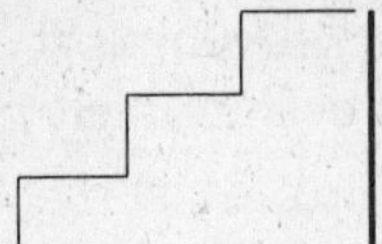

BRAIN-BUILDING SECRET #30
Stop the Noise in Your Head So Your Brain Power Can Work

Inside your head—and everyone's head—there is a great deal of "noise" that gets in the way of the natural activity of your brain power. Noise includes the constant stream of thoughts, evaluations, emotions, tension, agitation, churning, repetitive notions, judgments, memories, dream fragments, sensory impressions, desires, random images, and ideas.

Imagine, if all this unproductive debris were floating around in a swimming pool, how hard it would be to swim or even enjoy the water. Or imagine that this vast collection of unorganized mental activity were visible in the clear blue sky as a kind of awesome pollution, obscuring the sun and the natural clarity of the sky.

If you're trying to concentrate on a problem, background noise can be disruptive, irritating, and a definite obstacle to any mental work. Mental noise interrupts and distorts the clarity of your mind, the flow of information into and out of your brain, and your ability to process data.

On the other hand, when you can reduce your mental noise, you'll find your mental clarity increases noticeably and with it your ability to wield your mind like a sharp sword against a clear blue empty sky.

HOW TO GET THE NOISE OUT OF YOUR HEAD

Here is a simple noise-removing exercise that involves concentration and breathing.[4]

- ▼ Sit comfortably in a chair with your back straight, both feet on the floor. Take off your shoes and glasses; close your eyes.
- ▼ Breathe calmly and slowly; pay attention to your breathing, watching it rise and fall; inhale and exhale until you feel relaxed and attentive.
- ▼ Spend 5 minutes taking an inner inventory of the kinds of mental noise you are aware of in your mind. Categorize these different kinds of noise as if you were making a list.

- Pretend that your entire physical form is a hollow tube; where there used to be inner organs, bones, and muscles, now there is empty space.
- Inhale slowly, calmly, and with attention, except imagine you are inhaling air from the ground below you. Feel the breath rise up through your feet, legs, pelvis, intestines, stomach, chest, back, shoulders, neck, face, brain.
- As your breath rises through your body, remember that it passes through an empty hollow tube. As it does so, it makes a "swishing" sound like an air current sweeping through a round chamber.
- Allow the uprising air to sweep away all signs of tension, agitated feelings, random thoughts, repetitive memories—all the mental noise you became aware of at the start of this exercise.
- Relax and let go of everything as you exhale. Let your breath out slowly, as if you were watering a lawn with a hose that has a sprayer at the tip. Water the inside of your hollow tube with your exhaled breath.
- Repeat these steps and the breathing rhythms for another 5 minutes.
- Note how much quieter it has become in your head, how much of the mental noise has gone away. Note also how relaxed and calm you feel. You have just voluntarily slowed down your brain wave activity.
- If you have a mental task to do, such as calculations, planning, writing, analyzing, do it now while the noise level in your mind is much reduced.

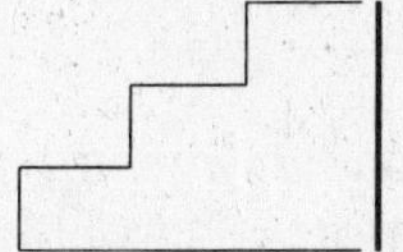

BRAIN-BUILDING SECRET #31

Managing Your Brain Power Rhythm—When to Think and When to Take a 20-Minute Break

It may surprise you to learn that as far as your brain function is concerned, all moments are not created equal. Your brain power, just like everything else in nature, has its own rhythms; this means there are better and worse times for calling on your brain to deliver its maximum power for the job at hand.

The secret here is knowing when your brain is going off duty and when to take a 20-minute break.[5] In other words, there are definite times during the day when your (left) brain essentially refuses to keep computing, analyzing, verbalizing, and generally thinking things out logically; it would rather be at the (right brain) beach.

When your body tells you it wants to take a break in the middle of the day, you'd be smart to listen. Don't be concerned that your friends might call you a slacker; these brain power rhythms are deeply set in the overall energy pattern of your body. Your observance of them is a key to more brain power.

HOW TO RECOGNIZE THE NATURAL SIGNS BY WHICH YOUR BODY AND BRAIN TELL YOU IT'S TIME FOR A 20-MINUTE BREAK

Stage One: Watch for These Recognition Signals

- ▼ You want to stretch, loosen your muscles.
- ▼ You yawn, sigh, experience drooping eyelids, dilated pupils.
- ▼ Your body becomes quiet, still, relaxed.
- ▼ You want a snack or need to visit the toilet.
- ▼ You remember happy thoughts and memories; you have blissful feelings.
- ▼ You stare vacantly into space; you doodle.
- ▼ Your reflexes slow down, hearing is impaired, mild clumsiness sets in.
- ▼ You experience a mild numbness in feet, hands, elbows, elsewhere.
- ▼ You feel a sense of confidence, satisfaction, introspection, easy intuition.
- ▼ You feel friendly; have interesting fantasies and daydreams; experience age regression; are disinclined to work and would rather focus inward.

Stage Two: Accessing the Deeper Breath

- ▼ Notice that the rhythm of your breathing is slowing down, smoothing out, getting deeper.

- Your body shifts into a relaxation mode.
- Find out where the sense of comfort is strongest in your body.
- Help this comfort feeling spread throughout your body.

Stage Three: Mind-Body Healing

- Let yourself float, drift, and enjoy the moment.
- There is no need to make a conscious effort to do anything; your mind and body are healing and rejuvenating themselves at their deepest cellular level.
- Practice *not-doing*—don't do anything, just be.
- Allow the creative, intuitive side of your mind to come alive; maybe solutions to problems or new ideas will pop up.
- Simply witness quietly and objectively what's happening inside you.
- Allow your mind the luxury of simply *wondering*.

Stage Four: Rejuvenation and Awakening

- As the 20 minutes end, reestablish contact with your normal waking state of mind.
- Note how relaxed, supple, smooth, comfortable, serene, and well you now feel.
- Shift your focus from inside to outside and go back to work.
- Do this at least once a day for optimal health.

WHAT THESE NATURAL RHYTHMS MEAN FOR YOUR BRAIN POWER

About every 90–120 minutes, your body goes through a rhythm that involves cell division, gene replication, hormone secretion, brain chemical release, and brain hemisphere dominance. These are rhythms that occur many times every day. During a typical 90-minute energy cycle, your brain will experience both a peak of heightened alertness and high performance followed by a trough of mental fatigue and the desire to take a break.

These peaks and troughs affect your performance in a wide range of mental activities, including your ability to concentrate, focus, learn, use short-term memory, perceive and be creative, as well as your athletic ability, hand-eye coordination, reflexes, dexterity, and general energy level.

In other words, during each 90- to 120-minute ultradian rhythm, you will experience a 20-minute period in which your brain power seems to diminish considerably, no matter how smart you are.

These 20-minute lows of right-brain functioning happen automatically. In fact, nearly all your major mind-body systems that are self-regulating—such as the nervous, endocrine, and immune systems—participate in this 90- to 120-minute cycle of rest and activity. Mental skills rise and fall according to these rhythms.

There are 90-minute rhythms in mental style, or the overall way in which we use our brain power. Every 90 minutes your verbal and spatial skills alternate with each other in dominance.

Here are some of the psychological and physiological processes that are affected by this 90-minute rhythm:

- gastrointestinal acivation
- sexual arousal
- urinary output
- heart rate
- body temperature
- rate of eyeblinks
- muscle tone
- appetite
- fantasy
- memory
- perception
- sense of time

MAKING YOUR BRAIN RHYTHMS WORK FOR YOU

This information has an immediately practical angle: don't expect your maximum brain power if your ultradian rhythm is in the trough phase of any of the key brain power categories.

In fact, if your mind and body are signaling it wants to relax into the 20-minute break, all the bodily processes that support mental activities are also going into a low energy point. Try to recognize this natural, recurring rhythm throughout the day.

When you do, you will realize that those moments when you feel sluggish, mentally dull, and not very smart, probably indicate that you are in the middle of a brain power low point and that this state of mental affairs is not a true reflection of your natural intelligence. Then the key is to learn how to use your ultradian highs and lows to best advantage.

Don't try to do your finest mental work when your body has enterd the 20-minute rest and rejuvenation phase; wait 20 minutes and see what a difference there is in your brain power.

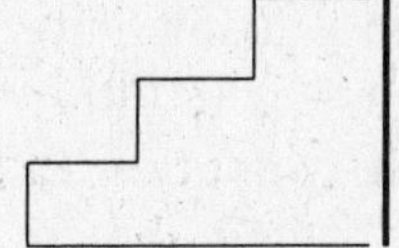

BRAIN BUILDERS! WORKOUT #20
Mapping Your Memory
Fitness

- Study this map for 3 minutes. Set your kitchen timer to be sure of the time.
- Close the book or look away from the map. Set the timer for 1 minute.
- Redraw the map from memory, including street names and locations.
- Keep practicing this until you can redraw the map accurately in 60 seconds or less.

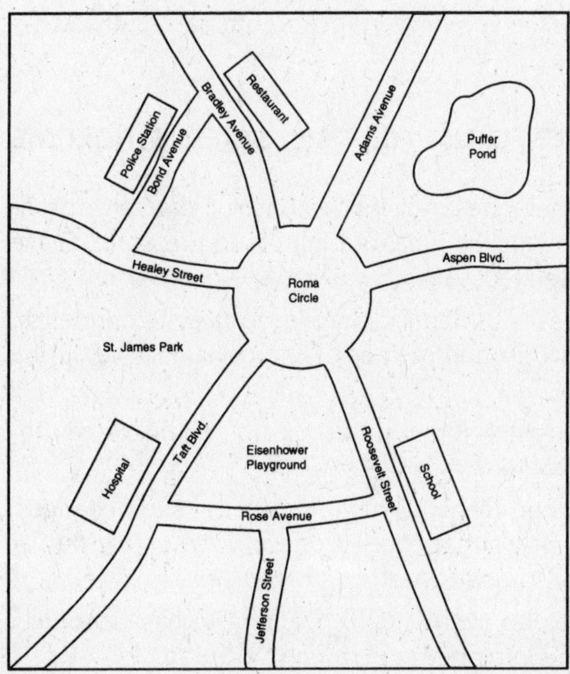

Diagram 3-1

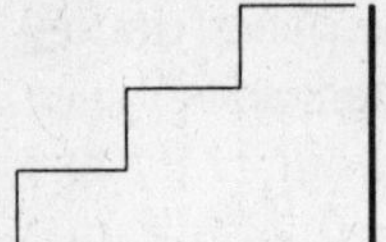

BRAIN-BUILDING SECRET #32
Eliminate Daily Stress Syndrome and Reclaim More Brain Power

You may be a hard-working person who has not been aware of these rhythms and you may have pushed yourself a little too far. Now, if you happen to ignore on a regular basis your ultradian rhythms and their natural demand for rest and rejuvenation at the cellular level, you may develop daily stress syndrome, which might be the basis of all psychosomatic illness.

If this happens, then you will have more problems with accessing your natural brain power. Your memory, learning ability, recall, and generally positive self-attitude will decline, and you'll drop function IQ points like marbles. The more important the need to have brain power for a job, the greater the need for balance in your daily brain and energy rhythms.

The idea of ultradian rhythms of course is a new one to most people, so it is quite likely that to some degree you are probably suppressing or ignoring your body's own natural signals for a 20-minute brain power break. So it is very important to eliminate daily stress syndrome from your life.

YOUR 10-POINT CHECKLIST FOR DAILY STRESS SYNDROME

- ▼ Do you have backaches, tension headaches, digestive problems, skin problems, asthma, or high blood pressure? These may be stress related.
- ▼ Do you have waves of depression, a drop in self-confidence, an increase in worry, and periods of emotional fatigue during the day?
- ▼ Do you find you often forget names, words, or misplace otherwise familiar objects?
- ▼ Do your moods go through frequent but transient changes, such as irritability, impatience, sadness, even crying during certain times of the day?
- ▼ Do you seem to be overeating or wanting to eat too much, especially in the late afternoon or early evening?

- ▼ Do you have addictions such as overusing stimulants, coffee, sugar, chocolate, alcohol, or other possibly harmful substances?
- ▼ Do you find yourself engaging in nervous gestures such as nail biting, hair pulling, or foot tapping?
- ▼ Is there stress and conflict in even your best relationships? Are you misunderstanding people and mistaking social cues even from friends?
- ▼ Do you seem to be prone to accidents, bumping clumsily into things, knocking them over, spilling drinks, making a lot of errors in detailed work after only a couple hours on the job?
- ▼ Does it take you a long time to fall asleep? Does your mind keep churning over thoughts, emotions, and experiences from the day? Do you wake up often in the night or wake up in the morning unrefreshed and tired?

If you've answered yes to four or more questions, most likely you have daily stress syndrome. You are losing valuable brain power every minute of the day you allow this condition to continue.

For a time and to a degree, your body can compensate for your habitual ignoring of these break signals. It will release more hormones and give you a second wind; you may fly high on coffee during the workday to give your brain power the extra needed boost. But soon you'll hit Stage Three: "malfunction junction." This is a downhill slope to illness and serious discomfort.

WHAT HAPPENS WHEN YOU HAVE DAILY STRESS SYNDROME

- ▼ You will bump into objects frequently, misspell common words, be prone to accidents, be clumsy.
- ▼ You will make untypical mistakes in judgment and bad decisions despite the fact that you know better.
- ▼ You will repeatedly make unnecessary errors in spelling, calculation, typing, computing, grammar, even speech.
- ▼ You will have major memory problems, lapses, failures to recall, even difficulties in remembering the object of a current sentence or thought.

- You will make embarrassing slips of the tongue, slur or mispronounce words, use words incorrectly or inappropriately, as if you were intoxicated.
- You will commit costly oversights in planning, miss crucial implications of your mental work, fail to understand jokes and word play.
- You will demonstrate frequent flashes of irritation and impatience.
- You will commit social mistakes, gaffes, misread people, misinterpret subtle cues between friends and colleagues.

From here, your brain power is on a steady roll downhill, shedding IQ points like dust on your descent into Stage Four: "the rebellious body." Here you may start doing permanent damage to your natural brain power. We know that a basic source of chronic stress comes when you suppress your mind-body's natural urge to take that 20-minute break for rest and rejuvenation at the cellular level.

Excess, chronic stress actually destroys brain cells that deal with memory and learning. So, if you have the signs of daily stress syndrome, start eliminating it today. Get onto the brain-building 20-minute break program as soon as possible and your brain will thank you.

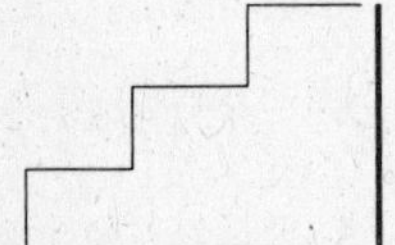

BRAIN-BUILDING SECRET #33
Let Your Nose Signal Your Optimal Brain Power Moments

Dr. Rossi's research, the investigations of other chronobiologists, and the ancient Hindu practice of yoga all have another brain power secret for you. It has to do with your nostrils and your breathing.

USING THE BRAIN POWER SECRETS OF YOUR NOSE

Here's how to find out the brain power secrets of your nose; you'll need a small hand-held mirror for this exercise.

- ▼ Sit comfortably in a chair, your hands on your lap, your eyes open; breathe calmly and normally for a few moments.
- ▼ Hold the mirror up close against your nose. Exhale normally. Note which nostril makes a bigger moisture pattern or mist-blot on the glass.
- ▼ Here's another way to check nostril dominance. Close your right nostril with your thumb on the side. Make a short, sharp exhalation through the left nostril and note the sound the air makes passig through the nostril.
- ▼ Do the same with the left nostril. The nostril that makes the higher-pitched sound on exhaling represents the more congested nasal passage.
- ▼ You might also try this test: Without plugging either nostril, exhale rapidly many times in succession. You will note a cool sensation in the nostril that is open.
- ▼ If you're still not sure, try this next. Take your right index finger or thumb and block your right nostril. Inhale through the left nostril. Note whether the nostril is open or blocked in terms of how much air can pass through it. Then take your left index finger or thumb and block the left nostril. Inhale through the right nostril.
- ▼ Note whether this nostril is open or clogged. Which nostril is more blocked up, which more open?

NOTICING THE FLOW OF ENERGY THROUGH YOUR NOSTRILS

Let's say your right nostril feels blocked up when you inhale and your left nostril is wide open, allowing plenty of air to move through it. This means that at this moment the *right hemisphere* of your brain (the part that handles spatial, intuitive, visual, holistic, emotional, and creative functions) is operating at full throttle and that your *left hemisphere* (the part that handles your logical, analytical, verbal, rational, and mathematical functions) is more dormant.

But within the next 90–120 minutes, this will shift to the opposite; your right nostril will open up and your left nostril will become clogged. In fact, this alternation between right brain and left brain dominance fluctuates every 90–120 minutes of your life.[6]

In other words, your nasal cycle fluctuates regularly every 90–120 minutes from having your right then your left nostril free and open for the passage of air; at the same time, one hemisphere and then the other of your brain is active and dominant during this same period. When your left nostril is open, your right brain hemisphere is active, or if your right nostril is clogged, then your right hemisphere is dominant.

Thus your regularly alternating nasal cycle is a reliable window into brain function. Your breath has a profound effect on how your body functions since it is the link between the body and mind.

LIFE UNDER YOUR BRAIN HEMISPHERES

Here is a quick review of what parts of your life fall under either the right or left brain hemisphere.

Left Hemisphere

- *Left nostril clogged, right nostril open.* Speech, writing, abstract thinking, verbal skills, time orientation, logic, discussions, details, talking, sociability, long-term memory, problem-solving, planning, analysis.

Right Hemisphere

- *Right nostril clogged, left nostril open.* Nonverbal memory, visual and spatial skills, intuition, emotional or musical sensitivities, the ability to make images, ability to synthesize information, to perceive holistically, seeing whole patterns, artistic creativity.

The ancient yogis knew that the science of nasal cycles is also the key to the technology of the mind. Or as one biological scientist put it, your nose is a tool for changing the cortical activity of your brain. You can synchronize your dominant nostril to be in accordance with your specific daily activities, depending on whether they are mostly verbal/analytical or spatial/creative.

This information about the brain-breath connection has a distinctly practical application. Say you have an important executive meeting, examination, writing assignment, or accountancy work and your left nostril is open and your right nostril is clogged, meaning your right brain, controlling spatial, intuitive functions, is dominant. (See Diagram 3-2)

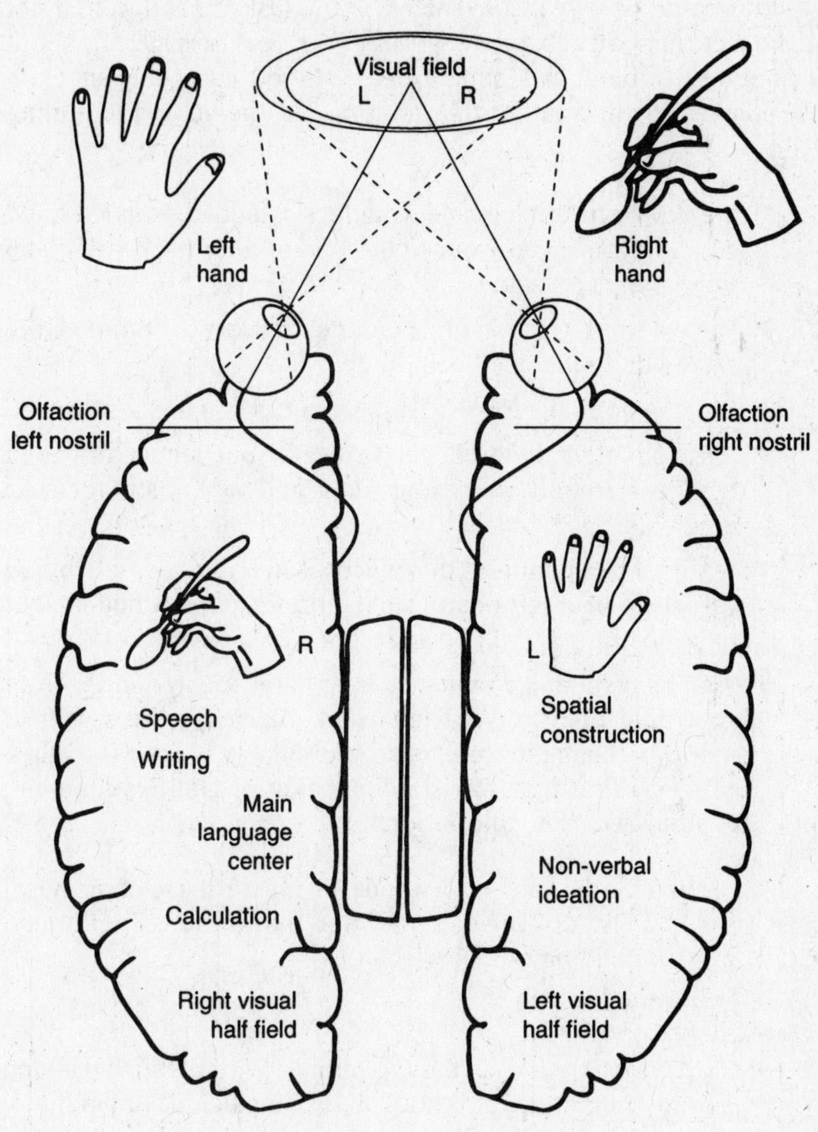
Visual field
L
R
Left
hand
Right
hand
Olfaction
left nostril
Olfaction
right nostril
R
L
Speech
Writing
Main
language
center
Calculation
Right visual
half field
Spatial
construction
Non-verbal
ideation
Left visual
half field

Diagram 3-2

GETTING YOUR NOSTRILS TO SHIFT ON COMMAND

This could be very inconvenient for the task at hand were it not for the fact that you can actually *change your nasal dominance* in about 10 minutes. Through this simple exercise, you can get your brain hemispheres to shift, rather than waiting out the 90 to 120 minute cycle.

- Lie down on your left side, your legs extended, your left hand cupping your head, your right hand at your neck—as if you were going to sleep.
- Place a small cushion under your left armpit to stimulate the nerves on that side of your body.
- Breathe normally for 3–10 minutes until you feel a shift.
- Use your right index finger to close your left nostril then breathe forcefully out of your congested right nostril for a few moments.
- Within 5–10 minutes, the mucosal membranes and blood vessels in your left nostril will start to expand, while in your right nostril, they will begin to open up.
- Your hemispheric dominance is simultaneously shifting from your right brain to your left brain. You may note a shift in mood, a change in the direction or quality of your thoughts; you may find that you start planning or crafting complete sentences or new calculations.

The yogis of India know a lot about the practical use of the nasal cycle. Here is a list of everyday activities that are best performed when the corresponding nostril is open.

Left Nostril Open

- *Right hemisphere dominant.* Long-term activities, starting a long journey, beginning of school study, singing, playing a musical instrument, planting, gardening, getting married, lending money, buying clothes or land, meeting relatives, treating illness, spiritual observance, opening a bank account, meditating.

Right Nostril Open

- *Left hemisphere dominant.* Performing short-term activities, making a short journey, studying difficult skills, writing manuscripts, sculpting or carpentry, borrowing money or accepting charity, practicing medicine, driving a car, giving orders, eating, drinking liquor, working with numbers and accounts, expressing anger.

GETTING YOUR NOSTRILS RIGHT FIRST THING IN THE MORNING

Here is one final way to make this information about your brain-breath connection practical.

- Immediately when you wake up in the morning, check your breathing to see which nostril is dominant. Make a note of this.
- Check your nasal cycle 120 minutes later to see if your nasal dominance has shifted. Make a note of this time.
- During the day, continue to note the changes every 90–120 minutes and make a note of the kinds of activities you are busy with at each time.
- At the end of the day, study your list. Get familiar with your brain-breath cycles so that you can put them to best advantage as another brain-building secret.

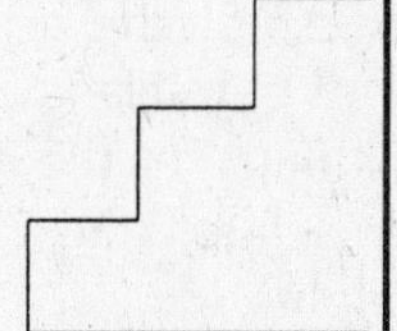

THE ANATOMY OF BRAIN POWER #4
Why Your Environment May Be Poisoning Your Brain, Making You Hyperactive and Making It Hard to Learn

Why is there such a high incidence of hyperactivity, learning disorders, and general behavioral problems in children and adults? It may be caused by poisons in their living and learning environment.

Since the 1950s, an enormous number of synthetic chemicals have been developed and put into products that surround us. There are now about 70,000 chemicals used in commerce, agriculture, building products, and foods produced in annual quantities of at least 170 billion pounds. Several hundred are *neurotoxic*—poisonous to your brain.

Scientists call them *volatile organic compounds* because they can evaporate and contaminate the indoor air of buildings and homes and they tend to get deposited in human fatty tissue because they are fat soluble. The prime organ of accumulation is your brain.[7]

WHY YOUR BRAIN FOG MAY BE DUE TO POISONOUS CHEMICALS

What happens when these compounds get deposited in your brain tissues? You experience symptoms typical of brain power drain like these:

- headaches
- forgetfulness
- dizziness
- mental fogginess
- inability to concentrate
- poor coordination
- inexplicable anger or depression
- anxiety
- memory and learning impairments

The effects are even more pronounced in children, who are about 10 times more vulnerable to the negative effects of these chemicals than adults. That is why a growing number of physicians suspect that the high level of contamination is directly linked to the high degree of hyperactivity and behavioral problems in schoolchildren. The classroom itself may be contaminating their brains.

Your typical office may be hazardous to your brain power, too. The fumes and evaporation products of synthetic materials, pesticides, fumigants, cleaning agents, sprays, copying machines, and numerous other sources all concentrate in the indoor air that everyone breathes.

Symptoms that typically result include these:

- lethargy
- concentration problems
- personality changes
- fatigue
- hyperactivity
- memory difficulties

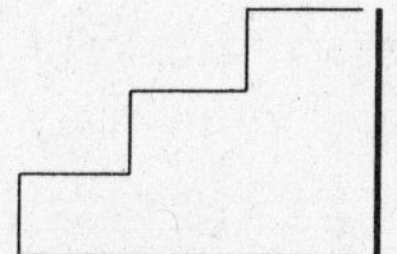

BRAIN-BUILDING SECRET #34
Smarten Up Your Attention, Memory, and Thinking—With Flowers

Starting today, you can take quick, simple, effective steps toward increasing your brain power using flower essences. Whether it's greater attention, focus, clarity of mind, memory, recall, mental vigor, or creativity you're after, the world of flowers has an essence that will work for you.

For example, a California mother in her forties named Camille decided she would launch her own marketing business so she could work at home and take care of her children. She knew she would need a great store of concentration, focus, and sharp mental abilities. To help hone these skills, Camille selected a series of flower essences. "I chose them to help me stay awake and remain focused during my work day. I've been able to notice the results ever since I started."

CHECKLIST FOR GREATER BRAIN POWER FROM FLOWERS

Here is a checklist of possibilities for greater brain power through flower essences. Study this list and decide which five conditions apply most directly to you; then put these in a list of priorities, putting the most important or pressing condition at the front of your list. Now that you have identified which mental ability you want to work on first, select the appropriate flower essence and start taking it every day for two weeks.

Note any changes in your brain power as the flower essence goes to work. When you note that this ability—greater mental clarity, for example—has improved, start working on the next brain power item on your list. Continue with this brain-building secret throughout the rest of your brain power program.

FLOWERS FOR MENTAL CLARITY

Do you feel foggy, mentally lethargic, dull, sluggish, and forgetful? Try *peppermint* for mental vibrancy and clarity and for more alertness. Peppermint helps rebalance your metabolism so that you can "digest" more ideas and think more clearly. Peppermint frees up your mind for more clearheaded thinking by giving the brain more energy that is usually tied up in digestion.

Do you want to be able to keep several mental tracks going at once, juggling details from different problems at the same time? Do you want more mental flexibility? *Rabbitbrush* is your answer. Rabbitbrush will help give you a more alert, mobile, active, and flexible state of mind. It might also help you develop a two-track mind. You will be able to focus better on details while at the same time having a broader perspective on the full picture.

Are you easily distracted, find it hard to concentrate, or feel mentally dull, spacey, and listless? Try *madia* for precise thinking, a longer attention span, and a new discipline in your focus and concentration. This flower essence will pull you back into your mental center where your mind will focus pinpointedly on any subject.

Do you have a hard time seeing the big picture, organizing ideas and details into a whole that makes sense? *Shasta daisy* will help you change this. This essence will help give you greater insight, to see the broader meaning amidst all the details; it's particularly recommended for people involved with intellectual work, such as writing, research, teaching.

Do you come across as disorganized, unfocused when you talk, or is your speech overexcited as you try to express too many ideas at once? *Cosmos* may help you slow down and integrate your ideas with how you talk so that you'll start sounding much more clear and coherent. Cosmos will help you speak slower and make more sense as you communicate more of the ideas that dance around your mind.

Maybe it's simply a matter of having enough mental vitality. When it's time to start an intellectual project, do you find yourself procrastinating, mentally sluggish, unresponsive, like you're dragging your feet and you left all your mental energy at home? Try *corn* to stir up enthusiasm and initiative, for the energy to bite off more than you can chew—and to chew it.

FLOWERS FOR SHARPER THINKING

Do you want strength and clarity in your thinking and a mind that is no longer clouded by negative thoughts? *Mountain pennyroyal* will help here. It sometimes happens that if your mind is too full of negative thoughts, chaotic thought patterns, or even the thoughts of others, this can congest your brain and cloud your thinking. Mountain pennyroyal will help clean up your mind, as if vacuuming up negative thoughts and images; this restores your mind's natural energy and vitality and soon you'll find yourself thinking sharper.

Does your mind turn the same idea over and over again, as if obsessed with a single thought? *White chestnut* will break up this fixation. Repetitive, obsessive thoughts can drain your brain's vitality, cloud your thinking, and literally give you headaches and insomnia. White chestnut helps to quiet your chattering, churning mind, ridding it of worrisome, agitated thinking.

Do you often finish other people's thoughts for them and are you impatient and hasty in your own thinking? *Impatiens* will help correct this. You may be quite mentally agile and have a lot of brain power at hand, but inner tension and agitation can get in the way and start to burn out your finer mental abilities. Impatiens will literally help you become less impatient in your thinking.

Perhaps, if you're a student or teacher, your thinking is too sharp at times and you have overextended your brain? *Nasturtium* will help restore bodily vitality to fuel your intellectual activities. If you are too much in your head, nasturtium will bring you back to Earth and give your mind warmth and new vitality.

Do you miss details, forget important points, go along without concrete purpose or direction with a kind of mental fuzziness? *Avocado* flower essence may sharpen up your mental focus, school your memory for details, get you back on track with a newfound sense of life purpose, even give you some joy in accepting the brain power challenge of puzzles, examinations, and new intellectual tasks.

FLOWERS FOR CONCENTRATION AND FOCUS

Do you want to be able to keep your focus taut even when you're surrounded by a great deal of activity? *Indian pink* will help you keep it together amidst the bustle and stress and will help you coordinate different activities at the same time. This flower essence will help you build a feeling of equanimity and centering in the middle of intense activity.

Do you find yourself daydreaming, going spacey, drifting off when you're trying to focus on a mental task? *Clematis* will give your focus an edge and ground it in practicality, blowing away the dreamy mists. If you find yourself preoccupied with your inner life, with imaginings and impractical ideals, clematis will put your focus back on the ground.

Is your memory taking the week off and does your thinking function in general seem to be on holiday? *Rosemary* will get both back on the job. Rosemary will help to awaken your memory and ability to recall while eliminating your forgetfulness and absent-mindedness.

Does your thinking keep bringing up the past even while you're trying to concentrate on present problems? *Honeysuckle* will help change your nostalgia and emotional attachment to the past into a fuller presence in the present moment. Once you understand your past events, relationships, or places, you can release your attention from them and have lots more energy for mental tasks.

Do you frequently go out of focus when you start thinking about other people or even identifying with their thoughts and feelings? *Pink yarrow* will help you define the boundaries between your mind and your friend's; you'll no longer keep picking up their emotional confusion or mental disharmony; instead you'll be able to strengthen your own concentration. Your mind will start feeling more self-contained and objective.

Are your senses overwhelmed and is your mind overstimulated, even congested, from too much input? *Dill* will chill you out. If you live in a city or work in a busy office or watch a lot of television, quite likely your mind is overfed with sensations, experiences, and images.

From your mind's point of view, this can be like overeating, and it will slow down your mental functioning. Dill helps you navigate with clarity and focus through the typical sensory overload of modern living.

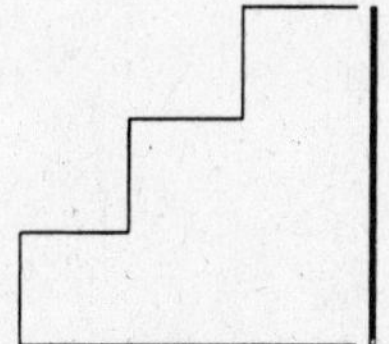

THE ANATOMY OF BRAIN POWER #5 More on Why Your Environment May Be Poisoning Your Brain, Making You Hyperactive and Making It Hard to Learn

HOW A SICK BUILDING CAN ROB YOUR BRAIN POWER

Too little attention is paid to the way enclosed spaces may be hazardous to your health and brain power. This is especially so with modern office buildings, department stores, shopping malls, and other enclosed spaces where we spend an enormous amount of our time.

Carpets. Carpets can be neurotoxic. A chemical analysis of the gasses released from a common office carpet revealed the presence of numerous toxic chemicals, including formaldehyde, benzene, and others. Similar outgassed products can come out of vinyl floor tile.

Insulation. Urea foam insulation containing formaldehyde is bad news for your brain health. The subtle fumes released by the outgassing of this product produce all the familiar symptoms of brain fog:

- ▼ depression
- ▼ fatigue
- ▼ poor memory
- ▼ cloudy thinking
- ▼ concentration difficulties
- ▼ a sense of unreality
- ▼ spaciness
- ▼ headache
- ▼ flushing
- ▼ dizziness

Bear in mind that you are likely to encounter formaldehyde in a variety of circumstances, such as a normal house, office building, mobile home, hospital, shopping center, permanent press clothes, paper products.

Copy machines. The gas emitted by copy machines can produce these symptoms:

- ▼ confusion
- ▼ poor attention
- ▼ fatigue
- ▼ slow reaction time
- ▼ numbness and tingling
- ▼ inept coordination
- ▼ headache
- ▼ dizziness
- ▼ impaired decision-making ability
- ▼ drowsiness
- ▼ confusion

So the next time you're scratching your head wondering where your IQ went to, look around you. It may have been drained off by your toxic environment.

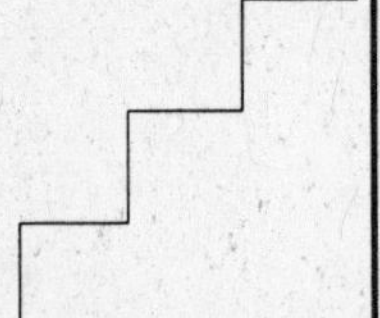

BRAIN-BUILDING SECRET #35
Be More Awake, Overcome Learning Problems, and Enhance Your Creativity with Brain Power from Flowers

Flower essences can help sharpen your brain power in the areas of attention, learning difficulties, and creativity.

FLOWERS FOR AWAKENESS AND ATTENTION

Would you rather be back in bed, buried under the covers, unconscious to the world? Is staying awake during the work day a real chore? *Milkweed* will transform your desire to escape from wakefulness and self-awareness into a strong, self-reliant state of attention. If you find yourself drifting toward ways of blotting out your awareness through food, drugs, excessive sleep, or frequent illness, milkweed will be especially helpful.

Would you like to be filled with vitality and freshness and have your brain power rolling at the top of the world without the use of stimulants? *Morning glory* is your answer. Many people feel dull, "hung-over," even toxic in the morning and generally unable to start the day without a stimulant jump-start. This state of affairs obviously will impair your brain power.

Do you work long hours in front of a video display terminal or computer screen and find your eyes get tired, your head aches, and you feel depleted? *Yarrow special formula* can help reverse this depletion. The small amounts of radiation or electromagnetic pollution in your work environment may drain your body energy and thus deprive your brain power of its necessary energy.

Do your nerves feel depleted, even worn out from too much mental work? *Lavender* will soothe the synapses and snap you back into a smooth wakefulness. Here the problem is that you are high-strung and wound-up; you're wide awake but overstimulated; perhaps you have headaches or tension in your eyes, neck, and shoulders. Lavender will help you relax and feel soothed, even sedated, without losing your wakefulness.

FLOWERS FOR OVERCOMING DIFFICULTIES IN LEARNING

Perhaps, if you're a student, you find yourself bored, apathetic, or indifferent to your course of studies yet you need to pull through and complete them. If so, then *California wild rose* may help change this, giving you a new round of enthusiasm, will power, and commitment.

Do you have difficulty learning lessons and often repeat the same mistakes? If you find that you keep repeating the same regressive patterns of thought, feeling, or experience, then *Chestnut bud* may help stimulate your brain power to finally grasp what is going on and to master the experience. This, in turn, will enable you to learn faster, deeper, and with more endurance. If you're trying to master a new and difficult academic subject but are making no progress, chestnut bud may help break you free into new insight.

Or maybe your feelings are too volatile and you are emotionally overactive and find this interferes with your ability to concencrate and study. C*hamomile* will produce an inner serenity and calm and chase away your moody irritability and release your emotional tension. When your moods don't fluctuate so widely and so often and when your "inner weather" is less turbulent, you'll find your natural brain power will emerge like the sun.

Are you experiencing a physical or mental handicap through birth or by accident that makes learning difficult, causing you to need an extra dose of fortitude to keep going? Or maybe it's a sudden shift in your fortunes, and you're recovering from a shock or loss yet you need your mental abilities in top form? P*enstemon* will help you find that inner strength to persevere even though you're undergoing rehabilitation or a long training. Penstemon helps put you in contact with new inner resources of courage and resilience.

FLOWERS FOR GREATER CREATIVITY

Maybe it's just that you don't feel inspired or creative—you have thinker's block. I*ris* will help revitalize the inner Muse and give you a fresh start on beginning and fulfilling new intellectual or artistic projects. Let iris help you get over attitudes about yourself that limit your own ability to be creative and artistically expressive.

Do you sometines have a great idea but can't marshall the will power to make it happen in the world—to express it? B*lackberry* will help you change your goals, ideals, and insights into concrete action; it will help you set your plans into priorities and inspire you to start moving on them.

Do you keep seeing things in fixed categories, in cliches, and you can't break free of these stereotypes into fresh, original perceptions and ideas? S*agebrush* may help you break through to a deeper layer of your creativity. You become aware of what is essential and basic while letting go of the mental props that impair your creative expression.

Do you want to combine thinking with imagination and to experience a new degree of creativity that uses both hemispheres of your brain? H*ound's tongue* will show you what holistic thinking and creativity feel like. This flower essence may give you a new sense of wonder and the ability to think specifically and clearly.

Do you stifle your spontaneous creative expression from lack of self-confidence or self-censorship? *Larch* will give you the inner confidence to express yourself spontaneously and creatively in new, even risky ways. You may find larch loosens your throat and you can communicate more openly, easily, and fully.

HOW TO USE YOUR BRAIN POWER FLOWER ESSENCES

Flower essences are completely safe with no unpleasant side effects. Once you've selected your first essence, take one dropperful four times daily, that is, when you awake, at midday, teatime, and then at bedtime.

If you have a day that is particularly stressful and you feel the issue you are working on (for example, focus and concentration) needs more help, increase the dosage to one dropperful every three hours. At the standard dosage, your bottle should last about one week. Continue for at least two weeks or until you can notice the changes.

Bear in mind that flower essences are a subtle vibrational medicine; they work quietly, deeply, and over time. See the Resources at the back of this book for complete information on how to obtain your essences.

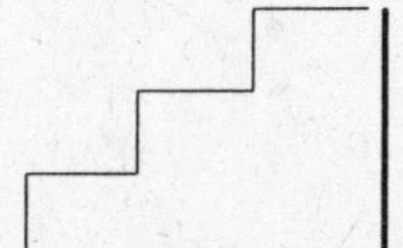

BRAIN-BUILDING SECRET #36
More Brain Power—At Your Fingertips

It may surprise you to learn that you have access to more brain power at the tips of your fingers. No, there aren't neurons or neurotransmitters buried secretly under your skin, but there is a simple hands-on technique from the field of the healing arts that enables you to give your brain a massage.

That technique comes from the natural therapy called reflexology and involves manipulating and massaging points on your feet and hands to stimulate your organs, muscles, nervous system, and brain. According to reflexology, which was developed about 80 years ago, there is a complete energy map of your body on the bottom of each foot and the palm of each hand.

The theory may be hard to prove, but for decades reflexologists have been gently massaging the numerous body points on the feet and hands to send healing energy to all the regions, systems, and parts of the body, including the brain and its functions. (See Diagram 3-3)

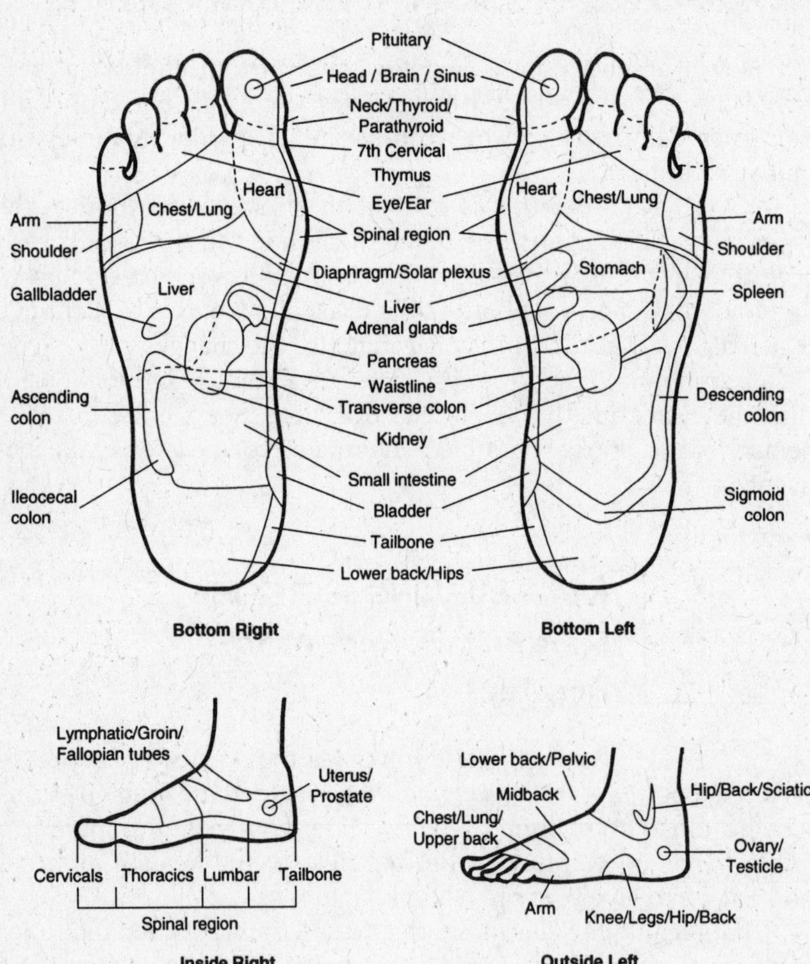

Diagram 3-3

THE KEY TO MORE BRAIN POWER LIES IN YOUR BIG TOES

The reflexological key to your brain and the doorway to more brain power lies in your two big toes. There, on the soft padded side of each big toe, from the back of the toenail to the first joint, are the reflex points for your brain, pituitary and pineal glands, the hypothalamus, temples, sinuses, and neck (see the accompanying illustration for detail). These are highly important parts of your brain.

The pituitary gland is your body's master gland, controlling the function of all your other endocrine glands and their hormone secretions which influence growth, metabolism, blood sugar content, and energy level.

The hypothalamus regulates your autonomic nervous system, which in turn controls your emotional reactions, appetite, body temperature, and sleep patterns.

The pineal gland plays an important role in controlling all your bodily rhythms, sleep and wake cycles, and possibly the function of insight and creativity. If you can keep these vital brain organs in top working order, clearly this will enhance your brain power. (See Diagrams 3-4, 3-5, and 3-6)

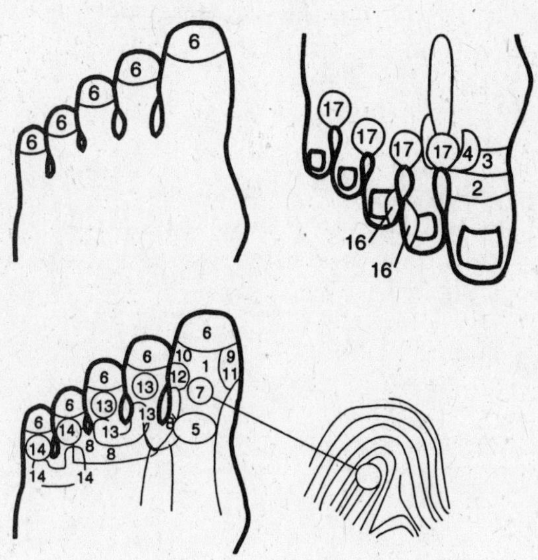

Diagram 3-4

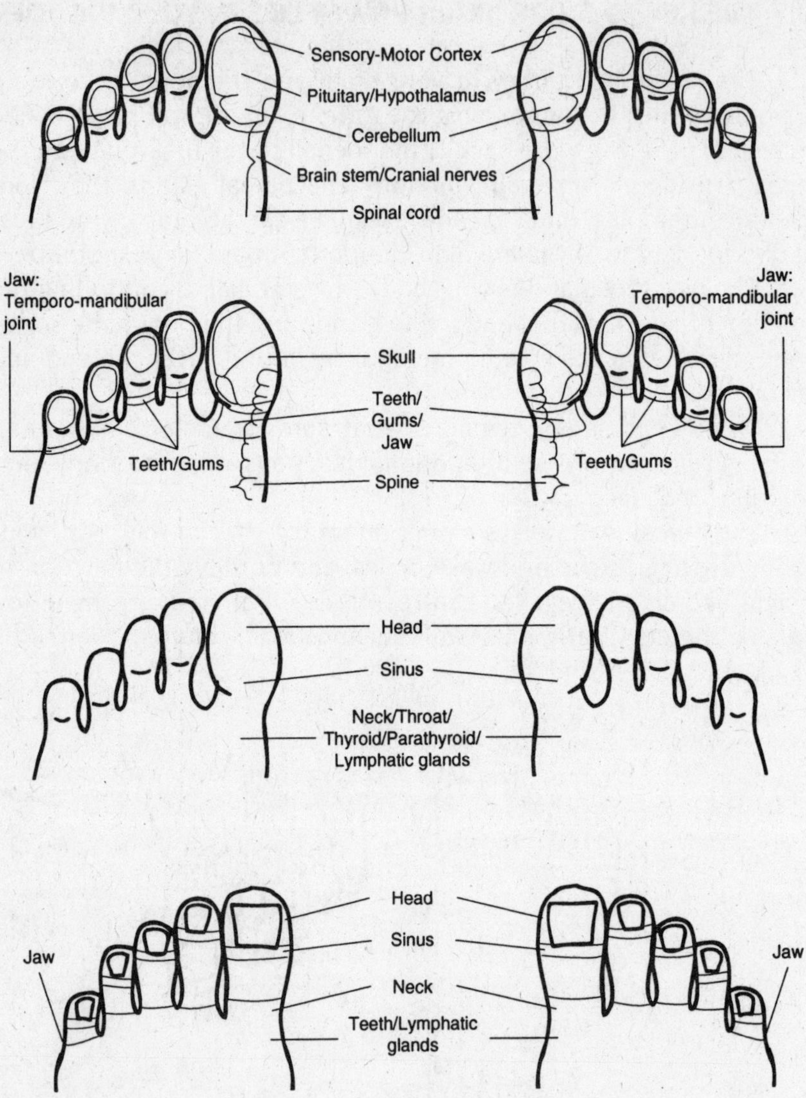
Sensory-Motor Cortex
Pituitary/Hypothalamus
Cerebellum
Brain stem/Cranial nerves
Spinal cord
Jaw:
Temporo-mandibular
joint
Jaw:
Temporo-mandibular
joint
Skull
Teeth/
Gums/
Jaw
Teeth/Gums
Teeth/Gums
Spine
Head
Sinus
Neck/Throat/
Thyroid/Parathyroid/
Lymphatic glands
Head
Sinus
Jaw
Jaw
Neck
Teeth/Lymphatic
glands

Diagram 3-5

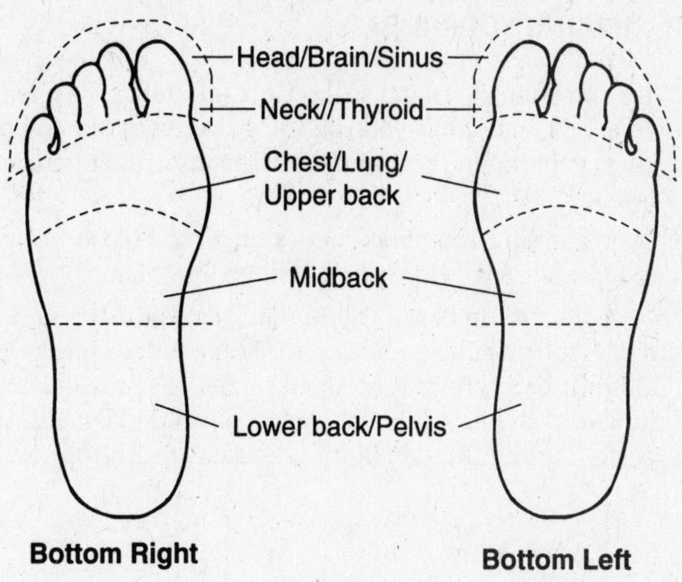
Head/Brain/Sinus
Neck//Thyroid
Chest/Lung/
Upper back
Midback
Lower back/Pelvis
Bottom Right
Bottom Left

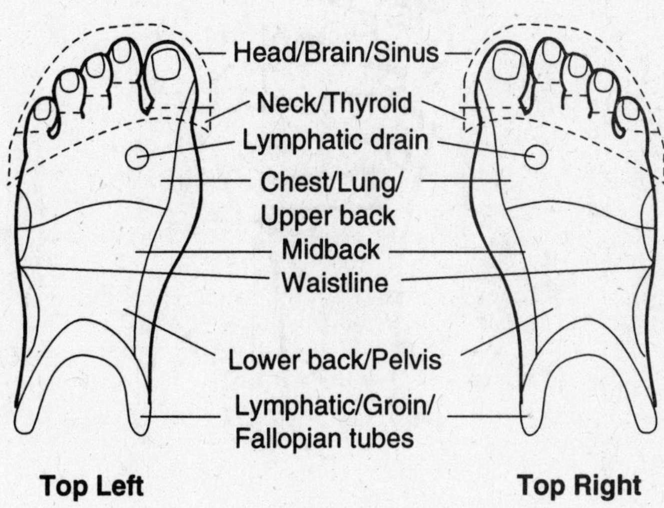
Head/Brain/Sinus
Neck/Thyroid
Lymphatic drain
Chest/Lung/
Upper back
Midback
Waistline
Lower back/Pelvis
Lymphatic/Groin/
Fallopian tubes
Top Left
Top Right

Diagram 3-6

HOW TO STIMULATE YOUR BRAIN BY RUBBING YOUR TOES

- Take off your shoes and socks, sit comfortably in a chair or on your bed, and cross your right leg over your left so you can hold your right foot with both hands. Don't strain. (See Diagram 3-7.)
- Use your right thumb and index finger to hold your right big toe. Stabilize your right foot with your left hand.
- Using your thumb, roll your thumb across the top of your big toe, just below the toenail on the soft padded side, and apply a firm, steady pressure in small circles. (See the illustration.) Roll your thumb while applying a pinch and squeezing type of pressure to the skin; if it hurts, ease up a little.

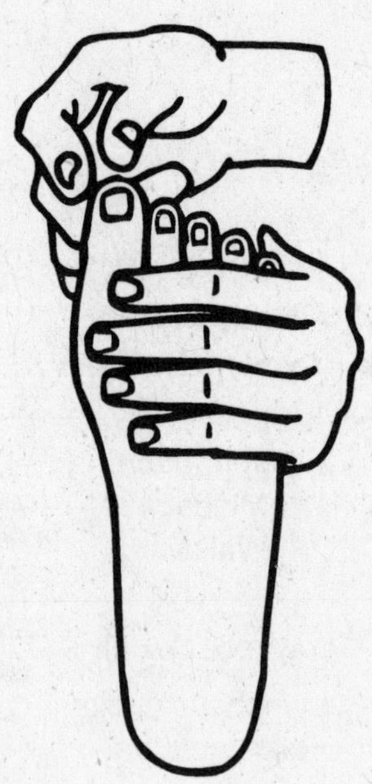

Diagram 3-7

- ▼ Continue the firm rolling motion down the outside of the right side of your toe, then down the left outside surface.
- ▼ Starting at the point just below and behind your toenail, continue the rolling pressure down the center of your big toe. Remember, this is on the backside of your toe, on the side opposite your toenail.
- ▼ Spend about 3 minutes massaging the brain reflex points on your right toe. Now repeat the rolling massage with firm, steady pressure on the soft padded backsides of your right foot's four little toes. There are brain reflex points here as well. Spend about a minute on each toe.
- ▼ Now reverse positions and follow the same sequence for your left big toe, then the four little toes on your left foot.
- ▼ Repeat the reflex toe massage on both big toes two more times.
- ▼ Try this brain power toe massage 15 minutes before you need an extra burst of brain power for a mental task, examination, meeting, or speech.

RUB YOUR THUMBS, TOO, FOR MORE BRAIN POWER

- ▼ In fact, while you're in the meeting, here is an extra, secret brain power reflex massage you can do on your fingers. You'll find the same brain reflex points on your thumbs and tips of your little fingers, so instead of fidgeting or tapping your pencil, give your brain a boost with your fingers.
- ▼ Hold your right thumb with your left index finger and thumb. Using your left thumb, repeat the firm rolling pressure you used on your toes to massage the top of your right thumb, the sides, and the soft padded backside, down to the first digit.
- ▼ Continue this rolling massage on the tips and soft undersides of the four fingers of your right hand. Reverse positions, and repeat on your left thumb and fingers. Practice this exercise for 5 minutes on each hand; continue longer if you enjoy it.

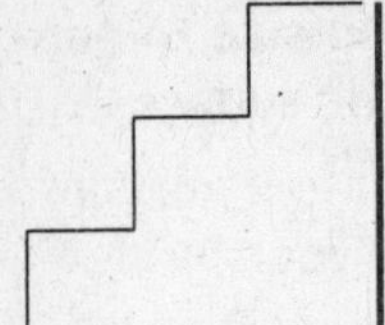

THE ANATOMY OF BRAIN POWER #5 Maybe It's Not Brain Loss: Other Factors That Can Make Your Brain Seem Older Than Its Time

Brain experts conservatively estimate that somewhere between 10 and 20 percent of elderly men and women with the apparent signs of Alzheimer's actually have *reversible* conditions. In other words, their supposed brain decline may be caused by other factors. Even more encouraging, there are positive steps you can take to speed up this reversal.[7]

REVERSIBLE CONDITIONS THAT MIMIC THE BRAIN LOSS OF ALZHEIMER'S

1. *Imitation senility*. Somewhere between 10 and 30 percent of supposedly senile patients are only pseudosenile, meaning their loss of brain power is due to something other than true brain decline.
2. *Water on the brain*. For example, common or at least treatable medical conditions can present symptoms resembling senility, such as a hormonal imbalance, an infection, or hydrocephalus, "water on the brain."
3. *Kidney infection*. In fact, there are at least 100 reversible physical conditions that affect the brain before any other bodily organ but are not senility. One example is undiagnosed kidney infection, which can make an otherwise brain power healthy individual seem like a schizophrenic.
4. *Low blood sugar*. Hypoglycemia (low blood sugar) produces symptoms, including weakness, dizziness, and confusion.
5. *Nutritional deficiencies*. Other reversible conditions, such as anemia (low iron content in the blood), exposure to environmental pollutants (carbon monoxide, lead, mercury), malnutrition, and vitamin deficiency (shortage of B12 or folic acid), can also imitate senility in the elderly.

6. *Medications.* There is also the brain-confusing effects of certain powerful drugs commonly given to the elderly. Confusional states are actually common among the elderly as adverse reactions to their medications.[7] In many cases the fastest way to restore the elderly patient to full brain power was to take them off the drugs giving them the bad reactions. Consider this example of fake senility.

   Two middle-aged men were referred to a psychiatrist. The first man had trouble coordinating his muscle movements, he could no longer calculate numbers, his memory of recent events was faulty. The second man had slow motor and mental responses, frequently got disoriented regarding time and space, couldn't concentrate, and often didn't recognize his own handwriting. Were they senile? Not at all.

   It turns out that both men for years had been taking methyldopa and a popular tranquilizer called haloperidol to treat their hypertension. As soon as they were both taken off the tranquilizer, all their symptoms disappeared within 72 hours.

7. *Depression.* This is a highly important factor that can produce symptoms of difficulties in attention, loss of memory, and a decline in the use of your brain power. Review Brain-Building Secret #14 for a full discussion of this factor.

8. *Using it too late.* And don't forget that if you start on the brain-building secret program at an early age, none of these conditions of old age and diminished brain power may ever apply to you.

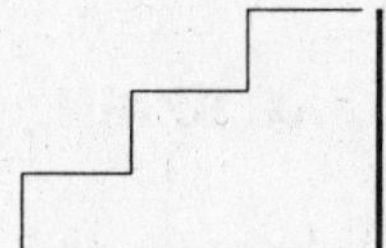

BRAIN-BUILDING SECRET #37
Massage Your Brain Hemispheres to End Forgetfulness

Not only does reflexology give you access to your brain at large, but you can fine-tune your approach to stimulate either the left or right hemispheres. This means that you have at your fingertips a key to stimulating either the logical, analytical, rational hemisphere or the intuitive, spatial, creative side.

LEFT HEMISPHERE BRAIN WORKOUT

If you want to sharpen your verbal, rational, and thinking skills, massage the reflex points for this brain hemisphere.

- Follow the instructions explained in Brain-Building Secret #36 for massaging the brain reflex points in your *right* big toe. Your right toe and its brain reflex points will "talk" to the left side of your actual brain.
- Continue with this exercise by working the brain reflex points on the four little toes, as well as your *right* foot.
- Repeat this exercise on the tip and underside of your *right* thumb and then on the tips and undersides of the fingers of your *right* hand.

RIGHT HEMISPHERE BRAIN WORKOUT

If you want to access the creative, intuitive, spatial part of your brain, you need to massage the brain reflex points for your right hemisphere.

- Follow the instructions explained in Brain-Building Secret #36 for massaging the brain reflex points in your *left* big toe. Your left toe and its brain reflex points will "talk" to the right side of your actual brain.
- Continue with this exercise by working the brain reflex points on the four little toes, as well as on your *left* foot.
- Repeat this exercise on the tip and underside of your *left* thumb and then on the tips and undersides of the fingers of your *left* hand.

ANTIFORGETFULNESS AND MEMORY-ENHANCING BRAIN WORKOUT USING REFLEX POINTS

Your memory may not be working at full capacity because you are under stress, your attention wanders, or you don't have enough brain energy.

Try this reflexology brain workout when you are studying, writing a paper, trying to master a new subject or language, or before any activities involving your left brain hemisphere.

Do the brain workout on your feet in the order listed. Consult Diagram 3–3 on page 152 to see where the brain workout reflex points are located.

1. *Solar Plexus.* Work the solar plexus and diaphragm reflex points on the bottom of your *right foot*. This exercise will help you feel calm and relaxed as your abdominal muscles release their tension.

   Use your thumb and index finger on whichever hand is stronger and place your thumb on the reflex point, as indicated. Apply a firm, steady pressure with your thumb, squeezing and pinching the point. Make 16 clockwise circles with your thumb pressed against the reflex area.

   Repeat this exercise on the same reflex points on your *left* foot.

2. *Pituitary gland.* Work the pituitary gland reflex point, located at the center of the soft underside of your *right* foot's big toe. Apply a firm, steady pressure with your thumb, squeezing and pinching the point. Make 16 clockwise circles with your thumb pressed against the reflex area.

   Repeat this exercise on the same reflex points on your *left* foot. This will help stimulate this master gland to secrete all necessary hormones that are involved in all bodily functions—in this case, those relevant to brain power.

3. *Brain.* Work the brain reflex points on the big toe of your right foot and then on the little toes of the right foot; do the same on your left big toe and left toes. Follow instructions in brain-building Secret #36.

4. *Thyroid gland.* Work the thyroid and parathyroid gland reflex points located on the big toe of each foot. You will find these points below the first digit on your big toe and above the place where it joins your foot. Work the sides and the central area of your *right* foot. Apply a firm, steady pressure with your thumb, squeezing and pinching the point. Make 16 clockwise circles with your thumb pressed against the reflex area.

   Repeat this exercise on the same reflex points on your left foot. This will send energy to the glands that control muscle tension and the rate of metabolism.

5. *Adrenal gland*. Finally, work the adrenal gland reflex points located toward the soft center of the bottom of your *right* foot, around the instep or arch. Apply a firm, steady pressure with your thumb, squeezing and pinching the point. Make 16 clockwise circles with your thumb pressed against the reflex area.

   Repeat this exercise on the same reflex points on your *left* foot. This exercise will help stimulate the release of epinephrine (adrenaline), which will aid your alertness.

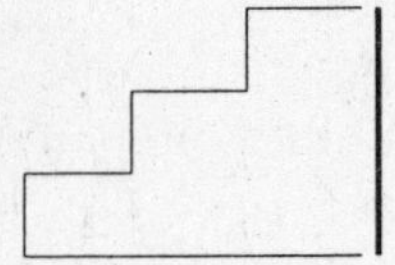

BRAIN BUILDERS! WORKOUT #21
The Face You'll Never Forget?

- ▼ Once a day, carefully study an object, picture, or person, chosen at random, for 2 minutes.
- ▼ Look away and draw what you have seen. Without consulting your first sketch, at the end of the day, redraw from memory.
- ▼ Do a different subject each day for a week. At this time, put all drawings away and redraw them from memory.
- ▼ Note the differences and discrepancies.
- ▼ Do this again for several weeks until your redrawings at the end of the week accurately match your individual day's drawings.

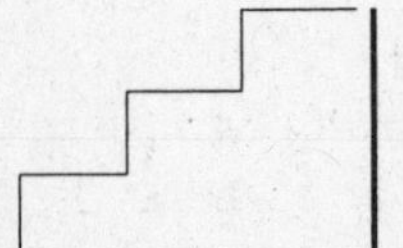

BRAIN-BUILDING SECRET #38
Priming Your Whole Brain Memory Muscles

Anthropologist Margaret Mead had a reputation for her vivid memory. She had seen, studied, and written about a fair amount of the world's native peoples and their environments during her long professional life, but what was most remarkable was her ability to remember in almost cinematic detail the different locales, climates, people, and events, as if they had happened only yesterday.

Possibly what made her memory so vivid and clear was the fact that the events were originally "encoded in her memory banks" as strong bodily sensations and lived images rather than as facts, figures, or abstract ideas.

This in fact was the idea put forward by one of our culture's foremost memory experts, an ancient Roman orator and writer named Cicero, who flourished in the first century A.D. He said that if you want to be sure of remembering events long into the future, you must commit them to memory clothed in images full of action, color, and sensation.

The key is to dress your experiences in "exceptional beauty or singular ugliness," with some kind of "ornament," either a striking image or a comic effect. Only in this way can you "well ensure your remembering them more readily."

REMEMBER YOUR CHILDHOOD AND BUILD BRAIN POWER

Here is an exercise based on the idea that as children we commit experiences to memory that are rich in detail and felt experience, that we store information that has "a freshness of perception and uncensored receiving of experience."[8]

Because the period of time involved in your childhood memories is so richly vivid, when you call these old memories to mind, it enriches memories you have stored away from more recent periods of your life. The process of remembering your childhood somehow charges all your "memory neurons" with the same kind of excitement you once had.

To do this exercise, you need to set aside about 45 minutes; you will also need either a partner to ask you questions or you can record your questions on a tape recorder, leaving long pauses for your answers. It's best if your answers are short, quick, and concise memories rather than detailed narrations. It may work best for you if you lie down on a sofa, bed, or floor mat and close your eyes, without falling asleep.

Breathe calmly and slowly; pay attention to your breathing, watch it rise and fall, inhale and exhale until you feel relaxed and attentive.

AS I REMEMBER IT, MY CHILDHOOD WAS . . .

Your partner will ask you these questions, allowing long gaps in between each question for you to respond. *Tell me from your childhood about*

- ▼ a very young boy
- ▼ an old lady
- ▼ your favorite foods
- ▼ a teacher you loved
- ▼ eating an ice cream cone
- ▼ your bedroom
- ▼ climbing a tree
- ▼ your favorite pair of shoes
- ▼ a family trip
- ▼ a favorite fort or hideout
- ▼ a balloon
- ▼ going to a store
- ▼ playing on the beach
- ▼ your favorite songs
- ▼ a birthday party
- ▼ a young girl you knew
- ▼ an old man
- ▼ your favorite TV character

Open your eyes, stand up, stretch, and see how you feel in your mind and body.

REMEMBERING WHAT IT WAS LIKE WHEN YOU . . .

Then sit down in a chair, close your eyes, and have your partner ask you these questions, leaving a minute's gap between each. *Remember what it was like*

- ▼ getting up this morning
- ▼ at your high school graduation

- doing what you did yesterday at this time
- when you heard President Kennedy was killed in 1963
- when you did something remarkable last summer
- the first time you fell in love
- your first day of school, ever

REMEMBERING THINGS YOU NEVER DID

The next set of memories will stretch your imagination because you did not, technically, experience them. Here you must call on your imagination to summon up pictures of historical events. Describe

- Abraham Lincoln giving the Gettysburg Address
- Leonardo da Vinci painting the *Mona Lisa*
- the building of the Great Wall of China
- erecting the stones of Stonehenge
- building the great pyramids of Egypt
- dinosaurs running through the marshes
- the creation of the Earth
- yourself in all your aspects—of body, mind, and soul—in this present moment

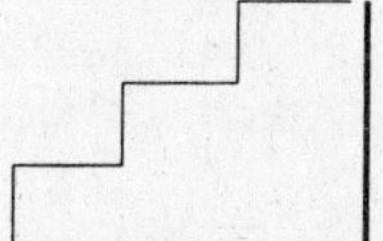

BRAIN-BUILDING SECRET #39
How to *Not* Chase the Bone While Giving Your Brain a Rest

It may sound ironic, but before you shift your mental abilities into high gear, you must first master the art of mental relaxation, which is a slowing down. Your mind can get quite active, even hyperactive, if you leave it unattended, a bit like a jungle monkey swinging from branch to branch with no goal in mind except constant motion.

But this hyperactivity (or "monkey mind") costs you physical energy, and one of the first places to be drained of this vital energy is your brain itself.

WHAT TO DO WHEN YOUR MIND IS LIKE A ROOMFUL OF TELEVISIONS, ALL TURNED ON

By way of metaphor, consider your mind as a roomful of televisions: each is tuned to a different channel, each is turned up loud. You can't hear yourself think over the racket of competing TV channels. You may also feel yourself growing anxious, on edge, unable to relax in this kind of environment. Often your life becomes like this as multiple sources of tension and stress all hit you at once—like a roomful of blaring televisions.

On the other hand, when you give your brain a rest, you walk into the room and turn down the volume *way down* on all the sets. Remember, this is your mind I'm talking about (my mind, too, for that matter).

That's why, periodically, you need to give your brain a rest—ideally, at least once a day. This happens naturally during sleep, except that when you dream your mind is actually quite active and is not at rest. The kind of brain rest I have in mind is something you do, voluntarily, during the daytime while you are awake.

HOW TO STOP THE DOG FROM CHASING THE BONE

The dog runs after the bone and tires out the mind. This is a peculiar expression Zen Buddhist teachers are likely to say. The dog is your attention; the bone is any thought that comes to mind and that you'd like to chew on; running is your chasing it and tiring out your brain and draining off its power.[9] You need four conditions for brain resting or evoking the relaxation response.

1. A quiet environment, such as a room free from household or outside noise
2. A comfortable bodily position, such as sitting in a soft chair with your shoes off
3. A passive attitude, or a state of mind that is at ease and relaxed, open to what may happen
4. An object for inner attention, something like the houseplant, flower, or affirmations from our earlier exercises.

The passive attitude is important here. It's a state of not responding to sensory stimulation, inner thoughts, feelings, and impulses, or the temptation to be distracted. There is an old saying that captures the essence of this nonresponsiveness: "The dog runs after the bone."

So pretend you are the dog; simply do not chase the bone (any thoughts, perceptions, sensations) when you see it. Remain seated, calmly focused, regarding the bone (thoughts, feelings, perceptions, impulses) with complete indifference. The real practice here is this: *The dog does* not *run after the bone*!

HOW TO PRACTICE "NOT CHASING THE BONE"

- Take the phone off the hook, turn off the TV or radio, and find a quiet room in which you will not be disturbed for 5 or 10 minutes.
- Sit comfortably in a straight-backed chair with both feet flat on the floor. Preferably, take your shoes off so your feet can relax.
- Don't slump or slouch or lean to one side, but sit up, erect but relaxed.
- Place your hands in your lap with the back of one hand resting in the palm of the other, like two saucers.
- Close your eyes. Become aware of your breathing. Note the rising and falling of your breath, the swelling of your midsection as you inhale, the emptying of your belly as you exhale.
- As you breathe out, allow a little smile to bloom on your face. Become aware of your whole body as you sit in this chair.
- Begin relaxing your body progressively, from head to toe.
- As you inhale, imagine your head filling with life-restoring energy. As you exhale, imagine you breathe out all the stress, thoughts, discomforts, and toxins from your head.
- Then do your neck, chest, arms, legs, and feet in the same way.
- Remember to smile on the exhale; this greatly enhances the relaxation response.

- Now with your body relaxed, give your brain a rest. As you inhale, count 1; as you exhale, count 2. Do this without losing track up to 10, then do it again. Do this for 10–20 minutes.
- You are basically numbering your breaths as a way both to relax and increase concentration. And don't chase any bones!

BRAIN BUILDERS! WORKOUT #22
Where Did I Leave My Office?

- Without being there in person, draw a detailed plan of your office, den, study, or workroom.
- Try to remember *everything* in there, down to individual paperclips and pencil stubs.
- Visit the room in question and see how accurate you were.

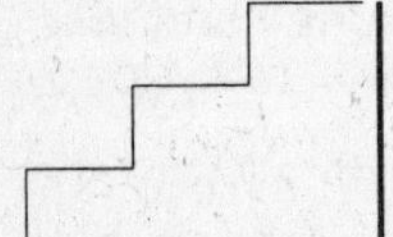

BRAIN-BUILDING SECRET #40
How to Quiet the Monkey Mind in Your Brain

It probably passes you right by, but one of the most striking features of your mental life (and mine) today is distraction. We are easily, continually, and chronically distracted every time we set our minds to focus on a topic or project. The trouble is that when you get distracted, you lose that mental edge so needed for the full use of your brain power.

Distraction consumes energy, and you may quickly find yourself too tired to keep on with a project or that your brain, like a muscle overused in exercise, is too fatigued to perform at its best level. In other words, because you are constantly distracted, you fatigue your brain and surrender vital brain power to the interests of the passing moment.

WATCH HOW QUICKLY YOUR ATTENTION CAN BE DISTRACTED

While all of us may wish for a mind we can use with focus, attention, concentration, and vigilance, we need only watch how quickly our attention gets diverted after a few seconds. Think of a jungle monkey chattering away as it swings through the branches; it is constantly moving, always chattering, and never still.

Our mind is often compared to this restless monkey. Our ease of distraction is often called the *monkey mind.*

Often your mind is like this monkey: superactive with thoughts, ideas, images, plans, and complaints, all tumbling through in chaotic succession, each clamoring for your full if fleeting attention. This wastes a great deal of energy, tires the brain, and keeps us all a little stupid from inattention.

Our brain-building secret on this point is simple but powerful: *Use your powers of inner visualization to reclaim your attention from the distractions of the monkey mind.*

HOW TO WATCH YOUR MONKEY MIND AT WORK AND PLAY

- ▼ Set a kitchen timer to ring in 5 minutes.
- ▼ Sit facing a blank wall.
- ▼ Put your hands in your lap; turn off the radio, TV, and record player; and take the telephone off the hook so there are no outside distractions.
- ▼ Do nothing until the timer rings; simply observe your thoughts.
- ▼ Pretend that in this 5 minutes everything that arises in your mind is somebody else's thought, is the dialogue for a television soap opera.
- ▼ See your monkey mind in action swinging from thought to thought.

HOW TO GET THE MONKEY TO PAY ATTENTION TO WHAT YOU WANT

Now we'll look at how to get more brain power from the petals of a flower. Let's challenge the monkey by setting our attention to focus on a different matter during the 5-minute period.

Here you can see how much energy the monkey claims and how this distracts you from what you choose to focus on. You can observe this directly by contemplating a flower. Here are the steps to follow:

- Set a kitchen timer for 5 minutes.
- Sit at a table with a flower before you.
- Resolve to do nothing for 5 minutes except gaze at the flower. Do not think about anything or pursue any thoughts that come to mind.
- Leave a little awareness free for monitoring your thoughts and watching the whole exercise as if you're viewing television.
- Note the monkey (your attention) swinging from branch (idea) to branch (thought) to branch (impulse).
- Every time your attention wanders from viewing the flower, refocus it on the flower. Keep bringing your attention back to the exercise.

WHY YOU SHOULD TRAIN YOUR MONKEY TO WORK FOR YOU

The monkey mind is a poetic way to describe a certain condition of the mind. Psychologists call it the inner monologue—that constant narration and commentary we hear every minute inside the head as if somebody is constantly talking, complaining, and chattering. It's easy to miss because it is so common and always present that you usually take it entirely for granted.

The constant chatter on television and radio only reinforces the notion that this is the way your mind is supposed to be. You get used to your mind being like a jungle. But the chatter actually wastes a great deal of valuable energy you could use for improving brain fitness. Silence saves energy and increases brain power simply because you no longer waste it.

But the monkey mind is one of the biggest obstacles to your gaining more brain power. Because the "monkey" is so easily and constantly distracted, you never gather the full attention and concentration that should be yours to focus on a problem and through which your natural high intelligence can flourish.

In other words, the monkey is stealing valuable brain power; on the other hand, if you can learn how to silence the monkey, at least for brief periods, you will find this mental silence quite energizing, giving you more brain power at the same time.

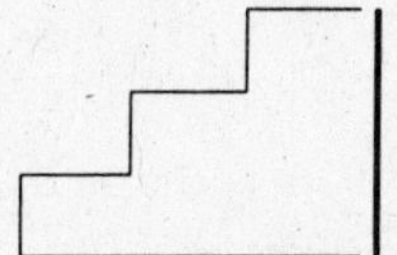

BRAIN-BUILDING SECRET #41
How to Look Carefully at a Tree with Your Eyes Closed

Knowing that the monkey mind robs brain power, schoolteachers in Japan devised a clever exercise to quiet the little beast. Customarily, they teach it to children to help them train the monkey mind at an early age. That way they encourage the habit of being attentive and focused, and through this the chattering monkey learns its place.

The Japanese grow *bonsai* trees, miniature or dwarf trees that have all the features of a full-grown, mature tree, except that they're only about 18 inches tall.

For the viewer, it's like looking in on a beautiful, miniaturized world from above, on a single majestic tree in the forest. However, you can substitute a handsome houseplant, preferably one with a woody stem, like a gardenia; a geranium plant will also work well. You want to use the houseplant's richness of texture and detail and its distinct shape and sections (leaves, branches, trunk) as a way to focus your attention.

HOW TO SEE THE PLANT INSIDE YOUR MIND

- ▼ Place the houseplant at eye level on the table before you.
- ▼ Study it; examine it; roam through its tiny leaves and delicate branches with your eyes; look at the plant so thoroughly that you can see it even when your eyes are closed.
- ▼ The goal here is to memorize the shape of the plant so you can remember it when your eyes are closed.
- ▼ When you feel you have completely memorized the shape of the plant and can remember it, close your eyes.

- Now picture the plant before you while keeping your eyes closed.
- Visualize the plant in your mind's eye with all its rich and subtle detail, as if you are painting it.
- Open your eyes and compare your visualized plant with the actual one before you. How closely do they match?

HOW HYPERACTIVE IS YOUR MONKEY MIND?

- Were you easily distracted during this exercise? Make a mental note of this; this is your monkey mind in action.
- What thoughts or emotions, specifically, leaped into your attention and struggled to pull you away from the exercise? This may hold valuable clues to other areas in your mind and body that may interfere with your natural brain power, as we'll discover later in this chapter.

This plant-gazing exercise helps you develop your powers of observation, short-term memory, concentration, mental imagery, and, most importantly, it teaches you—and the monkey mind—how to sit still with focused attention. You can sense the brain power that comes from silence.

Try practicing this exercise, which takes no more than 5 minutes, every day, as an opener for your new program of brain power calisthenics.

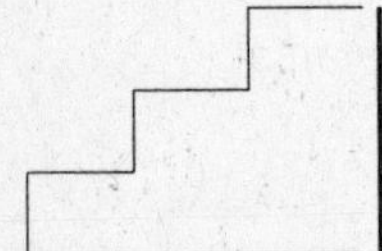

BRAIN-BUILDING SECRET #42
Do a Mindfulness Exercise First Thing in the Morning

One of the keys to being able to use your brain power is to be alert, attentive, and focused enough when it comes time to get your neurons on the job. What better time to set this up than the first thing in the morning when you wake up. Start the day mindfully, and the rest of your day will follow this keynote. Do it every morning for a month, and mindfulness becomes a brain power habit.

So try this tomorrow morning, the first thing when you wake up, before your coffee, newspaper, and your usual worries, anxieties, and duties assail you.

This exercise might take you 15–20 minutes at first but with practice you can probably reduce the time committment to 5 minutes.[10] The goal is to become aware of all your sensations in this moment.

PUTTING YOUR MIND IN THIS MOMENT—AND KEEPING IT THERE

- ▼ Sit up in bed, keeping your back straight but relaxed. You can do this lying down if you are sure you won't fall asleep. Close your eyes.
- ▼ Breathe calmly and slowly; pay attention to your breathing, watch it rise and fall, inhale and exhale until you feel relaxed and attentive.
- ▼ Focus your attention on your right foot. Notice any sensations to do with this foot. Is it warm, tingling, itchy, tense, relaxed, numb? Immerse yourself in the sensation data flowing to your awareness from your right foot.
- ▼ Now move your attention up to the lower half of your right leg, below the knee. As before, note all sensations in this area, including the simple, sheer fact that you have a lower right leg. Spend perhaps one minute here. Remember to keep a little awareness poised on your breathing.
- ▼ Move your attention up into your knee and right thigh, again noting all sensations. Spend about one minute here.
- ▼ Continue moving your sensing attention up the right side of your body in small steps, including your right hand, forearm, upper right arm.
- ▼ Now move across your body to the upper half of your left arm, then the lower half, then your left hand and fingers. Repeat the sensing procedure and continue with your awareness of breathing.
- ▼ Move your attention down your left thigh, across your left knee, over your left calf, and down to your left foot, spending about 60 seconds at each stop.

- Now broaden your focus and sense the feelings in both feet, both legs, then both arms and hands.

USING THIS MOMENT TO NOTICE WHAT'S AROUND YOU

- Keep your sensing attention on your feet and arms but also start listening to all the sounds in the room and in your environment, including your breathing, intestinal rumbling, stomach gurgling, or clock ticking.
- Don't judge or criticize any of the sounds; simply note them objectively.
- Gradually open your eyes while continuing to sense your arms and feet and the sounds of your immediate environment. Look around the room.
- Select an object, such as your clothes bureau, and actively, thoroughly examine it, for perhaps 20 seconds, as if seeing it for the first time.
- Then select another object and do the same close, active *looking*. Continue to listen to sounds and sense your body.
- You are now practicing a mindfulness exercise that involves sensing, looking, and listening. In fact, you are dividing your attention while keeping all your activities in focus.
- You are sensing your body, listening to your environment, actively looking at objects in your visual range, and keeping some awareness on your breathing—all at the same time. This puts you fully into the present moment.
- Practice this exercise anytime you need to regain your mental focus or before starting a big mental task, such as taking a test, writing a paper, doing calculations. Mastery of this exercise will train you to be better and more efficient at learning and have more focus and concentration at your command.

WHEN THE TIMER *DINGS*, REMIND YOURSELF THAT . . .

Here is another mindfulness exercise drawn from the Buddhist tradition. This is a simple but powerful way of becoming more aware in your daily activities; more awareness means more brain power available for perception, thinking, analysis, and presence of mind.

- You need a kitchen timer. Set this for 45 minutes and put it in a different room so you won't hear it ticking and you'll forget about it.
- When the timer rings, stop everything you're doing. Become aware of yourself, your body, your thoughts, your breathing, what you were saying or doing.
- Say to yourself: *In this moment I am aware of myself in the midst of my activities. In this moment I am mindful of all that is going on around me.*
- Repeat this every hour; practice for as many days as possible, ideally, every day for a month.

BRAIN BUILDERS! WORKOUT #23
What Is This Book All About?

- Select a book, such as a novel or biography.
- After each chapter, without consulting the book, write a one-paragraph summary of the contents, as if you were explaining the book to a friend unfamiliar with the book.
- When you have finished the book, summarize the entire story. Then without consulting your summaries, recount the book in reverse, explaining each chapter starting from the conclusion and working forwards to the beginning.
- Tell the story in reverse, as if you are retracing the steps of the characters in the opposite direction.

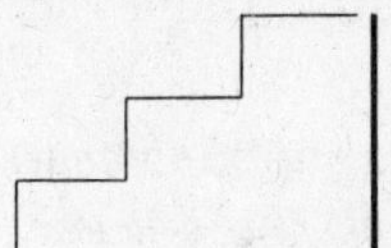

BRAIN-BUILDING SECRET #43
Spend a Mindfulness Day and Your Brain Will Thank You

Perhaps this brain-building secret will intrigue you: *Devote one day every two weeks for the next several months to practicing nonstop mindfulness in every aspect of your life.*

I guarantee that if you practice this exercise faithfully over a period of several months, you will note a dramatic improvement in your ability to learn, remember, and pay attention. It might be more practical for you to try this on a weekend, away from your job or ordinary weekday responsibilities.[11]

Mindfulness is the secret to being able to wield your brain power to maximum advantage when it comes to learning, studying, remembering, and generally being attentive to everything happening in your life—whether it's inside or outside your mind.

HOW TO BECOME THE MASTER OF YOUR ATTENTION ON THURSDAYS

If you can pay attention, holding your focus steady, you can learn and remember anything. So pick a day and vow to be the *master* of your attention for the entire day. Here's how to practice your brain power mindfulness day.

- Before you go to sleep, write yourself a note reminding you that when you awake, this is your special mindfulness day. Even the word "MINDFULNESS" in large dark letters placed next to your alarm clock will suffice.
- In fact, it wouldn't hurt to place a dozen of these signs around your house as surprise reminders. It may sound trite, but draw a happy smile under the word. Flashing a gentle half smile throughout the day will be part of your mindfulness technique.
- The minute you wake up, place your attention on your breathing. Lay there in bed, observing the rise and fall of your breath.
- As you awaken, deepen your breathing so that your breaths come as slow, long, and *consciously attended* breaths. There you are, right with the breath as it comes and goes.
- Try saying this: *Waking up this morning, I smile. Twenty-four brand-new hours are before me. I vow to live fully in each moment and to look at all beings with eyes of compassion.*[12]
- Don't jump, clamber, stagger, or fall out of bed. Move your legs and arms with complete awareness that this is an utterly novel experience that you are undergoing for the first time.

- Pay attention: make getting out of bed a rare event! As you do all your morning functions, give them your full, calm, intrigued attention. Remember to pay attention to your breathing. Try saying: *Attentive to each moment, my mind is clear like a calm river.*

THE SMILE ON YOUR FACE REMINDS YOU TO PAY ATTENTION

- Let a gentle half smile blossom on your face. This will help relax you and keep you focused.
- If possible, don't talk. Give your tongue a blessed rest. It's much easier to follow your breathing attentively if your mouth is shut and you're breathing through your nostrils.
- Follow your breathing and say: *Breathing in, I calm my body. Breathing out, I smile. Dwelling in the present moment, I know this is a wonderful moment!*
- Go about your morning household or home office chores, maintaining silence and an unwavering focus on your breathing and every motion your body is making.
- Vacuum as if for the first time. Pay your bills as if it is an absolutely novel experience.
- If you must talk, give it your full attention. Don't talk idly or unconsciously. Talk as if you're an actor reading a script. Be there with your full attention as each word flies off your lips.
- Set a kitchen timer to ring every 45 minutes. When it does, stop everything you're doing and refocus your attention on your breathing. Try saying: *Listen, listen, this wonderful sound brings me back to my true self.*
- At mealtimes, eat with complete attention, slowly, thoroughly, with complete interest and focus.

GETTING THROUGH DESSERT WITH YOUR MOUTH SHUT

- Don't think about dessert when you're having your soup. Be right here now in this moment with your soup only. Try saying: *Present moment, wonderful moment.*

- Take a walk, preferably in a park or garden. Walk very slowly with your attention on your breathing. Imagine that as you set your foot down on the ground, it imprints the earth with a lovely rose.
- Right foot down: a lovely white rose. Left foot down: a lovely white rose. Don't make a step without giving the ground a flower.
- When the telephone rings, take three mindful breaths before you answer it. You will notice a difference in what results.

OTHER MINDFULNESS TRICKS FOR YOU TO PRACTICE

- Consider practicing some of the other brain-building secrets during this mindfulness day, such as the lavender bath with relaxing music or the body scanning (Brain-Building Secret #44) and Tree Planting (Brain-Building Secret #41).
- Before going to sleep, spend 10–20 minutes following your breathing with full attention.
- Imagine that you are a smooth rounded pebble slowly sinking to the sandy bottom of a clear river bed. Drift gently down through the still water to the soft sandy bottom.
- Fall asleep with your attention on your breath.

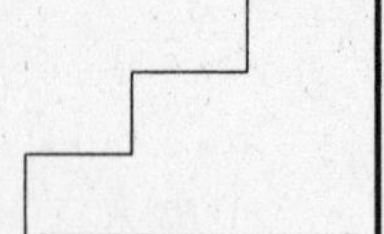

BRAIN BUILDERS! WORKOUT #24
Figure This Out For Yourself

Plot out all the steps you need to take to accomplish the following tasks:

- Training and keeping a seal in your house
- Building a conservatory off your kitchen
- Starting a daily newspaper
- Walking across Australia

- Taking apart and emptying a 6-story building with 32 completely full apartments

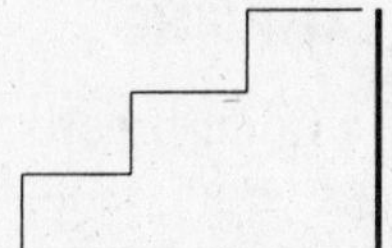

BRAIN-BUILDING SECRET #44
Body Scanning to Sharpen Your Concentration and Attention

This exercise is another technique for building mindfulness, which is one of the foundations of better brain power. Being able to pay attention for long periods is one of the prime brain-building secrets you will learn in this book.[13]

This technique helps you to reestablish mindful contact with your body and its sensations, thoughts, and feelings. In this case, you use your breathing as a means of focusing on different regions of your body. As a beginning, practice this for 45 minutes daily, 6 days a week for 2 weeks running.

HOW TO SCAN YOUR BODY FOR GREATER MINDFULNESS

- Start by lying down on a comfortable surface such as on your bed or a soft floor mat. Make sure you are not in an environment that will make you fall asleep. Also be sure you are warm and will be undisturbed. Close your eyes.
- Become aware of your breathing, of the regular rising and falling of your abdomen with each inhale and exhale. Follow this rhythm for a few minutes.
- Sense your entire body as a whole unit. Sense the "envelope" of skin in which you reside. Notice how it feels for your body to be touching the floor, where the actual points of contact are, and what sensations these contacts are sending to your awareness.
- Now focus your attention on the toes of your left foot. See if you can direct your breathing to this particular body region so that it seems you breathe in *to* your toes and out *from* your toes. This may seem odd and difficult at first, but pretend that either your toes are in your lungs or your lungs are in your toes.

- Note all sensations that arise from your toes as you breathe in to and from them. If you feel nothing, simply be aware of this "not feeling anything" experience. Spend a few minutes with your toes.

HOW TO FORGET ABOUT YOUR TOES WHILE EXHALING

- When you are finished with your left toes, take a fuller breath and exhale all the way down to your toenails. As you exhale, start forgetting about your left toes. Breathe with awareness but no object for a few cycles.
- Then shift your focus to the heel, ankle, sole, and top of your left foot. Repeat the technique of breathing in *to* your foot and out *from* it.
- When you are finished with your left foot, repeat the process in 2-minute increments, moving up your left leg, left thigh, to your pelvis.
- Then do your right toes, foot, calf, and thigh to the pelvis. Then move slowly up your torso, including your intestines, abdomen, upper back, chest, shoulders, and neck.
- Then breathe through the fingers, forearm, upper arm of each arm, one arm and one arm segment at a time.
- Continue the body scan with breathing including your chin, jaw, nose, cheeks, forehead, and scalp.

WHY HAVING A HOLE IN YOUR HEAD IS GOOD FOR BRAIN POWER

- When you move your breathing to the top of your head, pretend there is an empty "blowhole" there, the way whales have spouts. As you inhale, imagine you are sucking in air through this hole in the top of your head and sending it down through your body down to your toes, where it is exhaled.
- Reverse this and inhale through your toes, bring the air up through your body, and imagine you can exhale it from the top of your head.
- At the end of this exercise, which may well take you 20–40 minutes, depending on your style, you will probably feel highly relaxed yet focused.

- You will have seen how to use your mind like a laser focus fueled and directed by your own breathing. Your muscles will have relaxed and released a lot of their stored tension.

You have just performed a kind of purification on your entire body, detoxyifying it. Your body may feel light, even transparent, like a hollow reed through which the air you inhale and exhale is moving quietly. Your thoughts may have quieted down considerably; perhaps you have had a flash of insight regarding a current problem.

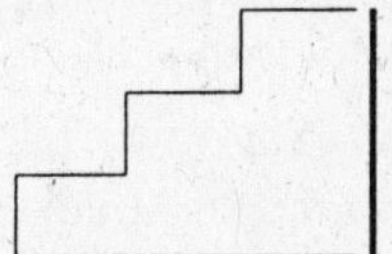

BRAIN BUILDERS! WORKOUT #25
Can You Imagine This?

Try guessing or estimating the answers to these somewhat fantastic scenarios:

- How many minutes would it take you to repaint your living room?
- What fraction of a ton does a single blade of grass weigh?
- How many eggs would weigh the same as the municipal garbage truck?
- How many ounces of water do you drink in a year, including the water contained in all beverages and all processed and whole foods?
- How many carbon atoms are contained in this book?

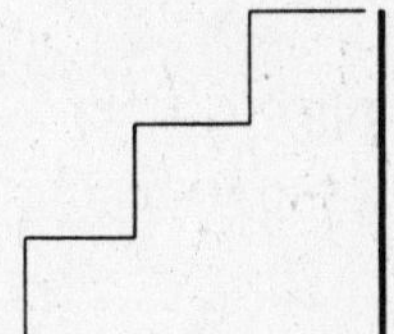

BRAIN-BUILDING SECRET #45
Priming Your Whole Brain Memory Muscles to Remember Each Day in Movielike Detail

This is a memory-building exercise you can practice every day, just before you fall asleep. If you practice this faithfully every night for a month, the results will astonish you.

- Once you are in bed and ready to go to sleep, either sit up in bed, with your pillows propped up behind you, or do this lying down if you're sure you can stay awake for 10–15 minutes.
- Relax yourself by following your breathing for a few moments.
- Start with the most recent thing you did today and remember it in full detail. This would include making yourself comfortable in bed and following your breathing.
- Then go back one step and remember what you did precisely before this. Perhaps it was climbing into bed. Then the moment before this. Probably it was brushing your teeth. Remember how you felt and what your thoughts were.
- Imagine your entire day is a movie reel that you are now running in reverse. It's almost like walking backwards or speaking in reverse, just the way it looks in a movie being rewound. In this case, you are the viewer (and recaller) moving back through every moment of your day, *in reverse*.

REVIEWING YOUR LIFE AS IF IT'S A HIGH-BUDGET MOVIE

Visually reconstruct or remember all your movements, such as

- I'm lying in bed starting to remember my day.
- I walked to my bed from the bathroom.
- I walked to the bathroom from my clothes dresser.
- I said such-and-such to my wife or husband as I stood by the dresser.
- I walked from the living room to my bedroom to stand by the dresser.
- I turned off the television and the lights in the living room.
- I was sitting in my favorite chair with my feet up watching "The Fugitive."
- Before this, I looked out the window at the full moon rising over the horizon . . .

Go back through your day, step by step, in reverse. You will probably find that the moments closer to where you are now in time you will remember in the greatest detail and the events from earlier in the day will be the quickest and shortest.

THE KEY TO MEMORY: YOU *CAN* REMEMBER IT

Something very interesting happens when you do this for a couple of weeks. You find yourself in the middle of your day, while doing different things, taking a mental snapshot of yourself doing this task so you will remember it better tonight. You are actually remembering in advance by being more aware in the moment of what you are doing. *This is the key to memory.*

If you are aware of your action in the moment you do it, then this same energy imprint remains later, even years later, to enable you to remember it. You have *preremembered* this event in your life.

In brief, the more you pay attention to your events in present time, the easier you can recall these events, as memories, in the future, or years later in a new segment of present time. Further, this exercise builds concentration, focus, mindfulness, alertness, attention to detail, and the skill of processing and storing information that becomes memory.

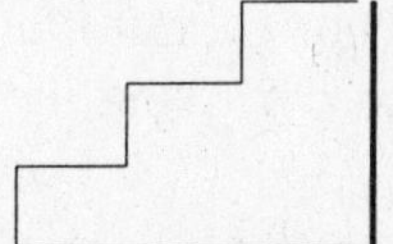

BRAIN-BUILDING SECRET #46
Priming Your Whole Brain Memory Muscles to Remember Your Life

This is another memory-priming exercise from a different source that may take you quite a long time to do. But it may be well worth the effort in terms of the steady calisthenics it gives your "memory muscles."

- ▼ Make a list of everybody you currently know this year, from your closest friends to people you barely know but have some feeling or attitude about, such as the postman, the person who delivers your heating fuel, your hairdresser.
- ▼ Structure your list according to categories, such as people from school, family members, people from work.

- Then expand the list to include everybody from last year, even though you don't see them anymore.
- Then expand the list to include people from the last 5 years.
- Then 10 years; then all the way back to adolescence, childhood, even infancy. It may take you a while to make the list.
- Then start at the top of the list and remember everything you can about each person and your feelings about them. Try to remember every interaction you had with them: fights, arguments, kisses, jokes, deep conversations, casual remarks, whatever.
- When you have completely remembered this person, erase their name from your list and dissolve your memory of them; then move to the next name and do the same. Try remembering one person a week.

MY LIFE: WHY REMEMBERING EVERYTHING FREES UP BRAIN POWER

Again, this is a long-term memory-building exercise, but the results can be remarkable. It may also free up a lot of mental energy and alertness, more than you would expect.

The theory here is that we lose a great deal of our overall life force energy, and thus energy available for brain power, by tying up old emotions in the past. Consider these scenarios:

- This person insulted me.
- This person hurt me.
- This person betrayed me.
- This person loved me madly.

In any case, you have energy tied up in your memories, probably far more than you could imagine.

When you recall the incidents, reexperience the energy involved, then erase the experiences from your memory again, you have freed up a great amount of brain power, and you have also given your "memory muscles" an astonishing long-term workout.

4 FEED YOUR BRAIN

▼▼▼▼▼▼▼▼▼▼▼▼▼▼▼▼▼▼▼

How Foods, Herbs, and Nutritional Supplements Can Boost Brain Power

Feed your brain. If you think you know what a big feeder looks like, think again. Your brain has an outrageous appetite for just about every nutrient known to food science and for about 20 percent of all the oxygen you inhale every day. You might think of your brain as a permanent adolescent: constantly growing, chronically hungry. Skillful use of nutrition, diet, herbs, and supplements can build more brain power.

In this chapter you'll be introduced to new brain-building secrets, all dealing with food, herbs, and nutritional supplements. Use these natural substances to build a strong organic base for your brain power. Because these brain-building secrets all deal with foods and edible substances, putting these ideas into practice should be very easy for you—we all must eat every day, so why not add a little *Gingko biloba* or vitamin E or extra choline to your diet. Your brain will thank you.

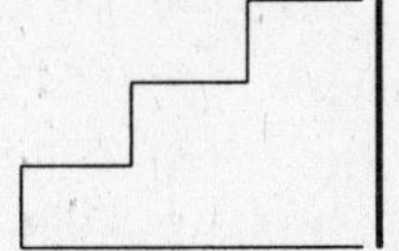

BRAIN-BUILDING SECRET #47
The Importance of Protein for Your Brain's Little Gray Cells

You have probably heard the expression, perhaps in the stories of British humorist P. G. Wodehouse or the mystery novels of Agatha Christie, that their heroes—with Wodehouse, the impeccable butler, Jeeves; with Christie, the fastidious Belgian detective Hercule Poirot—owed their considerable brain power feats to eating fish, lots of it, to build their precious little gray cells in the brain.

For that matter, why is it that many chess champions eat protein-based meals before their grueling stints at the table? An informal survy of several chess champions as to their pregame eating preferences revealed a fairly consistent tale. Whether it is shrimp, caviar, veal, or meat, the chess players confide, if you are expecting great things of your brain, give it plenty of protein.

WHY TWO PROTEINS RACE TO GET INTO YOUR BRAIN FIRST

As is often the case, when you peer beyond the popular expression, you tend to find a kernel of truth. Protein, and fish particularly, is definitely a brain food at the top of the list, but it makes a big difference whether you eat your fish or carbohydrate first when you sit down to a brain-boosting meal. "A land with lots of herring can get along with few doctors," says an old Dutch proverb.

It has to do with two competing amino acids found in proteins, tyrosine and tryptophan. In effect, these two substances vie against each other to reach your brain first and to exert their biochemical effects. Whichever one gets to your little gray cells first, gets to dominant the overall effect of the meal on your mental activities.

Tyrosine. Your brain uses supplies of tyrosine, which you present it through your diet, to make the neurotransmitters dopamine and norepinephrine, both of which are central to sharp thinking, long-term memory and recall, and a quality of general alertness. If tyrosine gets there first, it will stimulate your brain to stay at a peak level of focus and clarity for hours; if trytophan crosses your blood-brain barrier first, enjoy your after-lunch nap.

Tryptophan. The amino acid tryptophan, on the other hand, is used by your brain to make the neurotransmitter serotonin, which induces sleep and slows down overall nerve transmission and reaction time. Tryptophan arriving in your brain gets serotonin in gear, which then creates mental conditions of drowsiness, sluggishness, and for all practical purposes, a sudden—fortunately, it's temporary—drop in your functional IQ.

You'll find generous amounts of tyrosine in foods such as meat, poultry, seafood, and beans, where it basically acts as a nutritional brain stimulant; and you'll find adequate supplies of tryptophan in milk, dairy products, bananas, sunflower seeds, among other foods, where it tends to act as a brain power downer.

Our brain-building secret with respect to proteins is this: *eat your protein first before you touch the carbohydrates if you want to stay alert, focused, and awake after the meal. Simply put, fish first, potatoes second.*

THE BRAIN BUILDERS! SMART GUIDE TO EATING PROTEIN

In practical terms, if you are using your brain to earn a living and you need to stay sharp all day long, if not longer, have a high-protein, low-carbohydrate lunch, and eat whatever carbohydrates your meal contains (grains, bread, dairy products, potatoes, pasta) last. This also means that if you need lots of mental acuity in the morning, start your day with a high-protein breakfast and keep the carbohydrates in scant supply.

Conversely, if in the late afternoon or early evening, you need to chill out, wind down, and feel calm, now is the perfect time for a plate of complex carbohydrates. The timing of your protein or carbohydrate intake is the key to the effect the meal will have on your brain power.[1] Medical studies of the biochemical effects of tyrosine on brain function indicate that this amino acid can actually help a person overcome stress and depression.[2]

Fish oils. There is another reason for fish's remarkable brain-building effects. A fatty acid called omega-3 oils tends to concentrate in cold-water fish, such as salmon. The chemistry of omega-3 oils is such that it works to block disease processes at the cellular level, such as an excess production of substances that can produce damaging results when they are overproduced. Omega-3 fish oils can also block migraine headaches.

Among the fish highest in omega-3 fatty acids, containing more than 1 gram per 3.5 ounces of fish, are the following: mackerel, salmon, bluefish, tuna, Atlantic sturgeon, sablefish, herring, anchovy, sardines, and lake trout.

Shellfish. Shellfish stimulate mental energy, boost mood, and elevate brain performance perhaps even faster than the fatty freshwater fish. That's because shellfish are very low in carbohydrates and fat and are almost purely protein, which enables them to deliver a generous supply of tyrosine quickly to your brain. You get the quickest brain boost by eating 3–4 ounces of shellfish alone, as an appetizer. The downside of shellfish is that they tend to accumulate more oceanic toxins and pollutants than regular fish.

THE BRAIN POWER PROTEIN LUNCH—HOW MUCH DO I NEED?

How much protein do you need for maximum brain power? This depends on many factors, including your body weight, general level of mental exertion, the nature of your diet as a whole, and, to some extent, the kind of protein you eat. This is what I mean.

Many people in the last 25 years, including myself, experimented with vegetarian diets. There has been much discussion by nutritionists that on the whole Americans who can afford to eat well typically eat too much protein, specifically, too much red meat. Excess meat consumption has been correlated with a variety of health conditions, and generally the trend in the last 10 years has been toward reduced red meat consumption.

My experience has been contrary to this national trend. Over the last 10 years I have found myself eating more protein—not red meat, mind you—but more protein from soybeans, fish, and chicken. Looking back, I see this is directly related to my work, to how much work I am required to do; as my "work" is entirely mental in nature—writing and researching—my body has "told" me, through its various physiological channels, that it needs more protein, lots more, to keep the mind games rolling.

This may strike many readers as all too obvious, yet I suspect there are many others who may have been following rather protein-lean diets who are suddenly finding the old protein ways don't work anymore and brain power, which is increasingly the means of livelihood for many in America, needs more protein.

As Hercule Poirot never tired of telling his colleagues, his detective acuity depends on his "little gray cells," and as Bertie Wooster, the somewhat inept bachelor aristocrat fondly says of his all-accomplishing butler Jeeves, "The old boy eats a lot of fish."

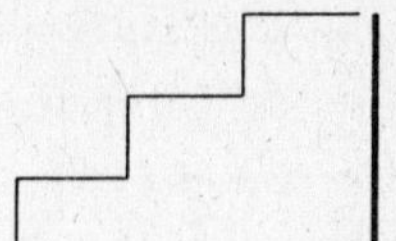

BRAIN BUILDERS! WORKOUT #26
Keep Your Eyes on Its Every Move

This exercise helps build better hand-eye coordination, which in turn helps your brain function more efficiently.

- Practice tracking moving objects with your eyes. Do this in a darkened room.
- Attach a pencil flashlight at both ends with string, then suspend it from an overhead hook. Allow it to swing back and forth, coming near and far. Follow it closely with your eyes.
- Better yet, have a friend hold the pencil flashlight and move it around in arcs, circles, squares, and zigzags.
- Track the light carefully with your eyes.
- As another variation, hold the flashlight yourself and move it around in different formations and shapes, following it with your eyes.

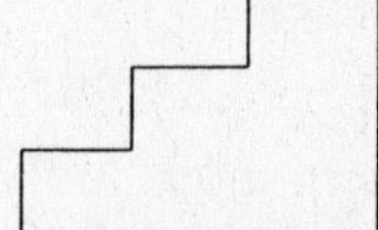

BRAIN-BUILDING SECRET #48
Ginkgo Biloba—A Brain Builder's Dream Herb from China

Ginkgo biloba is a 300-million-year-old species of tree, which makes it the planet's oldest. It has been used for millennia in China as a general brain tonic to increase mental alertness; increase oxygen flow to the brain; treat memory loss, depression, dizziness, and ear ringing in the elderly; and even help protect against the onset of dementia.[3]

Herbalists regard the leaves of *Ginkgo biloba* (also called "maiden hair tree") as the most effective agent for increasing blood circulation into the microcapillaries of the brain. In fact, something about the shape of the ginkgo leaf itself suggests its positive role in improving brain power. Its veins spread out in two directions, making the leaf appear as if cut into two halves, just like your brain's two hemispheres.

Recommended dosage: Use a liquid extract that contains at least a 24 percent concentration of the active ingredient, taken orally 120 to 160 mg daily, divided over three doses. For potencies lower than 24%, take up to 1 gm per day. No side effects from *Ginkgo biloba* are known even at daily dosages of 600 mgs at 24 percent concentration.

Although it can yield quick improvements in short-term memory, ginkgo is generally a slow-acting herb, so plan on 8 days before you see the first effects, 3 weeks before you notice real benefits, and 3–6 months to see significant and permanent effects. It's best to take it three times daily, dividing the total daily dosage into three parts; it stays in your system for only about 3–6 hours.

WHAT ONE OF THE WORLD'S MOST POPULAR HERBS CAN DO

It's not only the Chinese who use it. An estimated 1.2 million prescriptions per month are written out (worth $500 million annually) by European doctors for this herbal extract.[4] Here is a run-down of what it can do:

- works as an antioxidant to protect brain and liver
- enhances brain metabolism
- prevents hardening of the arteries
- stimulates the production of the "universal energy molecule"
- increases blood and oxygen circulation to the brain
- halts free radical damage to brain tissues, the nervous system, and liver
- improves the brain's ability to metabolize glucose, which is the primary sugar used as fuel and energy
- improves overall nerve transmission, so that electrical impulses move faster through the brain
- improves mental functioning in the elderly and helps halt the brain-aging process
- keeps the brain's arteries flexible so that they do not get clogged with blood platelets
- increases short-term memory
- enhances alertness and favorable learning states

- ▼ can stop early signs of mental decline if caused by depression or reduced oxygen flow to the brain

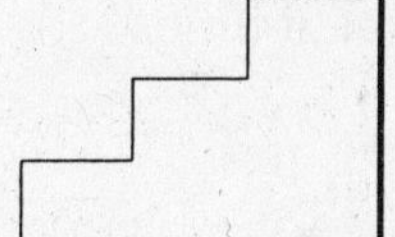

BRAIN-BUILDING SECRET #49 Ginseng—Your Brain Power's Elixir of Life

Ginseng, another herb of Chinese origin, is popularly known there as the "king of the myriad medicines" because of its qualities as a supplement for health and longevity. Its beneficial effects on the human system, recognized by the Chinese for at least 4,000 years, are as impressive as those listed for *Ginkgo biloba*. It is quite possibly the most widely used medicinal herb in the Orient as a whole.

Curiously, the ginseng root, which is the part of the plant used to make the tincture, resembles a miniature human, which perhaps is why the ancients referred to ginseng as the "root of eternal life" and "root of life plant." Its human-shaped form suggested that the divine spirit might in fact exist within this wonder tuber. Around 200 A.D., a Chinese emperor dubbed it *panax ginseng*, meaning "panacea from ginseng," and the botanical name has remained with the plant ever since.

Recommended dosage: You will find ginseng available as pills, extracts, tinctures, capsules, tablets, powders, pastes, as dried roots, granulated teas, even as an element in wines and liquors. Like ginkgo, its effects are cumulative; you should expect to take it for about a month before seeing major effects.

Doses of liquid extract or tincture in the range of 500–3,000 mg per day are generally advised, unless you have high blood pressure. If so, start with the low end of the ginseng dosage and work up to the higher as your blood pressure normalizes. If you start with a 500 mg/day dose, take it in three installments during the day.

Typically, ginseng comes in two forms as an extract: a reddish variety, which is stronger, more aggressive in its actions, and appropriate for use in winter; and a whiter form, whose action is milder and more suitable for summer use.

THE BRAIN-BUILDING BENEFITS OF GINSENG

- regulates heartbeat
- regulates blood pressure
- stimulates memory, learning, and other mental abilities
- improves digestion
- reduces fatigue
- enhances your ability to withstand stress
- acts as an antioxidant scavenger for free radicals in your system
- can heighten your body's resistance to stress
- generally normalizes and rebalances all your physiological systems
- works both as a calming tranquilizer and as an energy-booster
- sharpens your ability to concentrate, learn, and remember
- helps to increase blood circulation through the brain
- heightens the activity of the endocrine glands and the general rate of metabolism
- contributes to smooth, efficient mental processing
- sparks your concentration, level of alertness, and sharpness of thinking mainly through keeping your blood sugar level normal and balanced
- lowers any excess of glucose in your system

OTHER BRAIN POWER BENEFITS OF GINSENG

- *Brain chemicals.* Ginseng contains a family of chemicals called saponins (also called glycosides or ginsenosides), which influence the metabolism of certain brain chemicals you need for top mental performance.
- *Stress reduction.* Ginseng works to reduce the activation of your adrenal cortex and thereby inhibits the alarm stage of stress. When your adrenal cortex is working efficiently, it leads to the ability to remember better and faster, to learn more easily, and to have quicker access to short- and long-term memory.

- ▼ *Mood*. Ginseng improves mental performance, especially in conditions of stress, fatigue, and overwork because it increases the levels of a neurotransmitter called norepinephrine, important for mood and memory. Normally, stress depletes your brain's supply of this chemical, but ginseng shores it up, so that you don't go down with mind fatigue and loss of focus.[5]

TWO MORE CHINESE BRAIN-BUILDING HERBS

Ephedra sinica. In Chinese, ephedra is known as *Ma Huang*. It is derived from the stems of the joint fir tree and is the botanical model from which pharmacists developed ephedrine, which is used in amphetamines and in cold decongestants as a stimulant.

Among its many abilities, the herb ephedra can give you a cerebral lift reputedly worth several espressos, taken as a tincture or as part of a "smart foods" nutrient drink.

Common dosage: 1–2 cups ephedra tea daily. Do not use if you are pregnant or lactating, have high blood pressure, heart disease or arrhythmia, diabetes, glaucoma, thyroid conditions, or psychosis.

Epimedium sagittatum. Also called "horny goat weed," epimedium stimulates blood circulation through the smallest capillaries and is often prescribed in Chinese medicine as a remedy against being absent-minded and out of focus and having poor memory.

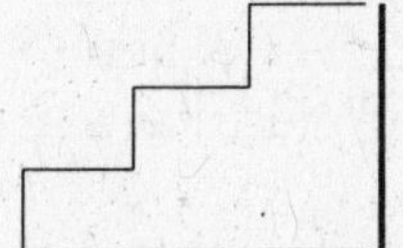

THE ANATOMY OF BRAIN POWER #6
Brain Chemicals— How to Send a Message Quickly Through Your Brain

If you saw the movie *Awakenings*, in which Robert de Niro plays a middle-aged man literally awakened from a lifelong trance by a "miracle" drug administered by the mild-mannered physician Dr. Oliver Sacks, played by Robin Williams (or if you read the book), you have already been introduced to the idea of a *neurotransmitter*. This is a special brain chemical whose job is to convey information between brain cells.

BRAIN CHEMICALS YOU SHOULD KNOW

- acetylcholine
- gamma-aminobutyric acid (GABA)
- serotonin
- dopamine
- norepinephrine
- endorphins
- tyramine
- taurine
- prostaglandins
- certain peptides
- the purine nucleosides

In the case of *Awakenings*, back in 1969 Dr. Sacks—he really is a doctor and this is a true story—gave his patients, who were nearly comatose, entranced, or hopelessly twitching with Parkinson's disease, L-dopa, a drug that is the precursor to the brain chemical *dopamine*. Dopamine, scientists now know, is 1 of about 50 messenger brain chemicals, or neurotransmitters, whose activity is vital to the life and well-being of your brain.

HOW INFORMATION IS PASSED ON THROUGH YOUR BRAIN CELLS

From a physiological point of view, neurotransmitters are the major players in your work of building more brain power. A neurotransmitter is a specific brain chemical that helps send electrical signals (or information) from one neuron to the next.

To understand neurotransmitters, we have to return to the neuron itself and how it conveys information. In every second of its life, your brain is like a self-contained universe with millions of tiny explosions flashing on and off like fireflies as your neurons release their electrical charge at the synapses. A neuron is simply a specialized nerve cell.

Each of the billions of neurons in your brain sends information or a bioelectric message to other neurons or to muscle fibers through an *axon*; neurons receive information through a *dendrite*, which resembles a tree with many branches. What is the information being sent? Primarily, thoughts, instructions, orders, and impulses, except that these are coded, not in words or gestures, but in terms of electrical charge.

Electrical charge is at the heart of your brain's communication system. This is like tiny waves of electrical energy rippling through the axon-dendrite network. Here's how it works. Most cells, including neurons, have a difference in electrical charge from their inside to their outside. It's a small but measurable difference, on the order 0.0075 of a volt. The overall flow of biochemical currents and changes in electrical charge inside and outside the brain cell is at the basis of your thought life.

THOUGHTS BECOME SPARKS THAT BECOME CHEMICALS

The meeting place for an axon and dendrite is called a *synapse*, and here the information leaps the minute gap and continues on. The smooth transfer of information across the synapse, or gap between axon and dendrite, is crucial to the smooth operation of your entire nervous system. However, a curious thing happens at the synapse. Electrical information is changed into *chemical* information, as tiny packages of specific brain chemicals are released.

These are the neurotransmitters, so called because they transmit the electrical information (thoughts and commands) between neurons. Technically, the speed at which this information is transferred across the synapse is not that fast. These impulses travel at about 100 meters a second, which is about 1 million times slower than an electrical impulse zips through a computer chip.

However, while the human brain may be slower than a human-made computer chip, it is far more flexible, with innumerable alternate pathways for information to flow, compared to a computer in which information flow often gets bottlenecked.

HOW BIG A STAFF OF CHEMICALS DOES YOUR BRAIN EMPLOY?

The estimate of how many neurotransmitters are at work in the human brain transferring information has grown in the last five decades, from 2 to 50, and some scientists push the number closer to 100.

This continuous flow of chemical messages or "words" underlies all your brain functions, including your thoughts, feelings, desires, impulses, and willed action. They are involved in such key life functions as alertness and excitability, sleep, dreaming, pain regulation, thoughts, moods, temperament. All states of mind—such as pain, memory, sex, moods, intelligence, even mental illness—are products of the interaction of the brain's messenger chemicals and their specific receptor sites in the neighboring dendrites. All the brain-building exercises in this book try to influence these brain chemicals and how efficiently they work.

In practical terms, here you can see the *physiological* dimension underlying memory, forgetting, information processing, quick recall, suppression, and other aspects of brain power. This is where you learn and forget, where you adapt and fall back into habits, where you can expand your IQ or lose valuable points.

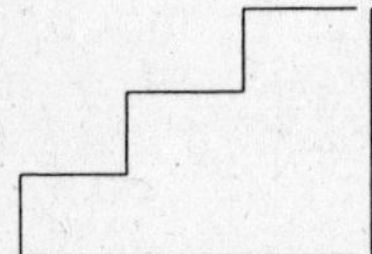

BRAIN BUILDERS! WORKOUT #27
Why Your Brain Likes to Swim Underwater Upside Down

Here are additional variations on the theme of exercising your midbrain and building better eye-hand coordination.

- At a swimming pool, swim around underwater in a circle. Do headstands in the shallow water.
- Stand on your hands in the deeper water. In general, whether you're in water or in a gym, spend as much time *hanging upside down* as you can.
- You might hang upside down, swinging and twirling, from vertical ropes, swings, or bars.

Recommended dosage of seeing the world upside down: 30–45 minutes, provided you have no preexisting health conditions that would make this exercise dangerous or unhealthy.

- Advantages to this exercise include increasing blood circulation to and through your brain and oxygenation of brain tissues plus stimulating neglected areas of your midbrain that deal with balancing and spatial orientation.

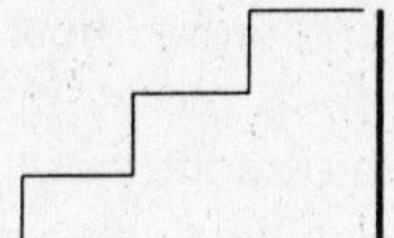

BRAIN-BUILDING SECRET #50
Brain Tonics and Mind Builders from Ayurveda

Ayurveda, which means "the end of the Vedas" is the oldest medical tradition in India and, according to some scholars, possibly the oldest in the world, even antedating traditional Chinese medicine, which goes back about 5,000 years. *Ayurveda* (pronounced EYE-Your-VAY-dah) is a complete body of thought and practices relating to the mind, body, health, and spirituality. Bear in mind that *Ayurveda* is a science and philosophy that recognizes the presence and effect of consciousness in all aspects of life, from food to behavior, weather to healing. Herbal recommendations and ideas presented in this discussion are based on the belief that the effects are slow building, subtle, and transformative at the level of consciousness. In this way, they can bring about the changes in brain power and mind state that Ayurvedic herbology promises.

This brain-building secret consists of a selection of suggestions dealing with herbs, foods, even gold and gemstones, taken from a variety of Ayurvedic sources, that share the common goal of improving your brain power.

GOTU-KOLA, THE HERB FOR MEMORY, MENTAL STAMINA, AND LONGEVITY

Gotu-kola, an herb commonly found in Asia and Australia, and often used to heal wounds, improve skin conditions, and reduce cellulite and varicose veins, is also recognized as a brain tonic and as an herb that can help build better memory and heightened intelligence while rejuvenating the entire system.

Ayurvedic herbalists also suggest that gotu-kola is effective in combatting aging, even senility. The leaf itself resembles the two hemispheres of the brain, which is perhaps why Ayurvedic doctors recommend this herb to relieve stress, calm the mind, and stimulate the flow of energy between the right and left brain hemispheres.

In a study with 30 developmentally disabled children, after taking gotu-kola for 12 weeks, they became more attentive and showed improved concentration. The herb contains a chemical substance called triterpenes that acts as a mild tranquilizer and that helps cut down stress and anxiety.

People in India take gotu-kola to live longer and improve their memory; the herb also gradually builds up mental stamina and brain power endurance and positively influences the health and smoothness of the brain's nerve response. Gotu-kola is praised for its ability to stimulate the brain, detoxify the system, and boost the energy level of cells.

Recommended dosage: As a tea made from leaves, one cup at bedtime, to promote peaceful sleep and alert awakening in the morning.

CALAMUS ROOT TO CALM THE MIND

This hot, penetrating herb (also known as Sweet Flag) is used to treat epileptic seizures, sedate convulsions, strengthen the memory, and stimulate the higher brain functions to bring clarity and calmness to the mind. Calamus helps to open up the flow of nerve impulses.

Its energy nature, in Ayurvedic terms, is *sattvic*, which pertains to clarity of mind and consciousness; this is why Ayurveda considers calamus to be one of the best mind herbs. Ayurvedic herbalists have praised calamus for centuries for its ability to purify and revitalize the brain and nervous system, to increase blood circulation to the brain, sharpen memory, increase sensitivity, and stimulate general awareness.

Recommended dosage: Ayurvedic physicians recommend taking a pinch of powdered calamus root (made from its rhizomes on the root) mixed with 1/4 to 1/2 teaspoon of honey in the morning and evening to help improve memory. Try mixing equal amounts of gotu-kola with calamus and honey (1 teaspoonful each) for a general nerve tonic. When using calamus alone in powder form, use 250–500 mg a day.

NUTMEG AND MILK FOR BETTER SLEEP

When you mix nutmeg with milk, it becomes a tonic for both heart and brain, claim the Ayurvedic physicians. Nutmeg, taken in quantities no greater than a pinch at a time, is also a relaxant and can help eliminate insomnia and produce restful sleep.

TRY GOLD AS A BRAIN-BUILDING TONIC

Don't hoard your gold but immerse it in water as a brain power tonic through gold-medicated water, Ayurveda recommends. Take an ornament made from gold—a ring, pendant, or bracelet—and boil in 2 cups of water until half the water evaporates.

According to Ayurveda, the energy imprint or "electronic energy" of the gold will pass into the water. Drink 1 teaspoonful of this gold-imprinted water three times a day to improve intelligence, memory, comprehension, general alertness, to strengthen your heart, soothe your nervous system, increase stamina, and impart discrimination.

WEAR BERYL OR RUBY FOR A SMARTER STATE OF MIND

Ayurveda recommends wearing the gemstone beryl, which comes in blue, green, or yellow hues, on a silver necklace or on the left ring finger, set in a silver ring, to subtly promote intelligence.

The gemstone red ruby is also believed to heighten concentration and promote mind power, especially if worn on the left ring finger set in gold or silver. Also, in terms of Ayurvedic color theory, *yellow* is associated with understanding and intelligence and the mind in general.

Consider wearing more clothes that are yellow, especially shirts and blouses, having more objects in your environment that are yellow such as flowers, pictures, lampshades, lights, or gemstones. The gemstones emerald, jade, or peridot are associated with the nervous system and may be worn on the body to good effect, says Ayurveda.

Other brain power gemstones include pearl or moonstone (calming the emotions), yellow sapphire or topaz to enhance wisdom, or blue gemstones for peace and detachment.

MORE AYURVEDIC BRAIN FOODS

- ▼ Oats, as in rolled oats, oatmeal, oat flour, oat "milk," are said to strengthen the brain and fortify the nervous system.
- ▼ Licorice, not the candy but the herb, is said to have a remarkable effect on strengthening the memory.
- ▼ Asparagus, the popular spring vegetable, is reputed to tonify the brain and nerves.
- ▼ Ghee, made from cow's milk, is credited with correcting mental disturbances caused by energy imbalances, improving the memory, and stabilizing the intellect.

- Foods worth including as general items in your brain power building diet, according to Ayurveda, include apples, oranges, quince, rose water, ginger, valerian, cloves, chicken, and goat's milk.

BRAIN PURGATIVES AND STIMULANTS

Incenses. Ayurvedic offers recommendations for herbs and foods that can cleanse and detoxify or "purge" the brain. Gently inhale burning incenses made from aloeswood, sandalwood, musk, and/or camphor to strengthen your mind and remove throbbing at the temples or a tendency to faint.

Chamomile tea. To "cleanse and purge" the brain, mix 1/2 teaspoon each of chamomile and marshmallow herbs, then boil in 1.5 cups of water for 5 minutes; cool, strain off the herbs, and drink.

Anointing with herbs. Herbs known to cleanse and clear the brain and its nerve connections include bayberry, camphor (in low dosages only), myrrh, turmeric, bay leaves, and mint—taken as teas. Try anointing your nose and forehead and top of your head with a mixture made of ghee plus calamus paste or gotu-kola to directly influence and clarify the brain.

MORE AYURVEDIC BRAIN-BUILDING HERBS

Basil. Taken as a powder (250 mg–1 gm) or tea (mixed with honey), basil heightens the acuteness of your senses, strengthens nerve tissue, increases memory, and promotes mental clarity.

Bhringaraj. An Ayurvedic herb (which happens to grow in the American Southwest) known as *bhringaraj* (also known as *kesharaja*, or in Latin, *Eclipta alba*) means "ruler of the hair" because it promotes hair growth. Yet perhaps its proximity of action to the brain accounts for its well-recognized brain-building features. This herb, used in a hot or cold infusion, mixed with ghee, as part of a medicated oil, or as a powder (250 mg–1gm), helps to calm your mind when it is excessively active, to bring on restful sleep, and to act as a general brain tonic.

Sage. Sage is recognized in Ayurveda for its ability to clear away emotional difficulties that hinder the mind and to generate calmness. You can mix sage with gotu kola or *bhringaraj*. Haritaki (*Chebulic myrobalan*, or *Terminalia chebula*) is a fruit (called the "king of medicines" in Tibet) is a rejuvenative that "feeds" and energizes the brain and nerves. Typically, haritaki is available as a decoction, powder, or paste.

REJUVENATIVE BRAIN TONICS

A branch of Ayurvedic herbology deals with the recipes for certain tonics that can rejuvenate the system and work directly on the brain. It's called *rasayana* and means "essence (*rasa*) of what enters (*ayana*)" by which Ayurveda points to substances or even energies that penetrate and rejuvenate the essence or basic nature of your mind and body.

Ayurveda's goal is to foster a daily revitalization of brain cells and a kind of immortality of the mind, so that, at least, it is as clear and open in old age as it once was in childhood.[6]

Generally, the rejuvenative brain tonics, prepared as teas, are prescribed according to basic temperament, which Ayurveda allocates according to the four elements of water, fire, air, and earth.

- For a *vata* temperament (very active, restless, speaking fast), use *ashwagandha*, calamus, garlic, and ginseng.
- For a *pitta* temperament (moderate in activity, determined, passionate, sharp in speech), use aloe vera, comfrey root, gotu-kola, saffron.
- For a *kapha* temperament (lethargic, calm, slow, self-contented, steady), use elecampane.

Other herbs used in this way include angelica, licorice, myrrh, oatstraw, onion, rehmannia, saw palmetto, sesame seeds, wild yam. It's best to take rejuvenative herbs or any Ayurvedic herbs targeted for the brain after meals, not on an empty stomach.[7]

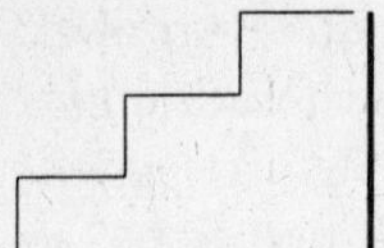

BRAIN BUILDERS! WORKOUT #28
Detectives and the Little Gray Cells of Brain Power—Part 1

For as long as I can remember, I have always been enthralled with detective and mystery stories. Hercule Poirot, Agatha Christie's vain Belgian detective; Sherlock Holmes, the restless sleuth of Baker Street; Perry Mason, the intrepid lawyer of Erle Stanley Gardner—I read them all.

Now, here is the first of five exercises in which you can put the skills of the detective to work to school your little gray cells.

- Read detective stories, murder and mystery novels, stories involving court and jury cases.
- There are many choices: Agatha Christie has the Miss Marple and Hercule Poirot series; Arthur Conan Doyle has a huge body of Sherlock Holmes and Dr. Watson stories; P. D. James has a half dozen Commander Adam Dalgliesh novels; Georges Simenon has his unflapable Parisian detective, Chief Inspector Maigret; and Colin Dexter has his chronically grouchy Chief Detective Inspector Morse.
- Here is an opportunity to exercise your mind. Pretend you are the detective. After each chapter, analyze the available information, draw up suspect lists, calculate probable motivations, try to figure out what the author is deliberately hiding from you or where he is trying to distract and mislead you, make a guess as to where the story is going.
- In short, try to outguess the author and be one step ahead of the guilty party. Your brain power will thank you, and you may come up with a better ending than the author. Find more *Detectives* exercises in Brain Builders! Workout #29, 30, 31, 32.

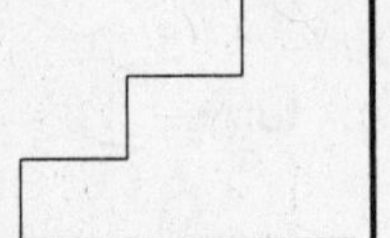

BRAIN-BUILDING SECRET #51
Brain Tonics and Mind Calmers from Traditional Chinese Medicine

Here is a selection of recommendations from traditional Chinese medicine (TCM) for using foods to calm and focus your mind. In TCM, energy and psychological states are seen as two aspects of the same condition. Organs, such as the heart, are more than the physical organ; they are complete energy systems that can occupy the entire body.

TCM sees mental hyperactivity, for example, as the result of too much *yang* energy (active, hot, sunny, bright, masculine, hard) in the heart flooding upwards into the head. When it does, you may experience irritability, headache, insomnia, fever, and mental disturbances. In such a case, TCM recommends dietary measures for strengthening the *yin* energy (passive, cooling, soft, moist, feminine, dark) of the heart.

- ▼ *Oyster shell.* These enhance heart *yin* energy and lower upward-rising *yang* energy; available as oyster shell calcium powder.
- ▼ *Whole grains.* Whole wheat, brown rice, and oats work gently but deeply to calm the mind.
- ▼ *Mushrooms.* Most mushrooms have positive cerebral effects, especially *reishi* (*ling zhi*), now becoming widely available in mushroom or supplement form. Reishi mushroom is known to soothe the spirit, nurture the heart, and calm your mind.
- ▼ *Silicon foods.* These include oatstraw tea, barley gruel, oat groat tea, cucumber, celery, lettuce, and juice made from celery and lettuce. These foods stimulate calcium metabolism and strengthen the nerves and heart tissue.
- ▼ *Fruits.* Lemons and mulberries calm the mind; mandarin calms the nerves, remedies insomnia, and aids memory, recall, and concentration.
- ▼ *Seeds.* These include jujube seeds, mandarin, and chia, which calm the spirit.
- ▼ *Herbs.* Consider regular use of chamomile, catnip, scullcap, or valerian as tinctures or herbal teas to soothe your nervous system or remedy insomnia. Dill and basil are used as calming agents in fresh form or powdered in teas.
- ▼ *Animal products.* Nonbovine growth-hormone-treated dairy milk, goat milk, and clarified butter nourish the heart energy, says TCM.

- ▼ *Minor mental depression*. Usually rooted in stagnant liver energy. Use brown rice, cucumber, apples, cabbage, fresh wheat germ, blue-green microalgae, kuzu root, apple cider vinegar. Try including at least one of these foods in each meal. For apple cider vinegar specifically: 1 teaspoon mixed in a little water, taken three times daily during depression.

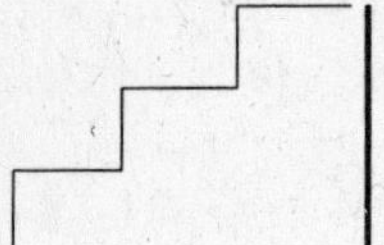

BRAIN-BUILDING SECRET #52 Antioxidants—Your Nutritional Strategy to Ageproof Your Brain

In 1956, a researcher at the University of Nebraska proposed a new theory of aging that has since come to dominate much of the thinking in holistic and alternative medicine. Dr. Denham Harman suggested that substances called *free radicals* in the human body might be the prime factors in causing a great deal of organ and system degeneration. The paradox is that oxygen is both essential to life and a poison to life.

Free radicals are electrically charged atoms within molecules that react easily and quickly with other compounds at the cellular level. They are distinguished by being incomplete, with a single unpaired or "free" electron available for bonding with other electrons, thereby creating strange, unnatural, and, ultimately, unhealthy molecular combinations.

A ROOMFUL OF FREE RADICALS READY TO HARM YOUR BRAIN

The result is, metaphorically speaking, a roomful of free radicals that collectively do serious damage to body tissues and organs. This sequence of free radical reactions is much like getting a strong dose of internal radiation. The results are many of the common signs and symptoms of aging and can include wrinkled, dry skin, age spots, arthritis, cataracts, senility, hardened arteries, cancer, Alzheimer's, memory loss, and strokes.

Aging may not be so much the result of an inevitable chronological decline as it is a biological process whose rate is determined by how fast free radicals destroy tissues and organs. Free radicals can mutate DNA, produce brain damage through oxygen deprivation, produce pigment changes and brown age spots that, in your brain as lipofuscin, can choke neurons to death.

Where do antioxidants come from? At one level, they are natural by-products of your body's own processes of metabolism where they serve a useful purpose. In fact, the normal processes of food digestion and exercise generate free radicals. At the cellular level, body-produced free radicals are necessary to defend cells against bacteria, viruses, pollutants, and toxins. Under normal conditions, your body's internal population of free radicals are kept in check by specific enzymes that scavenge excess numbers of these potent molecules. Unfortunately, given the nature of our contemporary technological, chemically polluted environment, there are now numerous new sources of *artificially* produced free radicals.

THE MODERN ENVIRONMENT IS FULL OF FREE RADICALS

New sources include X rays, microwaves, nuclear radiation, toxic heavy metals (such as aluminum and cadmium, found in public water supplies), smog, chemical food additives, cigarette smoke, exhaust from automobiles, and hydrogenated vegetable oils and artificial polyunsaturated fat substitutes, such as margarine, shortening, nondairy creamers, most bottled salad dressings, and commercial cooking oils.

The trouble here is that the minute you consume any of these products (and they are widely used in prepared, processed foods and in restaurant and fast foods), they "explode" into free radicals in your system. When these oils are used in high-heat preparations (deep-frying foods and French fries), the heat causes them to oxidize much quicker, releasing more free radicals. Where do most of these free radicals go? To your brain, which among all your organs is probably the one most vulnerable to the onslaught of free radicals that enter your body.

BRAIN-BUILDING ADVICE: FILL YOUR HEAD WITH ANTIOXIDANTS

Our brain-building secret with respect to free radicals is this: *Eliminate as many sources of free radical contamination from your diet and life-*

style as possible and start taking antioxidants to fortify your body against the damage that those already in your system might be doing.

Stop eating foods that contain or are based on artificial, unsaturated fat substitutes; avoid water that is contaminated with heavy metals (in other words, drink bottled water); avoid cigarettes and secondhand smoke; and start including antioxidants in your daily diet.

An *antioxidant* is a natural substance that acts as a free radical scavenger, literally consuming them within the cells of your body. Antioxidants include nutrients such as

- vitamins B1, B5, B6 (see Brain-Building Secret #57)
- vitamin C (see Brain-Building Secret #54)
- vitamin E
- betacarotene
- ginseng (see Brain-Building Secret #49)
- *Ginkgo biloba* (see Brain-Building Secret #48))
- amino acids taurine, cysteine, methionine
- zinc and selenium (see pages 205 and 206)
- enzyme compound coenzyme Q10 (see page 205)
- glutathione peroxidase and superoxide dismutase

GENERAL ANTIOXIDANT FORMULAS

A commercial antioxidant formula found in many health foods stores is *Maxi-Life CoQ10*, made by Twin Laboratories, available in powder or capsules.

If you'd like to make your own, this is an antioxidant shopping list formula.[8] Take this mixture two to three times a day for optimal free radical protection, most practically, by combining several multivitamin and supplement pills until you get the right amounts:

- beta-carotene, 25,000 IU
- vitamin E (mixed tocopherols), 800 IU
- vitamin C (as calcium ascorbate), 2 gm
- ascorbyl palmitate, 100 mg
- vitamin B1, 25 mg

- vitamin B2, 25 mg
- vitamin B3, 120 mg
- vitamin B5, 250 mg
- vitamin B12, 100 mcg
- folic acid, 800 mcg
- inositol, 100 mg
- zinc citrate, 30 mg
- copper (as coated gluconate), 2 mg
- selenium, 200 mcg
- L-glutathione, 500 mg
- L-methionine, 250 mg
- L-taurine, 250 mg
- coenzyme Q10, 30 mg

Coenzyme Q10. This naturally-occuring substance, also known as *ubiquinone*, is present in the human body where it acts as an antioxidant. One of its prime activities is to generate energy in brain cells while it simultaneously protects the neurons from the damage of free radicals.

Among food sources of CoQ10, polyunsaturated vegetable oils, such as soybeans, contain high amounts, and monounsaturated oils, such as olive, contain a moderate amount; other food sources include beef, roasted walnuts and peanuts, sardines, spinach, and white albacore tuna.

Normally, CoQ10 is made in your body from the amino acids L-tyrosine and L-methionine; however, stress, colds, illness, physical activity, hormone concentrations, and the use of prescription drugs can all act to lower CoQ10 amounts in the brain.

Recommended dosage: 10–90 mg daily.

Selenium. This antioxidant mineral works in combination with vitamin E to guard your system against free radicals. It is also a component of the natural enzyme antioxidant system glutathione peroxidase; selenium helps the level of this beneficial enzyme increase in your system.

Recommended dosage: 250–350 mcg daily. Selenium can be toxic if taken in excessively high doses such as 2,400+ mcg daily for a long term.

Zinc. As a mineral, zinc is required for many brain functions, including the activity of the antioxidant superoxide dismutase in which zinc works in tandem with copper to neutralize excess oxygen when it appears in its destructive form. Your brain normally contains a fair amount of zinc, which helps to guard brain tissues against lead contamination. Zinc supplementation should be undertaken in conjunction with copper, as too much zinc depletes your copper reserves.

Recommended dosage: 15–30 mg zinc daily; 1–2 mg copper daily.

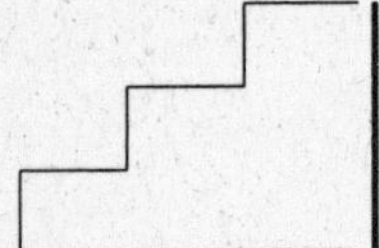

BRAIN BUILDERS! WORKOUT #29
Detectives and the Little Gray Cells of Brain Power—Part 2

Here is the second of five exercises in which you can put the skills of the detective to work to school your little gray cells.

I loved the stories and tried to outguess the detectives even before they closed in on their suspects. Sometimes I got it right; sometimes my solutions led to more elaborate plots than the author ever intended, so I supposed I had wandered off into my own unwritten thriller.

But what I didn't know then, but do now, is that everytime you read a detective story with attention—or even watch one on television—you are building brain power. Hercule Poirot frequently referred to his precious "little brain cells" as his most valuable asset.

- As a variation on your amateur brain-building sleuthing, read the final chapter of a good mystery novel first.
- Take Agatha Christie's *Death on the Nile*, for example. Carefully read the last chapter first until you understand who did the crime; now start the story from the beginning.
- Since you know the outcome, watch how Christie weaves her plot, dropping true and false clues, distracting you from the real culprits.
- Pay careful attention to all the details, the merest hints, the way the story itself is heading toward its conclusion.

- Here you can be a *literary detective* by analyzing the very way Christie (or any other author you select) puts together her edifice of mystery.
- Again, the pleasant effort of analysis, deduction, and extrapolation will build those precious little gray cells in your brain, the key to more brain power.

Find more *Detectives* exercises in Brain Builders! Workout #30, 31, and 32.

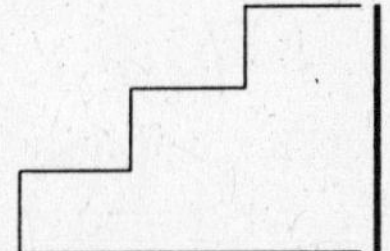

BRAIN-BUILDING SECRET #53
More Brain Power Herbs to Sharpen Your Mind

Here are two herbal recipes to build mental alertness and to counteract senility or brain drain in general.[9]

BRAIN POWER STAMINA FROM HERBS

You can combine these ingredients to make a tea or to stuff inside empty gel capsules. Mix equal amounts of

- peppermint
- Siberian ginseng
- skullcap
- wood betony
- gotu-kola
- kelp

This mixture will improve memory, heighten your ability to concentrate, produce more mental stamina, and generally help to overcome the negative effects of aging on your mental processes.

Recommended dosage: For general adult use, up to 12 capsules daily; for acute conditions, 3–4 capsules three times daily; for hyperactive children, 2–3 capsules in the morning, 1–2 capsules at dinner, plus 3-4 capsules of ginger root per day.

Here are the reasons these herbs were chosen to be part of this brain power herbal blend.

Peppermint. Peppermint works to prevent congestion in the blood circulation through your brain while strengthening and calming your nerves. This effect, in turn, improves concentration and focus on the task at hand. Students who have used peppermint before exams have scored better on tests.

Ginseng and gotu-kola. The brain power virtues of ginseng (see Brain-Building Secret #49) and gotu-kola (see Brain-Building Secret #50) have already been discussed.

Skullcap. Skullcap is a highly regarded nervine, useful in eliminating insomnia; its positive effect on mental abilities is probably due to the fact that it removes nervous tension, which can otherwise interfere with learning.

Wood betony. Wood betony is also a nervine known to reduce tension and nervousness, acting as a mild sedative.

Kelp. Kelp is a nutritionally rich sea vegetable that also has tension-reducing properties and may achieve this effect by insulating heart and nerve tissue from undue stress which would, if unchecked, wear them down faster and reduce their efficiency.

BRAIN-ENERGIZING FORMULA

You can combine these ingredients to make a tea or to stuff inside empty gel capsules:

- bee pollen, 125 mg
- ginseng, 100 mg
- gotu-kola, 100 mg
- myrtlewood, 75 mg
- alfalfa, 75 mg
- echinacea, 75 mg
- peppermint leaves, 60 mg
- Fo-Ti, 50 mg
- licorice root, 50 mg

- ginger root, 50 mg
- blue vervain, 50 mg
- sarsaparilla root, 50 mg
- cayenne, 40 mg
- kelp, 35 mg
- wood betony, 15 mg

Recommended dosage: Once a day.

BRAIN BOOSTER FROM WHEAT AND BARLEY GRASS

Making rich green juices from sprouts of wheat and barley grass has become popular in the last several decades among health foods advocates. You can buy fresh or frozen wheat grass juice in many natural foods stores and, if you buy the simple equipment needed, you can produce it at home. The juicing process somehow makes the otherwise inedible grasses digestible and assimilable. Bear in mind that these potent juices contain high amounts of chlorophyll, a powerful detoxifying, antibacterial, and antiradiation agent once it enters your system.

Recommended dosage: Twice a day.

BRAIN POWER FROM MICROALGAE

Probably the most popular of these single-celled green plants that grow in fresh water are spirulina and chlorella. Similar to wheat and barley grass, algae are high in chlorophyll, and among the microalgae, chlorella is the highest, containing about 76 percent chlorophyll. Not only are microalgae high in chlorophyll, but they contain more protein than beef and other meats and soybeans.

One form of algae called sun chlorella, grown in Japan, contains glutamic acid, which your brain requires to neutralize the metabolic waste from ammonia. It's also high in arginine, which is converted in your body to spermine; low levels of spermine are associated with memory loss and the onset of senility.

In general, chlorella contains a great number of nutrients essential to optimal brain function and for antioxidant reduction of free radicals. Various forms of commercially packaged chlorella and spirulina are commonly available in natural foods stores; follow product recommendations for daily dosage levels.

STAMINA FOR LEARNING FROM LEMON BALM

If you are a student cramming for an exam, a writer working late to meet a deadline, or a market analyst poring over statistical tables, an infusion of lemon balm (*Melissa officinalis*, or melissa, for short) may be your learning stamina answer.

An herbalist of the seventeenth century named John Evelyn once wrote of lemon balm, "Balm is sovereign for the brain, strengthening the memory and powerfully chasing away melancholy." In the Carmelite tradition from an earlier century, the renunciants used to make a water-based preparation with lemon balm, lemon peel, nutmeg, and angelica root as a balm against nervous headache and neuralgia.

Recommended dosage: Several strong cups daily, spaced several hours apart.

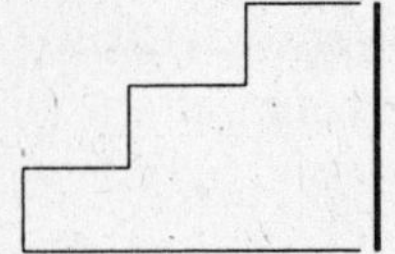

THE ANATOMY OF BRAIN POWER #7
A User's Guide to Your Brain's Neurotransmitters

- *Acetylcholine*. This neurotransmitter, made from acetate and choline plus glocuse and oxygen, within the axon, appears to be crucial to memory. It helps with the transmission of electrical current between neurons and thus increases your brain's ability to respond quickly to stimulation and new input. It is constantly being produced and taken apart, which requires a constant supply of energy (glucose) and oxygen in the brain.
- *Gamma-aminobutyric acid* (GABA). This brain chemical works to inhibit the transmission of nerve signals. This is important because with a potential of several trillions of nerve connections in your brain, you need something to keep the nerve firings from getting out of control. GABA is one of your most important *inhibitory* brain chemicals.

- *Serotonin.* This is another brain chemical that stops nerve transmission and helps to slow down the system; it may also be involved in producing sleep as part of the light-and-dark cycle. Serotonin, made from the amino acid tryptophan, also affects the general functioning and mood of your brain as well as regulating pain. Too much serotonin may produce depression; the popular antidepressant drug Prozac works by preventing serotonin from being reabsorbed by the brain from the synapses.
- *Dopamine.* This is the neurotransmitter that Dr. Oliver Sacks used to wake up his entranced patients in *Awakenings*. Dopamine is central to the activity and control of physical movement. When your brain's dopamine-producing center gets sluggish and stops operating, the result is most often Parkinson's disease, which is marked by erratic, uncontrollable movements, tremors, and twitches. Too much dopamine in the brain may lead to schizophrenia or physical convulsions.
- *Norepinephrine.* This brain chemical excites the brain, working like adrenaline or amphetamine on your brain's capillaries and may increase blood flow to the brain while arousing general brain activity. Norepinephrine is made in the brain stem then released to the brain at large. It is similar to adrenaline from the adrenal glands, which is needed for the "fight-or-flight" response and is a general brain stimulant, heightening brain activity and alertness. Norepinephrine appears to trigger long-term memory, such as memories of fearful outcomes to certain behaviors.
- *Endorphins.* This is one of the major drug's in your brain's "internal pharmacy" producing feelings of euphoria. Technically, endorphins are natural pain-killers, released during stress or when your body has achieved a desired goal. Endorphins reduce your brain's awareness of pain and irritation and generally make you "feel good" and, quite often, high; this improved sense of well-being can then inspire you to more work, creativity, deeper thinking, or more efficient mental processing.

On the basis of this brief discussion of only six of your brain's many dozens of neurotransmitters, you can see why neuroscientists speak in terms of "better thinking through chemistry." Part of this chemistry involves the foods and substances we put into our body to affect the brain. Amino acids, for example, form the precursors—early forms or building blocks—that your body uses to make the neurotransmitters, particularly acetylcholine and serotonin. This helps make it clear why, later in the book, as part of our brain-building secrets, you will see how combining the correct nutrients in the right combinations may actually help produce more neurotransmitters and thus enhance your brain power.

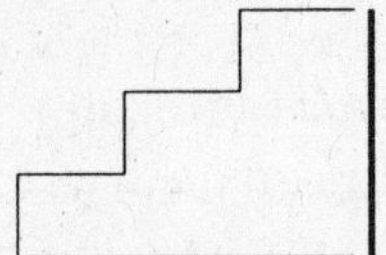

BRAIN-BUILDING SECRET #54
Prime the Vitamin C Brain Power Pump

We visited vitamin C (ascorbic acid) earlier in the book when we looked at the effect on your brain power of various nutrient deficiencies. Now I want to show you the beneficial effects of supplementing a nutritionally adequate vitamin C intake to maximize your brain power possibilities. Here we will consider the benefits and strategies for using vitamin C to boost your mental abilities.

Bear in mind that vitamin C plays an important role in your brain biochemistry as a major antioxidant. In fact, your brain needs up to 15 times more vitamin C to work as an antioxidant than the rest of your body; because your body does not manufacture vitamin C, you must get your supplies from outside dietary sources. Vitamin C works closely with another antioxidant, the amino acid *glutathione*, which works inside fatty membranes of the brain cells, in areas where vitamin C cannot penetrate.

Vitamin C also helps to boost supplies of vitamin E (see Brain-Building Secret #56), another brain antioxidant, which is otherwise depleted by the powerful actions of free radicals. Vitamin C reduces anxiety, promotes sleep, strengthens mental alertness, and is a potent detoxifier. As a circulating antioxidant, vitamin C bathes all your body's cells with protection against free radicals; once in contact with free radicals, the vitamin C molecule neutralizes them. In fact, this neutralization takes place some hundreds of thousands of times each second—provided you have enough vitamin C in your system. Vitamin C also seems able to boost IQ in the vicinity of 5 points.[10]

Recommended dosage: 1000–3000 mg daily, in 500-mg doses, through vitamin pills or powder; drink plenty of water to ensure proper absorption. Technically, vitamin C absorption is safe (meaning it won't produce diarrhea) up to levels of 10,000 mg, even in healthy individuals. Obviously when you are ill, your body's need for and tolerance of additional vitamin C intake rises dramatically. If you are a cigarette smoker, bear in mind that each cigarette you smoke robs your system of 25 mg of vitamin C. If you are older than 65, take 3–9 gm daily.

HOW VITAMIN C GETS PUMPED INTO YOUR BRAIN

Nature has provided your brain and spinal cord with a feature called the *vitamin* C *pump*. This is a medical concept that conveys the idea that vitamin C supplies in your body can be pumped and concentrated when needed to specific areas, such as your cerebrospinal fluid. The central nervous system has the highest concentration of highly unsaturated fats of the body; this means it is also the most vulnerable to the damaging effects of oxidation and free radicals.

In the "pump," vitamin C supplies are pumped out of the general blood supply and concentrated by 10 times the normal amount in the cerebrospinal fluid. The vitamin C pump then extracts vitamin C from this locale and sends it up to the brain, again concentrating it by a factor of 10.

Your brain cells are then bathed ("marinated," perhaps) in a sea of vitamin C that is 100 times more concentrated than you will find anywhere else in the body. You can see from this explanation how important it is to have an adequate, if not abundant, constant supply of bodily vitamin C.

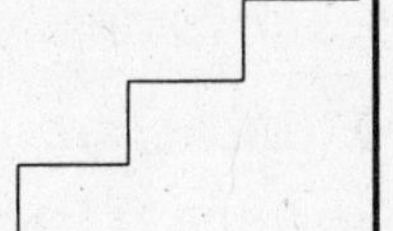

BRAIN BUILDERS! WORKOUT #30
Detectives and the Little Gray Cells of Brain Power—Part 3

Here is the third of five excercises in which you can put the skills of the detective to school your little gray cells.

Sherlock Holmes had such an apparent excess of the little gray cells that if he didn't have a first-rate mystery needing a resolution on his hand, he grew terribly restless and fretful. His brain was like a supertalented worker who had to be kept constantly busy or else he would grow surly and seek distraction or, in the case of Victorian Holmes, turn to the opium pipe.

Apply your detective's analytical ability to take the news and advertising apart.

- Act as if everybody is lying, misleading, or telling you only half the truth.
- Pretend that every ad you see is trying its hardest to make you think a particular idea even if it is not true or appropriate for the product.
- Try going for a week not taking anything at its face value. Look for the truth behind every appearance in the media.
- Do not let the information as presented work on you subliminally, that is, below the threshold of your awareness.
- Try to figure out the true story. Why is the true story not being told?
- Who stands to benefit?
- What is the hidden bias in the information being presented?
- What information is being left out? What is the "fine print" nobody wants you to notice?
- Does the ad make you feel better or worse about yourself?
- Does it make you want to think, act, or buy something out of character with yourself?

Find more *Detectives* in Brain Builders! Workout #31 and 32.

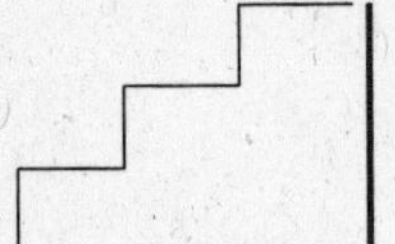

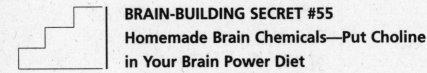

BRAIN-BUILDING SECRET #55
Homemade Brain Chemicals—Put Choline in Your Brain Power Diet

Acetylcholine, the neurotransmitter that scientists believe is essential to memory, is made from choline and acetate. Without adequate supplies of this brain chemical, your brain cannot competently store new information (memories) or function smoothly.

This is a biochemical fact that immediately lends itself to a new brain-building secret: Put choline and lecithin, available as supplements or in selected foods, in your daily brain power diet to ensure that your brain has enough acetylcholine.

Lecithin is a natural substance that is part of the structure of every cell in your body, particularly those in your nervous system and brain. In fact, lecithin accounts for about 30 percent of the dry weight of your brain; among other tasks, lecithin provides nutrition to the fatlike sheaths (called myelin) of nerve fibers and is the precursor to acetylcholine. Infants have high levels of choline in their system because it's needed to build the myelin sheaths around the nerves.

Recommended dosage: If you're taking phosphatidylcholine (which is 10 percent choline), you'll need to ingest it four times daily in doses of 2.5 to 3 gm per dose or up to 10 gm daily; if you're taking choline itself, then up to 1 gm daily; and if you're taking lecithin (which contains 20 percent phosphatidylcholine), which is released slowly and steadily once inside your system, you can get by with two daily doses. Nutritionists recommend trying this out for a 6-month period.

Take vitamin B5 (as pantothenic acid or calcium pantothenate) at the same time because your brain needs this substance to convert choline to acetylcholine. Start with low doses of choline; then gradually increase, to avoid possible diarrhea; people with a clinical diagnosis of manic depression should not take choline.

WHY YOUR BRAIN NEEDS CHOLINE

In all humans, choline is essential for the nerve transmission aspect of memory and information storage. In this vital activity, acetylcholine is a key player; this is the brain chemical that works to send messages between neurons.

As people age, their brains tend to have less acetylcholine because the enzyme that makes it becomes less active. Other biochemical changes in the aging brain also work to dampen the activity of this neurotransmitter or even to destroy it; the result, unfortunately, is typically a declining memory.

The good news is that choline, taken in through the diet, can cross the blood-brain barrier so that the brain can use it to make acetylcholine.[11] Researchers now believe that choline supplementation may improve memory in otherwise normal young people who have deficient memory abilities.

Scientists also speculate that it may be possible to permanently improve memory at an early age by increasing the choline intake of infant's during the crucial years of their development.[12] Administered at this formative stage of life, choline appears able to produce significant biochemical changes in the development of neurons, boosting memory and mental precision and slowing down age-related memory decline.

HOW EXTRA CHOLINE HELPED A POOR STUDENT EXCEL

The well-known nutrition writer Carlson Wade provides a vivid anecdote of how choline can straighten out learning difficulties and other deficits in brain power. He writes of a high school teacher named Oscar who started making many errors in his class; his students, too, were doing poorly on their tests.

When the principal sat in on one of Oscar's classes, he was dismayed to see that his teacher was confusing names and giving faulty answers and skewed interpretations. The principal recommended that Oscar seek a neurologist for a thorough evaluation; fortunately, this professional was also tuned into the nutritional side of brain power problems.

He found that Oscar was seriously low in choline and was beginning to be seriously deficient in the amino acids tryptophan and tyrosine. Consequently, he prescribed a nutrient-rich diet for Oscar and advised him to take 4 tablespoons of lecithin granules every day. The combination of these approaches would get the right nutrients into Oscar's brain and start shoring up the neurotransmitters that were in short supply.

Within 10 days Oscar was a changed man. Although he was 52, he felt as alert as a young man; finally, he could speak clearly and lucidly again, not jumbling his thoughts or tripping over his words. His memory had sharpened considerably too: he could now rattle off names, dates, places, and events with precision and speed. And he kept his job.

FOODS THAT ARE RICH IN CHOLINE

Food sources of lecithin include most seed oils and unrefined vegetable cooking oils, especially soybean oil, which contains 2 percent lecithin. Choline and lecithin supplements are also widely available as tablets, powder, granules, or in liquid form. To achieve the best results, your lecithin should contain at least 30 percent phosphatidyl choline, which is part of a compound called phospholipids, the technical name for lecithin.

Food sources with ample quantities of choline include

- wheat germ (1/2 cup), 2,820 mg
- peanuts (1/2 cup), 1,113 mg
- eggs (2 large), 800 mg
- calf's liver (3.5 ounces), 850 mg
- whole wheat flour (1/2 cup), 613 mg
- white rice (1/2 cup), 586 mg
- trout (3.5 ounces), 580 mg
- pecans (1/2 cup), 333 mg
- lecithin granules (1 tablespoon), 250 mg
- lecithin capsule (1,200 mg), 25 mg

TRY THIS CHOLINE COCKTAIL BEFORE YOUR NEXT BRAIN POWER DEMAND

Nutritionist Robert Haas frequently recommends his special homemade choline cocktail to clients who need "mental energy, memory enhancement, and antioxidant protection against age-accelerating free radicals."

Mix the following ingredients by crushing the tablets into powder and then blending with 2–4 ice cubes in a blender with fruit juice, until smooth:

- 1,500 mg choline
- 100 mg DMAE (see Brain-Building Secret #59)
- 100 mcg chromium picolinate
- 60 mg *Ginkgo biloba*

- ▼ 1–5 mg vitamin B1
- ▼ 1–9 mg vitamin B2
- ▼ 20 mg vitamin B3
- ▼ 100 mg vitamin B5
- ▼ 2 mg vitamin B6
- ▼ 1,000 mcg vitamin B12
- ▼ 1,000 mg vitamin C
- ▼ 400 mcg folic acid
- ▼ 15 mg coenzyme Q10
- ▼ 100 mg caffeine (green tea extract, preferably)
- ▼ 8 ounces fruit juice
- ▼ 400 IU vitamin E

According to Haas, within 30–60 minutes of drinking the cocktail, his mental abilities are markedly sharpened. You might try this in the morning in place of the habitual coffee and certainly before any important and demanding brain power task.

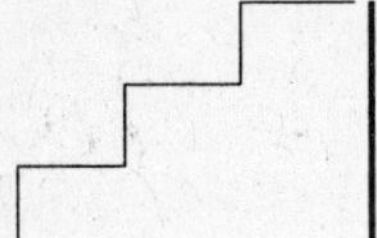

BRAIN BUILDERS! WORKOUT #31 Detectives and the Little Gray Cells of Brain Power—Part 4

Here is the fourth of five exercises in which you can put the skills of the detective to work to school your little gray cells.

I once spent one hour a week for 6 weeks watching a PBS Mystery Theater version of P. D. James *Devices & Desires*. I deliberately did not read the book so I would enjoy the suspense of not knowing for sure until the final episode.

It turned out that my solution was more complex than anything James had in mind. I had more twists and turns, more devious deceptions, and a grander conspiracy than James ever served up.

When the final episode came around, I was disappointed and believed my version was more satisfying and ornate. I wanted to see how elaborate a maze the author could construct and whether I, the amateur detective-rat, could figure it out before the author showed me the definite solution.

Take apart mechanical objects, study how they're put together, then reassemble them.

- ▼ This is another aspect of brain-building detective work. Depending on your boldness, you might try disassembling a watch, lawn mower, radio, tape recorder, washing machine, or car engine.
- ▼ It's better if the mechanical object is broken already, very old, and unwanted or inexpensive.
- ▼ If you're rich and can afford to take your Jaguar apart because you have two more in the garage, more brain power to you.
- ▼ This ambitious but simple exercise will hone your analytical powers even more, especially if you deliberately avoid consulting the owner's manual.
- ▼ See if you can work out the design principles by visual inspection and thinking.

Find more *Detectives* exercises in Brain Builders! Workout #32.

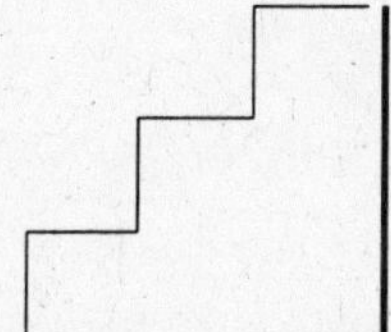

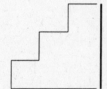

BRAIN-BUILDING SECRET #56
Keep Your Brain Power Pantry Well Stocked with Other Key Smart Mind Nutrients

Good nutrition is advantageous under any circumstances, but it becomes especially necessary when you are trying to build your brain power. In this section we'll look at certain important nutrients that must be in your brain power pantry in perhaps higher amounts than normal.

VITAMIN E, THE BRAIN POWER GUARD

Like vitamin C, this is an essential antioxidant and is part of a group of compounds called *tocopherols* that has eight members. Vitamin E is the most powerful fat-soluble antioxidant known to exist in nature; as such, it protects the membranes of neurons and brain tissue in general from the damages of free radicals.

You might think of vitamin E as a brain power guard; it doesn't so much add to your brain power as *Ginkgo biloba*, for example, but it enables you to preserve what you already have and not to lose it through the damaging effects of free radicals and the aging process. Vitamin E works cooperatively with selenium as antioxidant partners, so be sure to keep your selenium levels in good trim (see Brain-Building Secret #52).

Good food sources of vitamin E include the cold-pressed, unrefined oils of nuts, seeds, and soybeans, wheat germ, whole grains, nuts, eggs, and dark leafy vegetables. You can also obtain vitamin E through supplements, typically in the form of "natural mixed tocopherols," which will include natural and synthetic vitamin E plus a special "mycelized" form, in which the fat-soluble vitamin is broken up into little fragments to make them water soluble and thus quickly absorbed.

Recommended dosage: Daily intake of 800–1,220 IU (1 IU = 1 mg) and not to exceed 1,600 IU daily. Vitamin E is fat soluble, which means your body tissues can store it (unlike water-soluble vitamin C, which passes quickly through), so excess amounts can be harmful, possibly to the adrenal, thyroid, and sex glands in very high doses.

VITAMIN A, THE TOP-FLIGHT ANTIOXIDANT

Like vitamin E, vitamin A helps preserve intelligence by working as a fat-soluble antioxidant to protect neurons against free radicals in the brain. Beta-carotene is a precursor to vitamin A and is converted into the vitamin once it enters your body. Beta-carotene is unique among antioxidants for its ability to curtail the activity of a particular form of oxygen free radical called "singlet."

The singlet oxygen free radical is formed during normal processes of metabolism and as a result of your exposure to ozone or direct sunlight; you can also introduce it into your system from cigarette smoke, air pollution, and from other environmental toxins. Once inside the body, it can easily cross the blood-brain barrier and set to work damaging your delicate brain tissues.

Only beta-carotene can neutralize this especially damaging form of free radical. Good food sources for vitamin A include the liver of animals (beef, chicken), fish oils, carrots, spinach, kale, sweet potatoes, pumpkin, apricots, papaya—all yellow and orange vegetables.

Recommended dosage: For high-level wellness, most nutritionists recommend 10,000–35,000 IU daily; others suggest you can take 15-30 mg daily of beta-carotene, which is the equivalent of 25,000–50,000 IU. Be sure to keep your zinc levels adequate (20–25 mg daily) because zinc is needed to mobilize vitamin A out from its storage site in the liver.

It is preferable to take your vitamin A, either in supplement or food source form, in a meal containing fats. Do not overdo your vitamin A intake because high levels (greater than 500,000 IU or 300 mg daily) can produce a variety of mildly toxic symptoms; this is probably not too likely because nutrition estimates suggest that about 37 percent of Americans are vitamin A deficient.

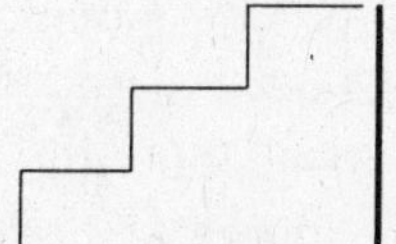

BRAIN-BUILDING SECRET #57 More Antisenility Nutrients for Greater Brain Power

Some of the vitamins and nutrients in this section you encountered earlier in the book in the context of possible deficiencies. The purpose here is to show the positive effects of using these smart nutrients to enhance your brain power at levels perhaps a little higher than standard RDAs. Regarding the B vitamins, it is best if you can take all Bs together in a single supplement that contains the minimum required amount for each nutrient.

VITAMIN B1 ENERGIZES YOUR NERVOUS SYSTEM

As we noted earlier in the book, if you are seriously deficient in vitamin B1 you will probably have some mental and neurological symptoms. These might include anxiety, depression, defects in memory, confusion, obsessive, repetitive thinking. And the symptoms tend to get worse when you're under stress. If you are a heavy alcohol consumer, you especially need thiamine supplementation.

Thiamine is also a strong antioxidant that contributes energy to nervous system function; in fact, it is a major player in the way your body converts glucose from food into usable energy.

Recommended dosage: 25–100 mg, or up to 250 mg daily divided into three doses spaced 5 hours apart.

VITAMIN B3 TO REVERSE MEMORY LOSS

This is an important member of the family of B vitamins, which are sometimes called the antisenility nutrients.[13] Niacin is credited with improving the ability of your red blood cells to carry more oxygen, which means your brain will get more "food" in the form of oxygen.

Not only can niacin restore damaged memory, but studies show it can enhance an already functioning one. Young and middle-aged healthy subjects took 141 mg of niacin daily for a month and demonstrated a 10–40 percent improvement in memory, according to standardized tests.

Recommended dosage: Niacin dosage for shoring up brain power and, presumably, for strengthening memory should be based on age, as follows: age 20–29, 100 mg daily; 30–39, 300 mg; 40–49, 500 mg; 50+, 1,000 mg. Generally speaking, the closer you are in age to the statistically typical age for the early signs of senility, say, 60 years and older, the better it is to start taking preventive measures, especially with nutritional supplements.

Niacin is absorbed best when taken right after a meal. Usually in dosages larger than 50 mg you may experience a sensation of flushing, itching, or tingling on your cheeks; this is harmless and will disappear once your body becomes accustomed to the regular intake of niacin.

VITAMIN B5 FOR BRAIN ANTIAGING

Vitamin B5 is a powerful antioxidant that can increase stamina and reduce stress. Your body also needs adequate supplies of pantothenic acid (B5) to convert choline into the essential neurotransmittter acetylcholine, which speeds messages from one brain cell to the next.

Vitamin B5 keeps the nervous system functioning normally. In laboratory studies with mice, scientists found that vitamin B5 may have antiaging properties. In one study, mice fed extra amounts of B5 lived 653 days compared to nonsupplemented mice, who lived only 550 days. Converted into human aging terms, this means extending your life from 75 to 89 years.

Recommended dosage: 250–750 mg daily.

VITAMIN B6 HELPS MAKE MORE BRAIN CHEMICALS

This vitamin is another antistress nutrient and is needed to make several key neurotransmitters. If you are deficient in B6, your body's ability to make these vital brain chemicals may be seriously curtailed, leading to symptoms of mental decline.

Recommended dosage: 2 mg daily for men; 1–6 mg for women, Do not exceed 500 mg per day without a physician's advice.

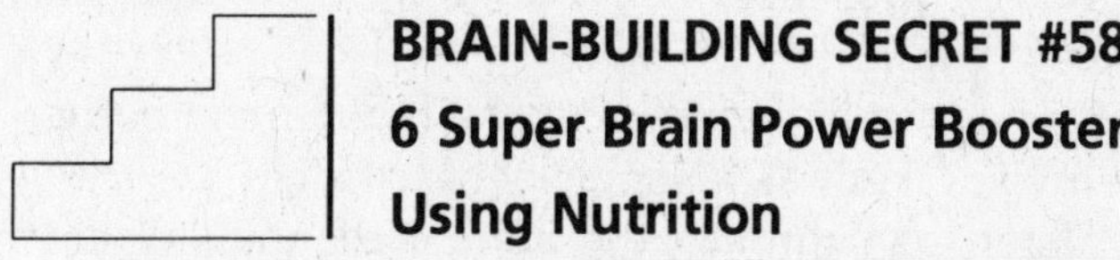

BRAIN-BUILDING SECRET #58
6 Super Brain Power Boosters Using Nutrition

1. PHENYLALANINE BOOSTS BRAIN POWER

This is an amino acid, commonly found in protein-rich foods, that you can take as a specific brain-boosting supplement, often in powder form. Phenylalanine is a key player in the biochemical process that builds the neurotransmitters (especially noradrenaline), but it is also an amino acid that gets used up quickly during moments of stress, danger, or excitement. Noradrenaline, by the way, is a neurotransmitter that boosts cerebral energy, enhances memory and retention, sharpens sensory perception, and improves concentration. There is ample evidence that phenylalanine can increase mental alertness and dispel depression.[14]

Recommended dosage: Nutritionists are not yet sure what the optimal daily dosage should be but generally recommend something in the order of 375–500 mg daily on an empty stomach. Other nutritionists suggest that if you take the D and L form of phenylalanine (called DLPA, which your natural foods store vitamin clerk can explain to you) twice a day, you are likely to experience mental arousal, a higher energy level, and a better mood.

Specifically, take 1,000–1,500 mg of DLPA in the morning before eating anything and then the same quantity again in the afternoon with 100 mg of vitamin B6 and 500 mg of vitamin C.

As a variant and for an extra brain power surge, supplement your phenylalanine powder with 2 teaspoons bee pollen, 2 tablespoons honey, 25 drops each of *Ginkgo biloba* and liquid ginseng, and a dropperful of DMAE. Stir together in warm water and drink first thing in the morning instead of coffee.

2. GLUTAMINE TO DEFOG AND ENERGIZE YOUR BRAIN

This is another brain-boosting amino acid that produces the brain chemical called glutamic acid. Glutamine has a reputation as a "brain fuel, brain energizer, and brain defogger" that makes your thinking sharper, boosts your alertness, and improves your overall mood.

Glutamine also has the ability to cross the blood-brain barrier, which means when you take it as a supplement, chances are it will reach your brain faster than through the normal channels of food digestion.

Once in the brain, glutamine is converted into glutamic acid, which then gets to work with detoxifying ammonia. If the ammonia level in your brain is too high (which can happen because it's the byproduct of protein metabolism in your brain), it can make you irritable and nauseous.

Also, if your brain's glutamic acid levels are low, the ammonia level rises, and this can produce fatigue, confusion, swings in mood, and a general inability to concentrate. As one nutritionist says, when you take glutamine it's like "almost plugging your brain into a free fuel source."

Better than coffee, which gives you only a brief energy boost, glutamine is a brain fuel that actually creates more energy in the brain. Students who take glutamine supplements before exams report feeling more alert, confident, and mentally clear.

Recommended dosage: Start with 250–500 mg daily; then build up to 1.5 gm daily.

3. ARGININE, AN AMINO ACID AGAINST MEMORY LOSS

Arginine is an amino acid that your body converts to spermine, which is found in semen, blood tissue, and brain cells. If you are significantly low in spermine, you may start to show the early signs of memory loss and senility.

On the positive side, arginine may be highly important as an antiaging, antisenility nutrient. A 1990 headline in *The New York Times*, not a publication given to exaggeration, declared: "Human Growth Hormone Reverses the Effects of Aging." This synthetically produced growth hormone costs $20,000 a year to take, which put it out of reach of nearly everyone. But it did inspire two progressive nutritionists to develop a much cheaper but equally effective alternative.

Durk Pearson and Sandy Shaw, authors of the best-selling book on nutrition and aging *Life Extension* (1982), came up with an alternative way to increase the levels of growth hormones in the brain.

To get a formula that enhances your mental abilities, among other benefits, combine

- arginine, 6g
- choline, 600 mg
- vitamin B5, 500 mg

4. GET MORE OXYGEN INTO YOUR BRAIN WITH GERMANIUM

This is a mineral that's gaining increasing attention as a successful brain booster ever since it was discovered in the 1980s. After he discovered it, Kazuhiko Asai, a Japanese scientist, figured out a way to synthesize it in the laboratory and then test it for its health benefits.

Germanium is normally found in minute quantities as a component in many medicinal herbs, including garlic, ginseng, chlorella, and others. Technically, germanium is a trace element found abundantly in the Earth's crust and is listed in the chemist's periodic table of the elements.

Tests have shown germanium's ability to stimulate the immune system and have positive effects against tumors, cancer, and viruses. Dr. Asai found that an intake of 100–300 mg of germanium daily had positive effects on the outcomes of numerous illnesses. More importantly for our purposes, germanium can increase bodily tissue's ability to accept oxygen, which is why informally it is sometimes called vitamin O, for oxygen.

STAYING UP LATE WITH GERMANIUM ON YOUR MIND

Dr. Asai's theory is that an inadequate supply of oxygen to any body part or system can be a cause of disease. Any substance that can increase oxygenation or even substitute for oxygen and bind with red blood cells clearly spells greater brain power.

A California scientist reports that when he needs to work late on a project and must keep his mind clear and focused, he takes several germanium capsules before getting started. This ensures that his brain will have enough oxygen for the brain power demands and that any to accumulated toxins that would otherwise interfere with his memory and mental abilities will be removed.

Germanium is also a powerful systemic detoxifying agent. For example, your mercury dental amalgams may be leeching toxic amounts of mercury into your system, or you may be getting similar contaminants from food fertilizers, mercury-poisoned fish, or PCB poisoning. Germanium has the ability to quickly capture any heavy metal deposited in your body and to remove it from your system in about 24 hours.

Recommended dosage: Per instructions on product, usually 30 mg daily as a preventive or brain-building measure, although some nutritionists recommend 60 mg daily; for minor problems, try 50–100 mg daily, and for pain relief 1–1.5 grams daily. But make sure it's *organic germanium sequioxide*, also called Ge-132. Food sources include aloe vera, watercress, pearl barley, comfrey, garlic, ginseng, angelica, shiitake and reishi mushrooms, onions, and the herb suma.

5. WHY OXYWATER CAN MAKE YOU SMARTER

The idea of boosting the oxygen supply to your brain has yet another application in addition to techniques like using germanium or exercising more. It's called *hyperoxygenation* (*oxywater*, for short), which means you drink small quantities of diluted food-grade hydrogen peroxide (H_20_2).

Like germanium, oxywater acts as a powerful agent against toxic substances, bacterial contaminants in your body, and general oxygen depletion in the brain. According to research studies, regular use of oxywater can improve alertness, reflexes, memory, and even intelligence. Patients with Alzheimer's and Parkinson's are responding positively to it. As one scientist working with it quips, "Oxywater may even cure stupidity."

Recommended dosage: Typically, you add 2–10 drops of food-grade hydrogen peroxide (diluted to therapeutic levels of 0.5–1.0 percent) to about 6 ounces of pure spring water and drink several times daily.

Various commercial formulas available include Dr. Donsbach's Superoxy, which comes in five flavors, and EQ 02, a safer oxygen electrolyte supplement available in liquid form.[15]

It's best to take antioxidant nutrients at the same time, such as *Gingko biloba* and vitamins A, C, and E, to counteract the hydroxyl radicals given off when your body metabolizes hydrogen peroxide.

6. SUPPLEMENT FORMULAS FOR SMARTER CHILDREN

A landmark 1991 California study lasting 12 weeks and involving 615 schoolchildren proved that IQ can be positively affected by meganutrient supplementation.[16] In fact, one-third of the students registered a 10-point IQ increase.

The dramatic improvements registered by the study also suggested that many supposedly "normal, healthy" children may in fact be nutritionally deficient even though they show no outward signs. Difficulties in mental function of course are among the first symptoms to appear when you are nutritionally deficient.

This is the IQ-boosting formula (100 percent of RDA) used in the California study:

- vitamin A, 5,000 IU
- B1, 1.7 mg
- B2 1.7 mg
- B3, 20 mg
- B5, 10 mg
- B6, 2 mg
- B12, 6 mcg
- vitamin C, 60 mg
- vitamin D, 400 IU
- vitamin E, 30 IU
- vitamin K, 50 mcg

- biotin, 300 mcg
- folic acid, 400 mcg
- calcium, 200 mg (only 20 percent of RDA)
- chromium, 100 mcg
- copper, 2 mg
- iodine, 150 mcg
- iron, 18 mg
- magnesium, 80 mg
- manganese, 2.5 mg
- molybdenum, 250 mcg
- selenium, 100 mcg
- zinc, 15 mg

THE ANATOMY OF BRAIN POWER #8
Testimonials That Brain Boosting Nutrients Work

- A movie producer who took a variety of smart drugs and nutrients (see Brain-Building Secret #59) including *Ginkgo biloba*, choline, hydergine, and piracetam, together and singly, reports that each of them, either alone or in combination, "has increased my mental clarity and stamina." He never gets writer's block, he can work quicker and be more articulate in his thinking, and he was able to write 20 episodes of a TV series in only 3 months. "I seem to be at peak efficiency constantly."[17]
- A client used choline, ginkgo, ginseng, and DMAE for 5 months. "I have noticed an improvement in short-term memory and long-term memory. Also, my friends have noticed an improvement in my general disposition."
- Another client reported that using ginkgo and DMAE helped her to shape her thoughts into complete sentences, a difficulty she had endured for years. The nutrients also gave her better control over her speaking.

- A client reported that after using choline, he could concentrate on many conversations at once, including his own, and keep track of them all. His eyesight became keener and his vocabulary and general thinking became "very concise."
- A computer programmer reports that taking choline with inositol or lecithin (300–400 mg with equal amounts of inositol every 3 hours during work) "significantly improves my short-term visual memory (I can 'hold more code in my head'). I could not perform at the same level otherwise."

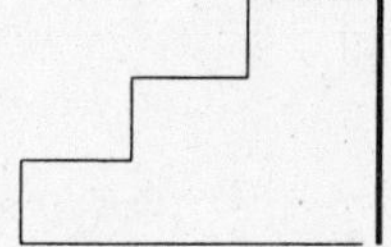

BRAIN BUILDERS! WORKOUT #32 Detectives and the Little Gray Cells of Brain Power—Part 5

Here is the last of 5 exercises in which you can put the skills of the detective to work to school your little gray cells. Apply your detective's keen powers of analysis and observation to take a movie plot apart.

- Perhaps you've seen Harrison Ford in *The Fugitive*. Unarguably this is a highly entertaining thriller, yet it is also a skillfully crafted story. As another exercise in developing your left brain powers of analysis, make a flow chart of the plot of this film.
- Pay special attention to how the clues are gradually dropped, whereby Inspector Gerard begins to realize that Dr. Richard Kimble might in fact be innocent.
- Similarly, you might chart the plot development in one of Alfred Hitchcock's more astounding thrillers, such as *The Birds*, *Vertigo*, *Rear Window*, *Northwest Passage*.
- Here the exercise is to notice the precise moments in which Hitchcock gradually increases the tension and suspense, deepens the sense of menace, and yanks the plot along like a dog on a tight leash.

- A Hitchcock plot will work on your mind and emotions unconsciously all the same. The brain power exercise here is to *see how the master does it*. This trains your powers of observation, deduction, and analytical thinking, and it may give you even more respect for the old master as well.
- If you've watched a Hitchcock movie, you know that he always finds a way to insert himself in the first 10 minutes of the film, as a casual, unimportant character who has about 5 seconds of screen time. There are two things you can do with this impish trick of Hitchcock's:
- First, watch 20 of his films and make a list of the different ways he inserts himself in the film.
- Second, think up another 20 ways he might have done it in these movies.

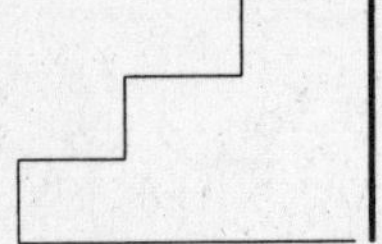

BRAIN-BUILDING SECRET #59
6 Smart Drugs and Nutrients for More Brain Power

In the last 15 years a new category of brain boosters called smart drugs have come on the market. They have generated a good deal of excitement and research, although they are still in the experimental stage and have not been officially approved by the FDA, which means for the most part you need to order them through specialty distributors. (See the Resources.)

In some parts of the United States, the enthusiasm for these smart drugs has led to the founding of special "brain cocktail bars" where you can sidle up to the counter and order special brain nutrient drinks called *Get Smart Think Drinks* along with your carrot and celery. Some of these are commercially available and present themselves with such exotic (trademarked) names as Blast, Rise and Shine, Memory Fuel, Energy Elicksure, Psuper Psonic Psyber Tonic.

While the ingredient lists usually include a healthy sampling of vitamins, minerals, amino acids, and trace elements, one of two elements is consistently found: either phenylalanine (which makes noradrenaline) or choline (which makes acetylcholine).

Are smart drugs safe? Probably, provided you don't overdo it. In general, they energize the brain by providing it with an optimal supply of oxygen, they shield the brain against free radical damage, they remove cellular debris from brain tissue, and they supply the raw materials necessary for the brain to make its essential neurotransmitters. Oxygen of course is the two-edged sword that both protects and cleaves your brain power.

On the one hand, oxygen energizes your brain, enabling you to think and recall more clearly and quickly; yet oxygen in the brain promotes neural damage from free radicals, which are derived form oxygen in the first place. The unique advantage of most smart drugs is that they put a great deal of brain-boosting oxygen into your brain yet simultaneously protect the brain from the potential damage wrought by free radicals generated by oxygen.

1. PIRACETAM—BRIDGING THE BRAIN HEMISPHERES

This is a synthesized drug, first developed in Belgium and often called Nootropil, that users say "wakes up your brain." It's part of a new category of drugs called *nootropics*, which means "acting on the mind" and includes most of the smart drugs available today.[18]

Piracetam, which is close in chemical makeup to the amino acid pyroglutamate, is known to

- ▼ improve memory
- ▼ strengthen general brain function under conditions of oxygen deprivation
- ▼ increase brain energy
- ▼ speed up the information flow between both brain hemispheres
- ▼ stimulate your brain to "grow" more receptor sites in its neurons for choline and related substance

A secretary who takes Piracetam daily (800 mg) found herself to be more alert, intelligent, and in a better mood. Another user says it keeps him alert while driving and helps him to formulate new and different ideas. A third person reported mixing Piracetam with choline, which was "one of the best things that ever happened to me." His extreme mood swings stopped, his concentration and speaking ability became much better, and he felt more self-confident.[19]

Recommended dosage: In the area of 2,400–4,800 mg daily divided into three equal doses.

2. HYDERGINE, THE ULTIMATE SMART PILL

This smart nutrient has been proven to strengthen various mental capacities and to slow down the aging process. Technically, Hydergine is derived (then chemically altered) from three substances called alkaloids that derive from a naturally occurring fungus found on rye grains.

Among its noted abilities are the following:

- increasing brain blood and oxygen supply
- protecting the brain from damage during times of reduced oxygen supply
- slowing down the deposit of age pigment in the brain, associated with Alzheimer's
- working as an antioxidant against free radicals in the brain
- increasing intelligence, recall, memory, and learning

At least 22 scientific studies have shown Hydergine's ability to act as an antisenility agent in the dosage range of 4.5–6 mg daily. Although the FDA has limited the use and dosage of Hydergine, European studies suggest that Hydergine can prevent and even reverse damage to brain cells.[20]

A son and his father took Hydergine (9 mg daily) together at Christmas. They wanted to see if it would stimulate their long-term memory; they had positive results within two days. The father, in his forties, could suddenly remember family events from his twenties with sparkling clarity; the son's memories went back to his childhood. "The everyday events truly had been stored away all these years; it just took some chemical prodding to jog them loose into the conscious mind."

Recommended dosage: 1 mg three times daily, taken as a tablet, liquid, or liquid capsule.

3. DMAE—FOOD FOR YOUR BRAIN

DMAE occurs in nature (fish, sardines, anchovies) as a chemical precursor to choline; small amounts of DMAE occur in your brain as well, where it works to increase the levels of acetylcholine. Taken as a supplement, DMAE gets your brain to synthesize more acetylcholine, which in turn improves your brain function.

It's considered one of the most potent of brain foods and is often placed at the top of the smart drugs list for its general ability to stimulate and uplift the central nervous system without the typical rush and letdown experienced with amphetamines. DMAE is regarded as a nutritional supplement, which makes it widely available.

Claims for DMAE (also known as Deanol) include its ability to improve memory and learning, enhance intelligence, uplift mood, and build physical and mental energy. DMAE is available as a powder, liquid, or in capsules. In the early 1980s, a drug company marketed a DMAE version called Deaner and published studies highlighting its effects.[21]

Here is one person's experience with DMAE: "When I take DMAE, I am more awake when I am awake, more sound asleep when I am asleep. Not only does my memory improve, but I have an easier time day-dreaming when I want to and concentrating on real-world tasks when I want to."

Recommended dosage: 250–1,000 mg daily, ideally in the morning; a sensible daily dosage to improve brain power is in the area of 400 mg daily, but because this is a relatively new dietary substance, you will need to find your own best levels. It will take several weeks of daily use to see the full brain power benefits; too much DMAE can produce insomnia, dull headaches, or muscle tension.

4. VASOPRESSIN/DIAPID, THE MEMORY EXPERT

This smart drug is actually a hormone naturally ocurring in your brain, released by the pituitary gland. Brain scientists believe that vasopressin helps you learn faster by imprinting new data (information) into the brain's memory centers.

If you want to learn something new, you can't do it without vasopressin; for that matter, if you want to remember items as well, you'd better be sure your brain is well stocked with vasopressin, which is available as a prescription drug called Diapid.

Studies in both the United States and Europe have shown that vasopressin can

- improve both short and long-term memory
- boost your ability to perform well on tests requiring concentration, recall, recognition, and information storage
- heighten learning ability and memory function in people with memory impairments
- reverse amnesia and protect against memory loss due to physical or chemical injury
- especially recommended for older people or patients who are already showing the early signs of mental decline

Recommended dosage: As a nasal spray, one spray in each nostril 3–4 times daily, which is equivalent to 12–16 U.S.P. posterior pituitary units, a formal measurement for this inhalant. Many physicians probably know of Diapid only as a substance used for treating frequent urination associated with diabetes.

It's best not to use vasopressin every day, as your system may develop a tolerance to it, which is to say, a kind of immunity. Better effects will be had from vasopressin when you use it for times when you need a quick mental lift and cerebral boost, such as before an exam or meeting or when your concentration powers are required.

5. LUCIDRIL—REJUVENATE YOUR BRAIN CELLS

Smart drugs experts call Lucidril the "garbage man of the brain" because it is able to remove the age pigment deposits (called lipofuscin) or cellular garbage that accumulates in your brain as a result of the normal processes of metabolism.

When lipofuscin deposits build up in your brain, they suffocate the neurons; when a lot of neurons are destroyed in this manner, your learning ability and general brain power start to decline. Bear in mind that these age pigment deposits are a supposedly natural, irreversible part of the aging process, which in turn spells a decline in your usable IQ. Any substance that can stop or even reverse this process is clearly a brain builder's best ally.

Lucidril is able to

- rejuvenate brain cells and thereby reverse the aging process
- repair the synapses or meeting points between neurons

- protect your brain in conditions of less than adequate oxygen, such as in strokes, heart attacks, or near drowning
- prevent aging and brain power decline produced by biological processes
- reverse generalized weakness and lack of vigor, confusion, and memory disturbances in the elderly

Here is an affidavit from a Lucidril user: "I had been having a problem with fatigue and depression, which disappeared when I started taking centrophenoxine. It also improved my memory and made me much quicker."

Recommended dosage: 1,000–3,000 mg daily. Lucidril, usually available in 500-mg tablets, is very quick acting; users report noticing an increase in alertness and a sense of stimulation soon after taking it.

6. DHEA

This is a naturally occurring adrenal hormone found abundantly in the human blood and in very high concentrations in the brain as well. In fact, there is 6.5 times more DHEA in your brain than anywhere else in your body.

Scientists know that DHEA blood levels decline seriously with age, probably leading to many of the age-related symptoms of mental decline, including senility. DHEA does not seem to do anything as specific as the other brain nutrients; rather, it is a general support for a variety of activities and mechanisms, particularly the manufacture of other steroid hormones in the body.

Recent studies suggest that DHEA has an ability to boost memory and generally improve cognitive activities. It may do this by improving the communication among nerve cells.[22] Studies also show that when you are low in DHEA, nerve degeneration begins to occur; on the other hand, in a lab study, adding low concentrations of DHEA to nerve cell tissue cultures actually increased the number of neurons present along with their ability to connect with other neurons and to grow more dendrites.

Recommended dosage: Like vasopressin, DHEA, which is exceptionally safe, is available by physician's prescription. DHEA levels for optimal brain power are in the range of 25–100 mg daily.

5 MOVE YOUR BRAIN

▼▼▼▼▼▼▼▼▼▼▼▼▼▼▼▼▼▼▼▼▼▼▼▼▼▼

How Exercise, Yoga, and Other Movements Can Boost Your Brain Power

Move your brain. While you cannot literally move your brain and exercise it in the same sense that you work out your leg muscles when you go jogging, exercise is still a vital key to better brain power. It gets more oxygen into your brain cells. Learn how to move your brain through exercise, yoga, Qigong, breathing exercises, and twirling.

This chapter presents brain-building secrets that have you moving, exercising, and breathing vigorously to get more oxygen into your brain cells. This is essential to optimal mental performance. You'll be practicing exercises drawn from classical yoga and the martial arts form called qigong, plus gaining a surprising insight into why the whirling dervishes twirl all the time.

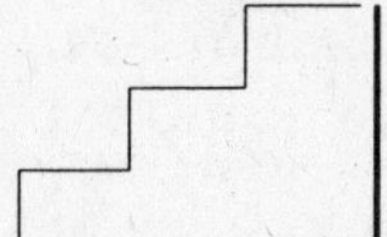

BRAIN-BUILDING SECRET #60
How to Creep and Crawl Your Way to More Brain Power

This brain-building secret will surely strike you as odd, but it is based on a major theory of brain development. This exercise works on what's called the *midbrain*, through which, as an infant, you first developed hand-eye coordination and with which you learned how to crawl and creep.

By practicing creeping and crawling again, you help to restimulate this important part of your brain through which you first developed balance and mastered the vertical dimension, that is (eventually), standing up and walking erect. The exercise also helps reknit your sensory-motor experience with your active brain power, so that you can perceive and relate to your environment, as an adult, in a more dynamic, brain-powered way.

This brain-building secret is easy to explain: *Get down on your hands and knees and spend the next 2 hours crawling and creeping around your house for the next 21 days.*

Sounds ridiculous, doesn't it? The strangest way imaginable to gain brain power? Yet, years ago, when you were an infant, you forged a working relationship between your midbrain, eyes, and hands by creeping and crawling around the house as a prelude to walking upright. This exercise *restimulates* that same midbrain.

START STIMULATING YOUR MIDBRAIN BY CRAWLING AROUND

- Start by moving forward across the floor on your hands and knees in any way that appeals to you.
- Eventually your body will find the "groove," and a rhythm and movement style that is comfortable and repeatable will suggest itself.
- Once your creeping pattern is established, put all your attention into the nuances of moving in this way.
- Note all the places where your body touches the floor and is moving across it.
- Note how the weight of your body is redistributed in this posture.
- Sense the extension of your muscles and bones; sense the texture and resistance of the floor.
- Note where your head and eyes are in relationship to the floor and your environment.
- Observe everything in your visual field—the chairs, tables, walls, and other objects. Your sense of visual perception is becoming *stereoscopic*, richer, fuller, more comprehensive. This will feed back to your brain and, in a sense, recharge your neurons.

OTHER FUN WAYS TO RECHARGE YOUR MIDBRAIN

There are a handful of related physical exercises that complement creeping and crawling and will similarly recharge your midbrain by working with eye-hand coordination.

They all involve fine tasks of close detail manipulation, such as

- Throw darts at a target.
- Unravel fabrics, thread by thread.
- Thread progressively smaller needles.
- Spin jacks.
- Do highly detailed sketches.
- Learn to tie complicated knots.
- Play string games, such as cat's cradle.
- Study a gemstone, rotating it slowly in your hands, observing it both close and far.

Other brain-building exercises along the same lines—providing you are up to them and have no preexistent health conditions that would make practicing them a bad idea—include yoga head stands, cartwheels, forward and backward rolls, or jumping rope.

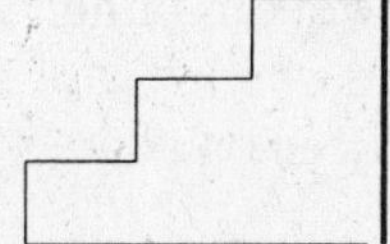

BRAIN BUILDERS! WORKOUT #33 How to Turn into a Rock

This is a concentration exercise using a sustained focus on physical objects as a way of heightening your ability to focus on any subject or object.

- Take a palm-sized rock or multifaceted crystal and hold it in your palm before you.
- Examine it thoroughly, noting all its physical qualities.
- Now pretend that you are exceedingly small, tiny enough to crawl inside this rock or crystal and become one with it.

- ▼ Now the crystal is your body. How does it feel? Do you feel heavy, light, empty, full?
- ▼ Pretend that as the rock or crystal you lay in a field. It's raining. Cows are walking about. How does all of this affect you, being a rock?
- ▼ Now the sun comes out and dries the moisture from your rock surface. How does this feel?
- ▼ When you have finished examining the life of yourself as a rock, count to 5, then return to your normal size and identity.

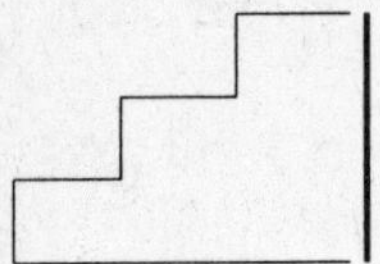

BRAIN-BUILDING SECRET #61
Working Out with Your Whole Brain—The 7 Links Between Moving and Learning

It may surprise you to learn that certain carefully constructed body movements can actually improve your brain power. Back in 1964, Paul Dennison scoured the fields of hatha yoga, kinesiology, acupressure, and behavioral optometry for practical techniques to help learning-disabled and dyslexic children improve their school abilities.

Dennison found that when certain movements were practiced that emphasized both sides of the body, both eyes and then both brain hemispheres would gradually be encouraged to work together. These exercises work *cross-laterally*, because, for example, the left arm will cross the right side of the body or the left eye will focus on something in the right field of vision.

When you do this cross-lateral type of activity, it encourages both sides of the brain to work together. And don't forget, your brain hemispheres already work cross-laterally—your right eye passes visual information along to your left hemisphere. The result of practicing these exercises can be an improvement in brain function. Not only does this improve the mental abilities of learning-disabled children, it can quickly improve a full range of brain power functions in otherwise "normal" adults.[1]

When practicing the exercises that follow, be sure to coordinate your breathing with your body movements such that when you extend your arms or legs, you do this on the exhale; when you draw your limbs back alongside your body, do this on the inhale. These exercises have immediate neurophysiological benefits while improving specific aspects of your brain function.

1. HOW TO MAKE A PRESSING DECISION

Stand up, with your legs about 18 inches apart. Place your index and middle fingers of your right hand about three fingerwidths away from your right ear and press firmly. Using the same fingers on your left hand, place them at your navel and press firmly. Hold both sets of fingers in position for 30 seconds, then release; reverse positions, so that you use your left hand to press against your left ear and your right hand at your navel.

This exercise resets your body's equilibrium, relaxes your eyes, and improves your body's general organization; because of these facts, it improves concentration along with the ability to make decisions and to figure out problems.

2. HOW TO PUT YOUR FINGERS ON MORE BRAIN POWER

Stand up, with your legs about 18 inches apart. Place your left hand, palm inward, against your navel. Find the hollow space under your collarbone on both sides, which is about 1 inch away from where the collarbone meets your sternum. Place the thumb and forefinger of your right hand in this hollow space on both sides, thumb on one side, forefinger on the other. For the next 60 seconds, rub these two spots vigorously; without moving your head, look to the right, then left, then right; keep doing this for the duration of the exercise.

This exercise stimulates the carotid arteries that oxygenate your brain. By stimulating carotid circulation in both brain hemispheres, this encourages both brains to work together, to "cross-talk."

3. HOW TO CROSS YOURSELF WHILE WALKING IN PLACE

While standing, march in place without moving forward. As your right knee comes up, touch it with the palm of your left hand; as your left knee comes up, touch it with the palm of your right hand. Do this for about 60 seconds, or for about the duration of 8–10 complete breath cycles.

This exercise works on both brain hemispheres at the same time; it also helps improve your brain's ability to coordinate visual and bodily information; this in turn improves your brain power in the areas of memory, listening, and reading.

4. THE LEFT HAND *DOES* KNOW WHAT THE RIGHT HAND IS DOING

You need a large sheet of blank paper, two pencils or crayons, and a table surface for this exercise. Hold a pencil in each hand. Start drawing shapes on the paper with both hands. Let the right lead the left in making large circular shapes; then let the left lead the right. You are making mirror-image doodles with both hands.

Track what both hands are doing. Make squares, circles, triangles, moving up and down the paper; make sure both hands are moving together and mirroring each other in their movements. Keep your hands moving; don't stop to sketch.

This exercise is obviously about developing your brain's cross-lateral abilities, plus orientation in space in relation to bodily balance. It also stimulates eye-hand coordination and eye-to-eye coordination. This, in turn, will improve your writing skills.

5. RELEASING BRAIN POWER ENERGY HIDDEN IN YOUR JAW

Stand up, with your legs about 18 inches apart. Place the fingertips of both hands against your left and right cheeks, just above the lower teeth and below the upper teeth. Press your right fingers into your right cheek, and your left fingers into your left cheek.

Gently massage your face as you make an exaggerated yawn, a very long and thorough exhale. Do this three more times, moving your fingers around your cheeks to find sore or sensitive areas.

This exercise has strong neurophysiological benefits. Approximately 50 percent of the nerve connections that go from your body into your brain pass through your jaw joints.

When you massage these joints, not only does it relax the jaw, but it stimulates those neurological connections and enhances brain power. In some cases, having a loose, relaxed jaw makes it much easier to express yourself creatively.

6. THE 8's MAY BE LAZY, BUT THEY'LL HELP YOUR BRAIN FOCUS

Stand up, with your legs about 18 inches apart. Extend your right arm out in front of you with your thumb sticking up toward the ceiling in standard American fashion to signal everything's okay.

Place your attention on the tip of your thumb. Now make a large sweeping figure eight ("lazy 8") with your thumb; don't move your head as you track your thumb with your eyes.

Make the point directly in front of you serve as the center of the figure eight. Repeat three times; then reverse hands and track your left thumb.

Then clasp both thumbs together and make three figure eights. Tracking figure eights in this way helps to integrate the visual fields of your left and right eyes while also improving bodily balance and coordination. It may also help your peripheral vision.

The exercise can have a direct effect on how well you can maintain mental focus in activities such as reading, writing, and general comprehension.

7. MAKING A POSITIVE POINT WITH YOUR EYEBROWS

You may do this exercise sitting down, but keep your back straight and your feet apart, flat on the floor. Use your fingers to probe about 1–2 inches above each eyebrow; there you will notice a slight indentation or hollow.

Place three fingertips from each hand at this spot over each eyebrow. Close your eyes and gently press the points, pulling lightly on the skin to make it taut. Hold this position for the count of 10 breath cycles.

These are acupuncture points that help release emotional stress and a sense of guarded defensiveness. When you massage them in this manner, it helps your brain shift from an emotional to a more rational, calmer state.

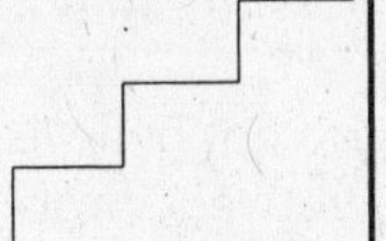

THE ANATOMY OF BRAIN POWER #9
Is Your Brain Really on the Top of Your Shoulders?

It seems like such common sense that nobody ever questions it—that your brain is inside your head, that all your mental activities happen inside the gray matter of your brain. Throughout the popular and clinical discussion of brain power, certain theories are consistently presented.

STANDARD THEORIES OF THE BRAIN AND WHY I DON'T AGREE WITH THEM

There is the *triune brain* idea, that states that the human brain is made of three main components, derived in effect from evolution. These include the so-called reptilian brain (brain stem, to do with sensory-motor functions, survival issues), mammalian brain (limbic system, emotions, pleasure and pain, memory, biorhythms), and neocortex (analytical, reasoning processes, language, higher intelligence).

Then there is the *split brain* theory with its model of a left hemisphere and right hemisphere, each with distinctively different functions. Your left brain handles analytical, logical, calculative tasks while your right brain is intuitive, spatial, and visual.

Another prominent notion is *brain geography*. This is the idea that your brain is a highly specialized organ; you can make a list of the top 30 brain power functions and assign each of them to a specific area in the brain.

A HOLISTIC—AND UNCONVENTIONAL WAY OF LOOKING AT YOUR BRAIN

Let me share with you a brain-building secret. I do not personally believe in any of these notions. I personally regard them as fundamentally limiting and demeaning. I think they are all insults to human brain power. Each of them views your human intelligence as a fragmented, compartmentalized, mechanical function. Perhaps there is a different, more holistic way of looking at the brain, mind, and intelligence.

Before we do, here is another heretical opinion. I do not believe the seat of thinking and mental activity is truly and definitively located in your brain. But if it isn't in the brain, where else in the body might it be? I propose that intelligence and the thinking activity are distributed throughout your body as a whole.

The views of Austrian philosopher Rudolf Steiner (1861-1925) give us a new starting point. Steiner was a highly influential seer in his time, developing new ways of conducting medicine, art, education, science, agriculture, and philosophy itself. He was widely regarded as being clairvoyant, with the skill of seeing energy fields around people and with having deep insight into the workings of nature, the human being, and reality in general. Among the many unconventional things Steiner taught, one is particularly relevant here.

YOUR BRAIN IS ACTUALLY ALL AROUND YOU

Surrounding each human being is an evanescent, constantly active energy field or aura, Steiner said. It is full of pictures and images, as if 20 movie projectors were beaming their movies onto this shimmering curtain all at once. These swirling, weaving images, said Steiner, represent the subtle basis of our thinking activity.

After all, most brain power experts today agree that you remember better, faster, and more thoroughly when you work with images, that your memory for visual information is nearly perfect.

What Steiner does is show us where all these visual images live—it's not in your brain, but rather all around your body like a picture membrane. Memories are stored here; in fact, everything you ever did in your life, or thought, is still present in this picture aura around your body, Steiner said. When you sit down to deliberately perform a mental task—think, calculate, solve a problem—it happens in your picture aura *first*, then, in your physical brain.

All the intricate biochemical activities inside your brain happen as a result of the energetic thinking activity that takes place first in your picture aura. This means that for all practical purposes your brain is not on the top of your shoulders but all around you, like a transparent, picture-filled film.

IT'S NOT SCIENCE FICTION BUT THE BASIS OF NATURAL MEDICINE

Of course this is stranger than science fiction, yet it ties into common sense from an interesting but unexpected angle. Health. Steiner, who was keenly interested in transforming Western medicine to include some of these ideas, taught that this same picture aura (which he also called the "etheric body") is the source of your health, vitality, and, when you are sick, healing and rejuvenation.

Just consider: Your thinking activity and your health take their cues from the *same* subtle energy field around your body. Here's where it all ties into common sense.

In this book, I present brain-building secrets that work with your attitude, your physical and emotional health, and your mental flexibility. They are all intimately connected. Changing your attitude affects your energy field; your energy field in turn affects the way you think, and it is the foundation for everything that happens in your physical body and brain. There is a seamless feedback loop at play between your physical organism, your brain, and your energy field, or picture aura. Changes you make in one place affect the rest of the circuit. The way you think will affect how your body runs; the kind of energy coming into your body from this energy field affects how you think.

That's because in this most peculiar model that Steiner gave us, your brain and your body are both somewhere else—around you, as an energy field, and your brain is most certainly not on the top of your shoulders.

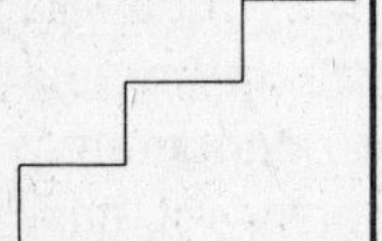

BRAIN BUILDERS! WORKOUT #34
The Little Black Circle of Remembering

Yogis use this exercise to develop photographic memory and, on a more practical level, to help remember items that have slipped away, such as names, locations, and information. The exercise will also improve the working relationship between the conscious and unconscious aspects of your mind.

- ▼ You need to practice this exercise in a quiet room where you will not be disturbed by people or telephones.
- ▼ For this exercise, lie *face up* on the carpet or bed, with the shades drawn and the lights dimmed.
- ▼ Close your eyes. Wipe away all thoughts or at least pay no attention to them. Visualize that all you can see is a warm screen of velvety black.

- ▼ Now picture a square of white paper 12 inches square set about 1 foot from your eyes and in the middle of this dark black screen. Keep this image steady and clear.
- ▼ With the white square framed clearly against the dark black background, place a black circle the size of a 50-cent coin in the center of the black square.
- ▼ Focus your attention on this black circle.
- ▼ When you can clearly see all three levels of this image, erase the scene from your memory as you would wipe a chalkboard. Other images may momentarily take its place in your attention.

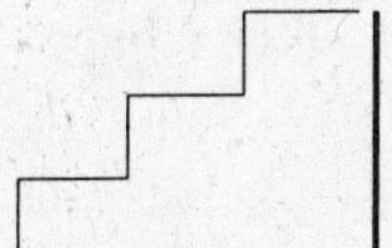

BRAIN-BUILDING SECRET #62
Brain Aerobics and Brain Breathing: 7 Exercises to Build Brain Power

It may be obvious to many that one of the best ways to build brain power is to give your body some vigorous exercise. But then maybe it isn't so apparent. Quite often I have to remind myself to leave my desk, papers, books, outlines, and writing and to shake a leg. I am not a particularly athletic person and have been called a "lazy exerciser," and I would rather read a book than climb a mountain.

But I have enough common sense (the minimum, some would say) to know that if I am stuck on a mental problem or worn out on a writing assignment, the best remedy is a brisk 20-minute walk. Once I lived on a lake, so in the summer months, I could run out of my office (I've always worked at home), trot about 50 feet across the lawn, and jump in for a 20-minute swim.

YOUR BRAIN DEMANDS 50 PERCENT OF ALL THE OXYGEN YOU INHALE

Quite often, sentences, ideas, and insights are shaken loose by this vigorous use of the rest of my body. The brain comes along for the ride and feels quite refreshed. Naturally, physical exercise improves blood and oxygen circulation, releases pleasure-producing endorphins in your brain, and helps you to relax—all of which are important for brain power.

Don't forget that even though your brain typically makes up only 2 percent of your body's weight, it requires 20 percent of your body's total intake of oxygen, and if you are a fast-growing child, it demands 50 percent of all oxygen inhaled. Vigorous exercise delivers stores of oxygen to your very demanding *oxygen-dependent* brain.

You have probably heard of "runner's high." This is the delightful mood elevation—the experience of spontaneous endorphin release in your brain—that comes as a reward for exercise. It fills you with a flush of well-being and a lovely high; endorphins, after all, are a kind of natural opiate produced by your brain. That's why exercise is a perfect antidote for depression; in a metaphorical sense, it shakes all your heavy, depressive thoughts loose and levitates them with a hit of endorphins.

SO GIVE YOUR BRAIN ALL THE OXYGEN POWER IT WANTS

Blood supply to your brain is crucial for full mental powers; medical studies show that cardiovascular problems contribute directly to a progressive decline in mental abilities in the elderly.

In fact, if you're between the ages of 33 and 61, unless you exercise regularly, your cerebral blood flow can drop by as much as 23 percent of what it was in your youth. Physical exercise stimulates your brain while physical inactivity numbs it. Sensory stimulation, physical movement, and deliberate thinking seem to produce an immediate increase in blood flow into the brain.[2]

HOW TO BREATHE WITH YOUR BRAIN AND BELLY

You breathe 20,000 times a day, but with each breath, are you sending the maximum amount of oxygen to your brain cells? Probably not.

- Stand up straight. Push your abdomen out and, placing your left hand against it, push even more, but without straining.

- Starting with your abdomen, inhale up into your chest while pushing it against your right hand. In other words, your left hand is pressed against your abdomen, your right hand against your chest.
- When you exhale, try to exhale fully.
- Repeat, slowly. Try to make your breathing rhythmic.
- When you exhale, see if you can extend the exhalation to a count of 8. Don't strain.

HOW TO SHINE YOUR SKULL

This is a brain-breathing exercise from the yoga tradition that reputedly gives your brain a "radiant brightness."

- You may do this sitting or standing.
- Purse your lips across your teeth, allowing only a small slit for air to pass through.
- Take a deep inhalation through your nose.
- Exhale strongly in short bursts so that the air squeezes through your pursed lips.
- When you have fully exhaled, breathe normally for a moment; then repeat twice.

RELAX YOUR BRAIN WITH YOUR NEXT BREATH

- Do this while standing.
- Bend your knees slightly, so they flex but do not lock into place.
- Place your feet 8 inches apart; bend your knees slightly so you feel the weight of your body resting on your feet.
- Your arms hang loosely at your sides. Keep your back straight and in alignment with your arms. Your belly can hang out; do not tense it.
- Repeat the brain-belly breathing exercise.
- Stay in this position for 2 minutes.

BUILD YOUR BRAIN WITH OTHER AEROBICS EXERCISES

These can include

- jumping rope
- playing squash
- handball
- racquetball
- swimming
- tennis
- aerobic dance or exercise
- using workout machines, such as treadmills, rowing machines, and stationary bicycles

Try to do one of these twice a week.

BUILD BRAIN POWER BY EXPANDING YOUR CAROTID ARTERIES

When the carbon dioxide content of your blood increases, the carotid arteries in your head expand to allow more blood to flow to your brain. This physiological fact is the basis for an exercise approach that gets more blood (and oxygen) circulating through your brain. Through specific exercises, you *permanently expand* the carotid arteries that feed your brain.

The idea is to use carbon dioxide enrichment to literally expand your brain's capillary (small blood vessel) blood flow. This, in turn, stimulates the *physical basis* of your brain power, namely, the supply of oxygen to the fine blood vessels in your brain. If you do this in a concentrated period of 1 hour daily for 3 weeks, your carotid arteries are more likely to stay expanded, supplying more oxygen than ever to your brain.

An added benefit to this approach is that with permanently broader carotid arteries, more toxins can be removed from your brain. **Caution**: If you have cerebrovascular problems or have had a stroke, do not do this exercise.

HOW TO BREATHE INTO A PAPER BAG AND DETOXIFY YOUR BRAIN

- Take a small paper grocery bag.
- Secure it around your nose and mouth by holding it in place with your hands. Inhale then exhale into the bag.
- For the next 30 seconds, rebreathe your exhaled air, which will be mostly carbon dioxide.
- Repeat this once every half hour for several hours. You may wish to have someone attending you.

BUILD BETTER CAROTIDS BY BREATHING UNDERWATER

While swimming, hold your breath and swim underwater for as long as you *comfortably* can. Try to increase the amount of time you can hold your breath underwater every day for a month.

Dr. Win Wenger, who practiced this exercise faithfully for long periods of time, increasing his underwater time to 4 1/2 minutes, recommends trying it for up to 1 hour every day for a 3-week intensive period.

That means practicing held-breath underwater swimming in comfortable segments (30–60 seconds, perhaps) that total 60 minutes. "An hour's total time under water, 2–3 minutes at a time, per day, over 2-3 intensive weeks, should add an eventual 5–10 I.Q. points to your intelligence and an immense increase to the richness and span of your awareness," Dr. Wenger claims.

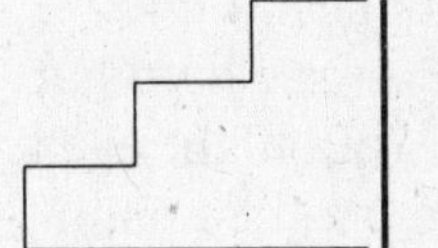

THE ANATOMY OF BRAIN POWER #10
Proof That Exercise Builds a Smarter Brain

Consider these examples that show the powerful brain-building effects of physical exercise, especially aerobics or any kind of stimulating movement that increases oxygen flow to the brain.

▼ *Jog to think clearly*. A number of men and women age 60 and older all suffered from cardiovascular disease. During a trial program, they either walked or jogged 6–10 miles a day for 26 days; they also had a health-promoting special diet during this time.

At the end of the month, they were tested: All of them scored higher on IQ as well as in certain key "psychological inventories" such as being able to think clearly, express themselves fluently, think efficiently, and perceive more details. Not only did the combination of exercise and careful diet improve their circulation, but it clearly improved their mental abilities, in only a matter of weeks.

▼ *Calisthenics builds intelligence*. In another example, 32 people took a series of tests for mental function and personality. Then they started a 10-week program of running, physical recreation, and calisthenics, and took the same tests again. All of them showed big gains in intelligence, performance speed, ease of learning, and general brain function, plus reduced levels of anxiety and depression—as a result of the exercise program.

▼ *Running lowers anxiety*. Even exercising twice a week can be enough to get the nerve endings stimulated and your synapses limber. Men who ran twice a week *regularly* showed 14–27 percent lower scores on tests that evaluated them for anxiety, hostility, and depression. It was not the number of miles run that made the difference, but the regularity of the running.

Incidentally, if you have an important mental test or task looming on the horizon, such as writing a book or taking the college boards or a law exam, you can taper your exercise program, doing progressively *shorter* workouts beginning 2–3 weeks before the big brain power demand. Exercise hard but not long, and quit before you're exhausted. You might even quit your exercise program 2 days before the brain demand.

- *Stay active to remember better*. A group of 48 women over age 65 were divided into two groups. One group comprised active women who had an exercise program three times weekly; the second group self-rated itself as sedentary. Both groups were tested on their ability to estimate the speed of a sequence of flashing lights.

The women who were physically active fared much better and were able to remember previous light sequences after 10 minutes; their ability to recall these details continued to be much stronger than the inactive women after 1 week and even after 40 days.

CONCLUSION: EXERCISE TO PROCESS INFORMATION MORE EFFICIENTLY

The conclusion: If you are sedentary, you may be able to remember items but at a much slower rate than if you are physically active. The more you exercise, the more you increase your speed of reasoning and recall and the faster will be your response time, regardless of age. In other words, exercise clearly increases your brain's *ability*, *efficiency*, and *speed* to process information and perform mental calculations.

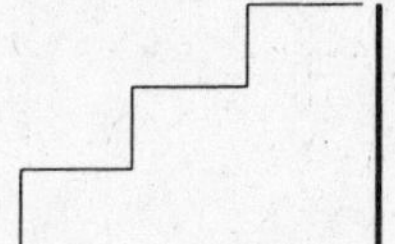

BRAIN-BUILDING SECRET #63
4 Dynamic Ways to Cleanse Your Brain by Breathing—Plus a Turtle

This exercise comes from another aspect of the Chinese tradition called Taoism. Taoism, which includes a complete philosophical model of the world, emphasizes longevity and thorough well-being through a series of body-mind techniques.

Brain-cleansing breathing is a basic technique from this tradition that enables you to breathe away stress from your mind. You learn how to empty your mind of useless, negative thoughts and to bring it into a state of balance. If you have troubles with your neck or are seeing a chiropractor regularly, *do not* do this exercise without professional approval.

HOW TO PRACTICE BRAIN-CLEANSING BREATHING

- ▼ Ideally, this exercise is performed while sitting cross-legged on the floor, with your knees close to or touching the floor.
- ▼ Many people are unable to do this without a long period of training, so you may also do this seated comfortably in a chair with your feet placed flat on the floor about 12 inches apart.

▼ Make sure your back is straight but not strained. Rest your hands lightly on your knees, clasping your thumbs securely in the midst of the fingers of each hand. (See Figure 1.)

FIRST YOU DO THE TURTLE TO STRETCH YOUR NECK

This is a preparatory exercise traditionally called the turtle to get you ready for brain cleansing. The turtle will stretch all the muscles of your neck and stimulate the thyroid and parathyroid glands and essentially all the nerves comprising the central nervous system that pass through this region. You start with the posture just described.

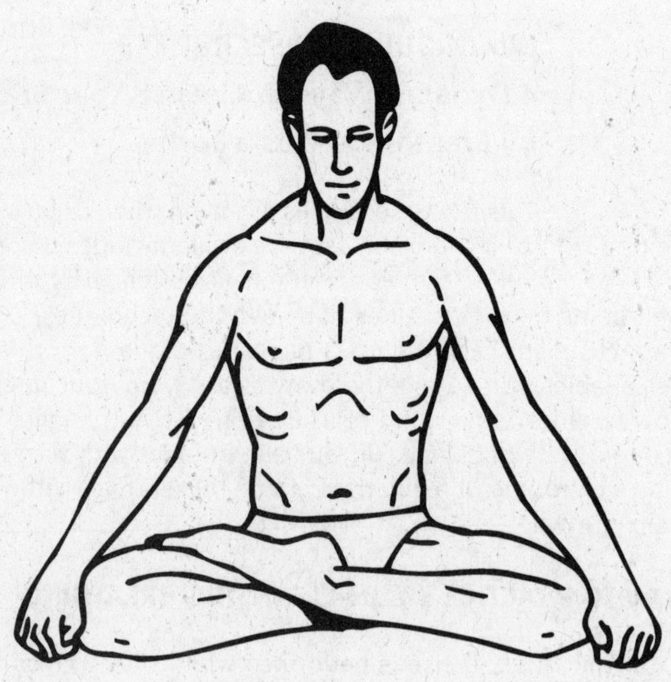

Figure 1

- You may either close your eyes or look straight ahead into muted, not bright, light.
- Put all your attention on your movements; think of nothing else. Keep your fingers clasped around your thumbs in a fist. This keeps all the qi within your body and in circulation.
- Slowly move your chin down into your chest while stretching the top of your head upward.
- Relax your shoulders downward. As you stretch your head upward, inhale. (See Figure 2.)

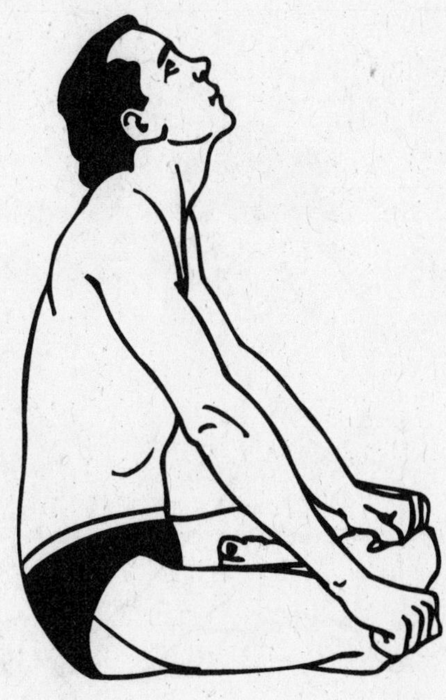

Figure 2

- ▼ Now reverse this movement. Slowly move the back of your head down to your shoulders, so that your chin comes up, stretching your throat and your shoulders upwards.
- ▼ As you bring your head down and chin up, exhale. Do not strain or force any movement. (See Figures 3 and 4.)
- ▼ Practice the turtle 12 times.

It may take a while before you feel comfortable with these unusual movements. When you get the exercise right, you will most likely feel a lessening of tension or fatigue in your neck. These two movements actually mimic the turtle, in whose honor the exercise was originally named, as it extends its flexible head and neck from out of its protective shell.

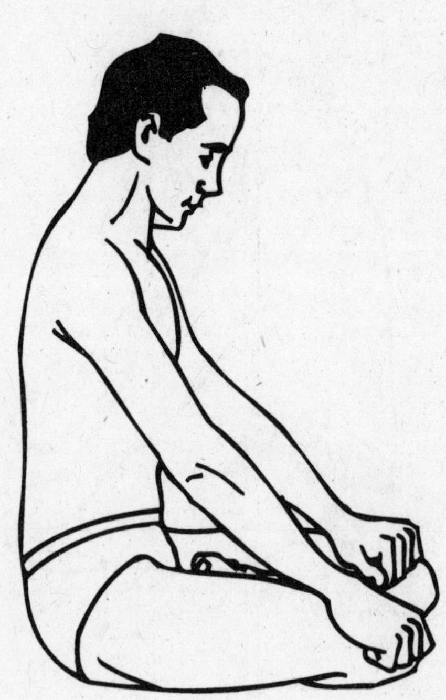

Figure 3

NOW THE TURTLE CLEANSES ITS BRAIN BY BREATHING

Now move your head into the second turtle position with your head titled backward, your chin up.

- Slowly, without straining, inhale. As you do this exercise, gently tighten your anal muscles. This is called a *bandha*, or lock, in classical yoga and is a way of keeping all the energy, or qi, within your system and intensifying the experience of the exercise.
- Imagine that as you inhale, the breath is like a boiling steam or misty fire or white smoke that slowly rises up from your abdomen through your inner organs and chest cavity to your head.
- This fire fills your head with white. Imagine that you cannot see anything, think, or even imagine, other than being aware of this white smoke in your head.
- Do this visualization as you inhale.
- When you have finished your slow inhale, then slowly, gently straighten your head and neck so that you are looking straight ahead again.

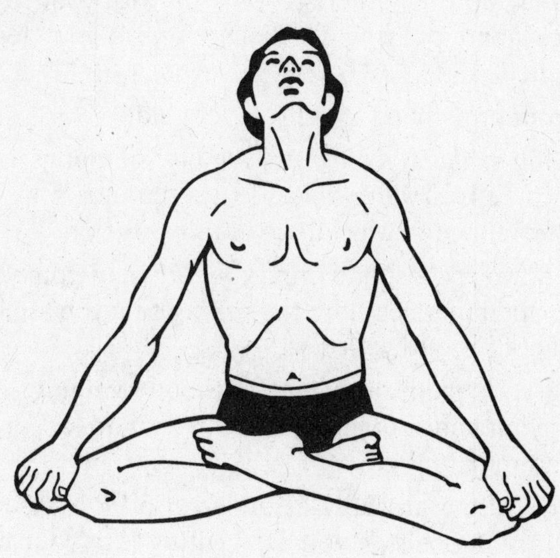

Figure 4

- Exhale all the white smoke from out of your head and body as if you are a fire-breathing dragon blowing out steam in slow motion.
- Feel your head as being empty. Visualize that the white smoke you are exhaling carries with it all your tensions, negative thoughts, worries, bad habits, and tendencies to be angry or irritable or anxious.
- Imagine, too, that as your head empties of these qualities, their place is filled with a clear, bright-blue sky that has no room for anything other than its fresh clarity.
- Visualizing the color blue in your head helps to cleanse and purify your mind.
- Repeat this fire-breathing exercise six more times, which is to say, for another six inhale/exhale cycles.

STAND AND CLEANSE! YOUR BRAIN WILL THINK BETTER

This is a variation or supplement to the exercise just described.

- You may do this either standing up with your legs about 18 inches apart or lying on the floor with your legs similarly extended.
- Let your arms hang loosely at your side.
- Do a full exhale to completely empty your lungs. Gently move your head backwards toward your shoulders (as you did in the turtle) and slowly inhale in this position.
- Expand your chest and bring your arms up from your body so that your fingers point to the ceiling or, if you are lying prone, to a spot beyond your head.
- Bring your palms together, without straining. If you can't bring your hands together, raise your hands as far as they will go and remain there.
- As your arms are fully extended over your head, visualize that in this position you are inviting into your body all the *yang* energy (active, sunny, warm, masculine, daytime, energizing) from the universe into your lungs, inner organs, and brain.

- You may visualize this as a bright white smoke, as you did in the previous exercise.
- When you have fully inhaled, hold your breath, with your mouth closed, lock your anal muscles again, and keep your arms in a raised position.
- Hold this pose, without straining, for as long as you can, for perhaps 10–15 seconds.
- Visualize that the white smoke is penetrating every cell and neuron of your body. You are unable to be aware of anything other than this all-enveloping white smoke inside you.
- As before, know that it is cleansing and purifying the contents of your mind.
- Now slowly exhale. Bring your head gently forward, separate your hands, move your arms slowly down to your sides again.
- But as you slowly move your arms down, visualize that all the *yin* energy (passive, watery, nighttime, cool, damp, moist, feminine) from the Earth comes up into your body through your fingers.
- As you exhale, imagine that all the white smoke inside you comes out and is replaced by the beautiful clear blue empty sky inside your head.
- Repeat the exercise six times or until you feel like quitting.

DRAIN YOUR BRAIN WITH A SHOULDERSTAND

This is an exercise from classical hatha yoga that will stimulate your brain, get a great deal more blood and oxygen into your neurons, and limber up your back and neck. In fact, this *asana* (or yoga posture) will invigorate your entire body and all its systems, as its name in Sanskrit, *sarvangasana*, meaning "all parts pose," clearly outlines.

The shoulderstand pose, like the turtle, will stimulate your thyroid and parathyroid glands as your chin presses into your chest. As with the two previous exercises, do not do this exercise if you have any neck problems without getting the approval of a chiropractor.

- Lie comfortably on your back on the floor, your feet spread about 12 inches apart, your arms resting loosely at your side, your hands palm down on the floor.
- Make sure you are wearing loose-fitting clothes such as a track suit, bathing suit, even pajamas. Also make sure the floor space behind you is clear for 5 feet.
- As you inhale, push down on your palms as you raise both legs in parallel fashion straight up above you. (See Figure 5.)

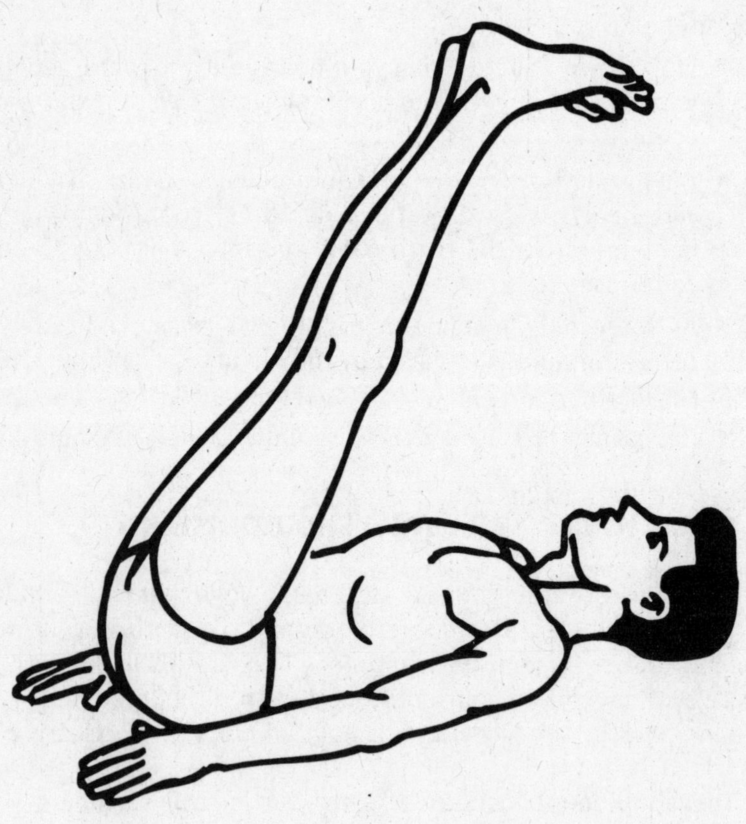

Figure 5

- ▼ Still inhaling, lift your hips off the floor as you roll your legs up and over beyond your head so that they are at a 45-degree angle to your torso on the floor. (See Figure 6.)
- ▼ As you start to exhale, move your arms up to support your hips, keeping your arms as close to your shoulders as possible.

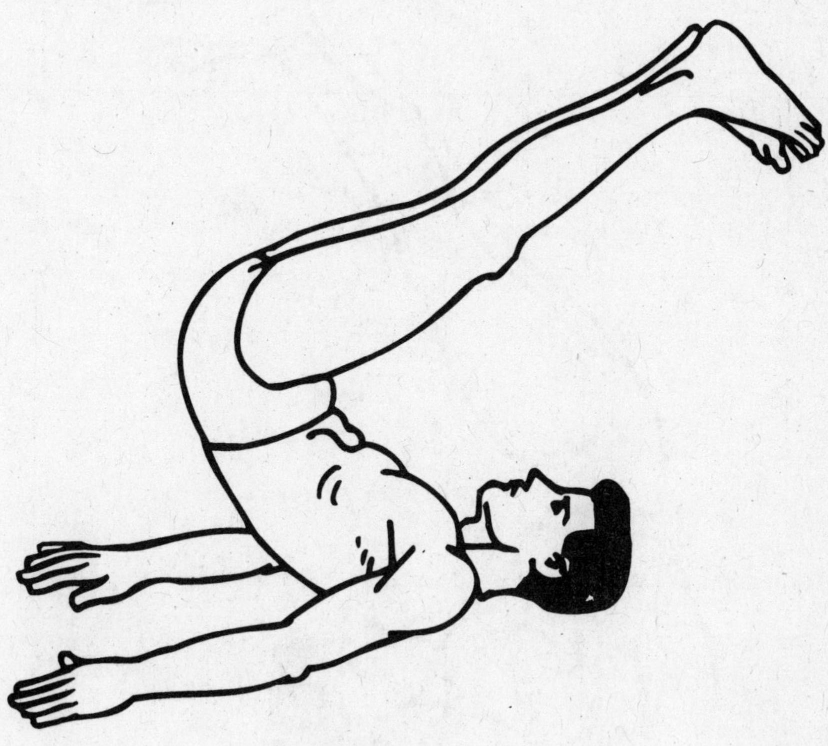

Figure 6

- ▼ Gently push your back up, lifting your legs so that your legs and feet point straight up to the ceiling. (See Figure 7.)
- ▼ Straighten your spine and slightly arch your back. Use your arms, with your elbows and upper arms resting flat on the floor, to support your body.
- ▼ Press your chin firmly against your chest, but do not strain.
- ▼ Breathe slowly and deeply while maintaining this pose.

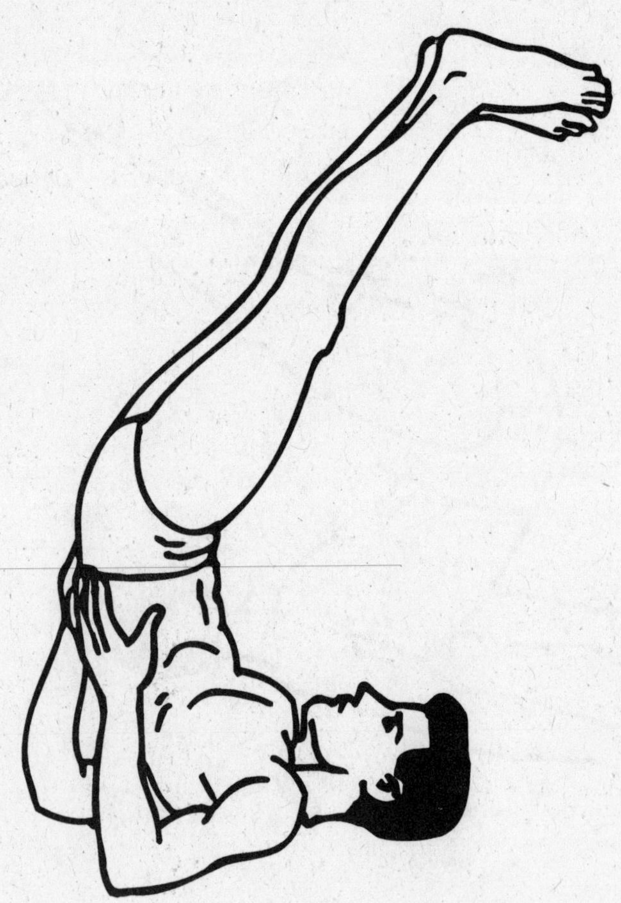

Figure 7

▼ Keep your feet relaxed. Hold this position for 10–30 seconds, or longer, depending on your comfort. (See Figure 8.)

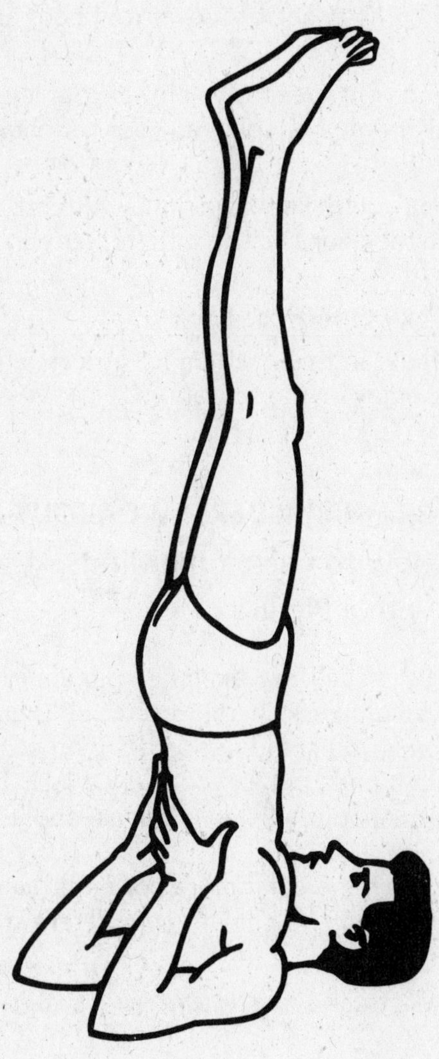

Figure 8

- To come out of the pose, slowly, gently lower your legs to that 45-degree angle over your body.
- Place your hands on the floor again, palms down.
- Slowly roll your back down onto the floor and bring your legs, keeping them together, back over your body and slowly down to the floor.
- Do not bend your knees as you lower your legs. You may hear a few pops from your spine as your vertebrae adjust themselves.
- Try to unroll your spine, vertebra by vertebra, as you let your back touch the floor, starting with the vertebra closest to your shoulders.
- Let your ankles touch the floor.
- Relax. Remain in this position for at least a minute, quietly breathing, enjoying the sensation.

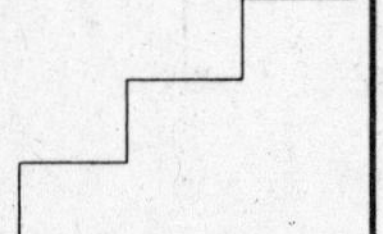

BRAIN BUILDERS! WORKOUT #35
How to Calm Your Mind with a Picture

By visualizing an inner picture, you will gain a condition of inner calmness in this exercise. There are different kinds of inner images you could use to bring on calmness, such as a walk in nature, in a park, in the woods, by a lake, to an art museum, or any setting that predictably brings about calmness and relaxation in you.

Remember, your mind is far more powerful than you ordinarily give it credit for being able to conjure up different states of mind at will.

- You are standing on a beautiful beach under the summery sun.
- You walk along the water's edge, listening to the sounds of sea birds and the lap of waves. The sand is warm under your feet, and you feel the delicate grains of sand trickling through your toes with every step.

- The blue sky above is outrageously pure and open; you can almost see the stars in the daytime behind the blue veil of space.
- The breeze blows lightly against your skin, ruffling your hair. It blows away your cares, worries, frustrations, doubts, and discomfort.
- You are marvelously composed and unshakeably present in the moment. Seagulls take up your concerns and fly off with them, dumping them in the deep ocean.
- The sun sparkles so brightly on the water that you need to blink and squint to keep your eyes from being dazzled. You sense what perfection feels like.
- Once you can feel the sense of beauty and peace of this inner image, you can summon it back virtually whenever you need it, without even going through all its steps.

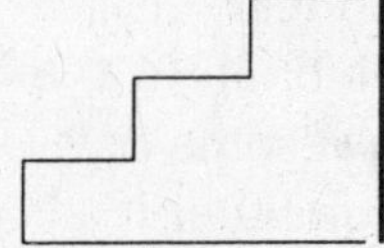

THE ANATOMY OF BRAIN POWER #11
Is Your Body Nothing More Than Your Brain's Humble Porter?

The inspiration for this perhaps odd rumination is a quotation from the preeminent American inventor, Thomas Alva Edison. "The chief function of your body is to carry your brain around," he once said. I wonder if he meant this in jest or in seriousness, for he was after all a man whose brain changed the technological face of the twentieth century.

SUPERINTELLIGENCE ON *STAR TREK*—TOO BIG FOR ONE BRAIN

You find this attitude increasingly in the way life goes on in the late twentieth century, and you find it prominent as well in a certain attitude that surrounds the subject of brain power itself. There are many books on developing brain power; I've looked at most of them and occasionally they irritate me.

Before I explain why, allow me to digress—entertainingly, I hope—to describe an episode from *Star Trek: The Next Generation* that is especially relevant to brain power.

The episode concerns the sudden transformation of a meek junior officer—not a man of superior brain power, articulation, or self-confidence—into a superbrain, a man who becomes all brain, surpassing even the ship's massive computer in intelligence and instantaneous computing ability. At the beginning of the episode, he stumbles through his lines in a minor drama performed for the ship's officers. Then an electrical shortage leaves him unharmed but oddly changed.

Suddenly, without thinking about it, he is able to figure out complex problems, even to suggest unique and successful solutions to vexing technical problems on board the *Enterprise*.

THE MAN WHO IS ALL BRAIN MEETS SOMEONE BRAINIER

Then, as usually happens in *Star Trek*, a disaster suddenly strikes and nobody can figure it out, except him. He wires his brain to the ship's computer and becomes a living interface to the awesome computing powers of this intelligence machine. Soon the computer itself and thus the ship depend on him for a way out of the disaster. Nobody on board particularly likes this unique form of mutiny and hijacking and try to unplug his brain from the computer. The story ends with an unexpected twist.

A far superior intelligence from another sector of the galaxy has manipulated the whole affair. This intelligence is literally all brain, all awareness, mind, or consciousness. It is exceedingly curious about the rest of the universe but is unable or too lazy to travel to find out; so it brings the universe to itself for friendly conversation.

Once the *Enterprise* arrives in this being's sector, they all "sit down" for a lively chat about life, the universe, and everything—and the junior officer returns to being a mediocre intellect. That's too bad, because he's tasted the elixir of unlimited intelligence, an IQ far beyond his mortal imaginings. He's momentarily experienced a feeling of total brain power, of brain power of the stature of the creator itself, so he thinks.

THERE'S MORE TO IQ THAN OUTSMARTING THE COMPUTER

The moral of the episode is that he is still a man, a human being, with a personality, a biography, feelings, and desires—yet it is this remaining part of himself that must carry the great intellect generated by the computer. His brain power may be great, but his wisdom is no match. He is all brain, but the driver is ill equipped to handle this awesome vehicle.

And behind it all is yet a greater mind pulling all the strings or, should we say, manipulating the computer chips. This manipulator is also all brain; it literally has no body but is all mind. Its intentions are good and friendly if a bit odd.

The reason I bring this up is that I do not agree with Edison's remark and I hope he made it in jest, because otherwise it can seriously mislead us all into believing that the brain is all, IQ is the goal, and brain power is simply the ability to outcompute the computer. It is indeed a seductive prospect: unlimited brain power.

After all, the possibility is at least theoretically "wired" into the structure of your brain itself. I'm talking about the estimated 1 trillion neurons in your brain. Until a few years ago, science's best bet as to how many possible connections these neurons could form was 1 followed by 800 zeros.

WHAT IS THE LARGEST NUMBER YOU CAN COMPUTE?

But in the 1970s, a Russian brain scientist upped the ante, gigantically, with a revised estimate. Dr. Pyotr Anokhin of Moscow University said that if you want to describe the brain's "ultimate" information-processing ability, you need a vastly larger number. Such a number is a map of your brain's ability to make new patterns and connections, which is the same as learning, storage, and IQ.

This number is so large, Dr. Anokhin declared, that to write it out in longhand you would need a line of numbers 10.5 *million kilometers long*. "With such a number of possibilities, the brain is a keyboard on which hundreds of millions of different melodies—acts of behavior or intelligence—can be played," he wrote. "No man yet exists or has existed who has even approached using his full brain." This of course is the idea behind the intriguing *Star Trek* episode of the man with the unlimited brain—on loan.

It is a highly seductive prospect. Unlimited brain power, to some, is surely the ultimate high, aphrodisiac, and goal of living. Yet your body—that is to say, the rest of your humanness—is not merely the humble porter to the great brain on your shoulders. If you think this way, you will surely run into serious trouble with the rest of your life. Brain power is good, but wisdom is even better.

YOUR SUPERBUILT BRAIN IN SERVICE OF THE WHOLE PERSON

Might I suggest that you always remember that brain power has its rightful place in your life, but only as an aspect of something greater—your wholeness. Superior intelligence does distinguish human beings from the animal kingdom, but there is something even more distinctive about our lot: it is the wisdom to use our considerable brain power appropriately.

This book is full of techniques for boosting your brain power and to avoid the effects that aging tends to have on our mental abilities. So, please, let us all pursue the highly desirable IQ points, adding more to our store, but let's do this in service to the *whole* of our life and the *whole* of ourselves.

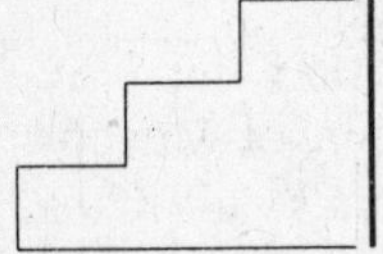

BRAIN-BUILDING SECRET #64
Qigong Can Boost Your Energy and Promote Intelligence

Traditional Chinese culture offers us yet another way to enhance intelligence and boost brain power. It's called qigong (pronounced *chee-gung*) and means "mastery of qi," which is your body's vital force and energy. Qigong is a series of exercises and movements that coordinate your natural qi and how you hold and move your physical frame.

It is a complex martial art that requires a skilled instructor to teach a student the full range of techniques. Yet there are simple, beginning exercises that you can master from reading about them in a book and without a live teacher.

But, first, let's consider a little of qigong's reputed benefits. Chinese masters in this ancient martial arts form explain that if you want health and longevity, you must achieve coordination and balance of your body, qi, and spirit. That qigong can deliver these benefits is made clear by the exceptional abilities long-time practitioners report.[3]

- They can learn how voluntarily to raise or lower their blood pressure.
- They can generate skin temperature changes in their palms by almost 4°C after only 15–20 minutes of practice.
- After three months, students can often show a dramatic increase in the "vital capacity," which is a measure of the largest breath your lungs can handle
- Athletes improve their running scores by 30 percent
- Qigong helps to stabilize the cardiovascular system at a healthier level of functioning.
- It improves the body's ability to metabolize oxygen.
- Qigong practice changes the dominant brain wave pattern from beta to alpha, which is the state of relaxation and inner focus.
- Qigong promotes relaxation, reduces anxiety, and heightens concentration, mental power focus, and clarity of mind.
- Schoolchildren benefit from including improvements in appetite, sleep, and attention span.
- Children are less restless, less distractable, and less prone to being hyperactive.
- Ability to do math calculations and to memorize information improves.

The following is a simple, easy, but effective qigong exercise that helps circulate your qi and rid your lungs of stagnant air. It's preferable to do this first thing in the morning.

HOW TO PRACTICE RISING EAGLE QIGONG EXERCISE

- Stand up straight with your legs about 18 inches apart.

- Keep your head and torso erect; allow your hips to gently slide forward; bend your knees slightly so that you feel your body weight distributed equally over both feet.
- Relax your shoulders and let your arms hang loosely at your sides with your fingers loosely extended.
- Breathe through your nose with your mouth closed.
- As you inhale, expand your lower abdomen, and as you exhale, contract the lower abdomen.
- Place your attention on a spot a little below your belly button, as if your center of awareness is positioned there.
- Keep this focus there as you move through the rest of this exercise.
- As you breathe in, let your wrists float slowly up to chest level, as if you are slowly raising them over your head.
- Stop when they reach chest level. Your elbows will be loosely bent, and your forearms will seem to dangle out in front of your chest.

YOUR WRISTS ARE HELD ALOFT BY INVISIBLE STRINGS

- Pretend there is a delicate string holding each wrist in place.
- As you begin to exhale, let your hands move forward until your arms are almost fully extended out in front of you, parallel to the floor and perpendicular to your body.
- Move very slowly, as if the air is as thick as water. Don't strain. Accomplish each movement with a minimum of effort.
- Now inhale again, slowly, and let your arms and hands float up over your head, again with the sensation that a delicate string is lifting them up.
- Exhale, let more of your body weight sink into your knees, as your arms float down to your sides again, extended at shoulder level out from the left and right sides of your body.
- Keep your knees bent, move your hands across your legs, so your right hand rests on your left thigh and your left hand rests on your right thigh.

- Your knees are bent to the degree you are starting to enter into a standing crouch.
- Let your hands swing apart again, while keeping your knees bent as in the previous step. Inhale.
- Allow your hands to swing apart and float palm up to chest level again, this time extended out to the left and right. Keep your knees bent.
- Reverse your hands so your palms face the floor.
- On the exhale, straighten up your posture so you are standing straight again.
- At the same time, push your arms down, as if by doing this it enables you to unbend your knees and straighten your back.
- Repeat the entire exercise 9 times.
- After you have done this exercise 10 times, remain in the standing position and notice your body's sensation of energized relaxation.

WATCH THE QI FILL THE BOTTLE OF YOUR BODY WITH ENERGY

- Your body may feel both transparent and full; or perhaps your fingers are tingling and your hands feel slightly swollen. This is evidence of qi filling your body much the way a mist fills a bottle.
- Visualize this qi mist as full of light, seeping into all your bones, organs, and tissues.
- For the next three swallows of saliva, visualize that this saliva travels all the way down your body to the point below your belly button, filling it with warmth and light.
- From here, this point of radiance spreads throughout your entire body like an ink stain on paper.

THE 8 BENEFITS TO PRACTICING RISING EAGLE QIGONG

Qigong teachers tell us that there are at least 8 benefits to expect from regular qigong practice. Remember of course that Rising

Eagle is only one (and a beginning exercise) of many dozens of qigong exercises.

Among the normal beneficial reactions to this enhanced circulation of qi through your system expect to have

- improved mental clarity
- much more saliva
- better sleep
- warm sensations in different body areas
- better digestion
- stronger appetite
- stronger body metabolism leading to faster growth of nails and hair
- a sense of mental and physical relaxation coupled with a feeling of harmony and ease

2 STORIES OF PEOPLE FOR WHOM QIGONG MADE A BIG DIFFERENCE

Peng Wenzhang was a 53-year-old man working as an official in a government office in China. His job required him to keep the minutes of important meetings, but he found himself unable to remember the names of the officials present; he had difficulties reading documents, he didn't sleep well, and he had poor control over his temper. Then he started practicing qigong.

His eating and sleeping patterns improved, and his memory function returned to normal. Not only was he now able to fulfill his secretarial function at meetings, he even started to write articles. A previous condition of puffiness disappeared and his walk became brisk and healthy.

Another man, age 64, a professor at Beijing Industrial College, had suffered from hypertension for 11 years, such that his blood pressure once reached 200/120 mm HG. After practicing qigong for only 2 months, his blood pressure dropped to 140/70 and stabilized at that level; he took no other medicine for his hypertension during this time.

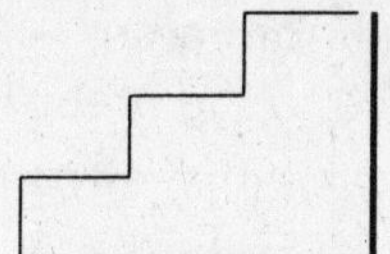

BRAIN BUILDERS! WORKOUT #36
Affirm Your Ability to Learn—Over and Over

Practice this in a relaxed, calm state of mind, with your eyes still closed. Making affirmations of your learning potential are especially effective when you are in this state of mellow relaxation.

There are numerous phrases you can choose from; the key is to select one whose positive tone matches your own sense of what's possible or that helps lift you up into that belief.

Repeat any (or all) of these affirmations silently 4–6 times. Concentrate on its meaning and sign your name to it with each repetition—in other words, *believe* what you say.

Try to recite them with a sense of rhythm, even bounce.[4]

- I can do it.
- Now I am achieving my goals.
- Learning is something I enjoy a great deal.
- Learning and remembering are easy for me.
- My mind works effectively and efficiently.
- I am supremely calm and confident.
- My memory is alert, my mind is powerful.
- I remember all I need to know as I need it.

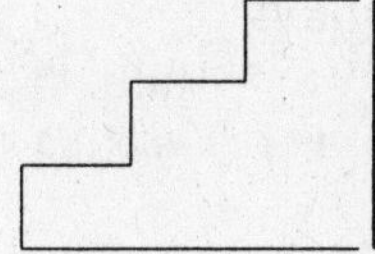

BRAIN-BUILDING SECRET #65
Why the Sufis Twirl and the Brain Benefits of Spinning

If you have ever seen a whirling dervish, or *Maulawiyah*, in action, you will have seen a person twirling rapidly for a long time, somehow miraculously without getting dizzy yet with complete concentration. Sometimes they spin several hundreds of times before stopping.

While this is a devotional act within the Sufi tradition (an esoteric aspect of the Moslem faith), it has distinct benefits to the brain. Children, of course, do it all the time, spontaneously, as part of their playing, spinning in circles, making cartwheels and somersaults, even rolling down hills.

HOW SPINNING AROUND MAKES YOUR NEURONS HAPPY

Physical movement, especially spinning or twirling, can "supercharge" your neurons; motion itself acts as a kind of brain nutrient.[5] Among other things, repetitive motion, such as spinning, has these benefits:

- ▼ stimulates the fluids and the millions of nerve endings in your inner ear, part of the vestibular system
- ▼ sends electrical impulses into the brain, stimulating parts of the limbic system known to be associated with both pleasure and learning
- ▼ "exercises" your brain by stimulating overall neural activity
- ▼ directly facilitates learning
- ▼ directly hikes your IQ up by as many as 30 points
- ▼ downshifts your brain waves to a state of pleasure and rest
- ▼ beneficially stimulates all body fluids, including lymph
- ▼ gives your organs and tissues an internal water-based massage

Twirling is a kind of brain-building exercise not unlike body building in its results. Spinning may even stimulate your neurons to "grow" more dendritic connections, which increases the already complex neuronal network and thus the physical basis for higher IQ.[6]

Our brain-building secret with respect to motion and learning is this: P*ractice this twirling exercise at least once a day, ideally before beginning a learning or study session*.

HOW TO TWIRL FOR BETTER BRAIN POWER

- ▼ Stand up straight with your legs about 18 inches apart.
- ▼ Extend your arms straight out from your body so they are parallel with the floor.

- Focus your vision on a point straight ahead of you at about eye level.
- Now start slowly spinning around from left to right, moving your entire body.
- Try to keep your feet in approximately the same place. Keep your eyes focused on that single point each time you come around.
- Spin around 6 times, then stop. You will probably be dizzy. Over the next several weeks, try to work your way up to being able to spin 21 times comfortably, without feeling dizzy.
- Say you are a student, professor, or executive preparing for an important exam or presentation. Consider practicing this twirling exercise an hour before the crucial brain power test.[7]

6 SOUND YOUR BRAIN

▼▼▼▼▼▼▼▼▼▼▼▼▼▼▼▼▼▼

How Music, Sounds, and Frequencies Can Boost Brain Power

Sound your brain. Did you know that music, sounds, even electronic frequencies are food for your brain? Your brain emits a spectrum of energies, or frequencies, called brain waves, and these change according to your activity. Feed your brain nourishing sound waves and watch your brain power grow.

In the brain-building secrets in this chapter, you will learn about the surprising relationship between certain kinds of music, specific sounds, and exact sound frequencies and how your brain works. *Sound your brain* means there is another kind of brain food besides smart nutrients, herbs, and vitamins. In this chapter, you'll learn how to use your ears and listening ability to master the *ear force* to give your brain the sound food it needs for *brain force*.

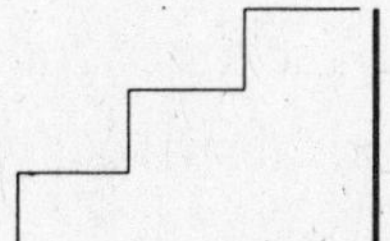

BRAIN-BUILDING SECRET #66
It Pays to Listen Well If You Want to Remember Well

When it comes to memory, print is not the only medium from which we take in information. Hearing, listening, the ears—these are major players in the information game. But according to brain power experts, on a scale of 100, the average listening ability for any of us is only 55. About 85 percent of people who take this test score average or less. There are various reasons why we do not hear well: distractions, boredom, immediate forgetting of what was heard, indistinct sounds.

Bear in mind that you probably spend 45 percent of your day listening to people, unless you are a writer and you spend 95 percent of your time listening to yourself and 5 percent listening to editors. If you are a student, epecially in elementary and high school, you probably spend a dismaying 60–70 percent of your time listening to teachers. The best approach under these circumstances is to develop new ways to hear, because you know they'll never let you run out of the room.

A QUIZ TO SEE HOW WELL YOU LISTEN

Here is a simple quiz to give you an immediate idea of where your skills fall in this spectrum of listening habits.[1] Choose one of these five possible answers for each question; then add up your score. Rating: Almost always = 2, usually = 4, sometimes = 6, seldom = 8, almost never = 10. Do you . . .

- Brand the subject uninteresting?
- Immediately find fault with the speaker's style?
- Find yourself overstimulated by a particular comment?
- Listen mostly for facts?
- Try to outline the contents as soon as you hear them?
- Pretend to be interested in the speaker?
- Allow yourself to respond to distractions around you or in your mind?
- Avoid or ignore difficult material as you hear it?
- Allow yourself to get riled by words with emotional sparks in them that upset and antagonize you personally?
- Wander off into daydreams in the middle of the speaker's sentences?

20 STEPS FOR BETTER HEARING AND MORE BRAIN POWER

As a remedy for the unimpressive score that most of us have, here are 20 steps for better listening.[2]

1. *Maintain aural health.* Make sure your ears are technically in order, not plugged with wax or biologically damaged.
2. *Train your ears.* Practice listening thoroughly to all the sounds in your environment while focusing on those most important to you.
3. *Maintain general physical health.* A healthy body makes for a healthy mind, so keep your general level of fitness high, through exercise and good nutrition, and your hearing will be correspondingly finer.
4. *Listen opportunistically.* This is like saying, Look under every stone, no matter how boring it is, in case there is a jewel amid the soil. See if there is something you might learn or benefit from, even a single sentence.
5. *Listen longer.* Don't pass judgment on the value of the speaker's message until it's finished and you understand it. When you have the picture, try to make an impartial assessment.
6. *Listen with optimism.* This means setting yourself up for a possible benefit from investing your time in listening. If you believe in advance that you may possibly gain from this interaction, it makes it more possible that something will be said to make this happen.
7. *Challenge your brain.* Expose yourself whenever possible to material that is more challenging than you are accustomed to, such as listening to an academic talk about Foucaultian deconstructionism.
8. *Listen with awareness.* Make your listening skills the state of the art, as important as any other brain power function. Be as awake as you can during the act of listening; remind yourself you are listening; don't fake it.
9. *Use all your senses.* This is called synesthesia and means to use your sight, sense of smell, bodily awareness, even touch in conjunction with your hearing during a listening situation.
10. *Keep your mind open.* Don't flinch when you hear words or concepts that trigger your emotions. Try to understand why the speaker is using them.

11. *Use brainspeed.* Did you know your brain can process information about five times faster than the speed of speech? This means keep the "staff upstairs" busy studying the speaker's body language, anticipating, organizing, and comparing the material as it comes to you. Pick a slow speaker to work with first to perfect this on-the-job analytical ability.
12. *Evaluate the content, not the delivery.* In this case, the medium is not the message—the message is. The speaker may have shortcomings as a presenter, but it is the information being presented that counts.
13. *Keen your ears for ideas.* This is like brain food. Try to grab whole ideas and themes from the speaker's river of words; link the facts to the larger picture and you will remember both.
14. *Make mind maps.* This is a different way of note taking based on the structure of the thinking process itself, involving both brain hemispheres.
15. *Ignore distractions.* This is like the dog chasing the bone when it should be sitting still. Keep your focus steady on the person speaking.
16. *Take frequent breaks.* Every 30–60 minutes take a break from the subject; your brain needs the time for integration, and the speaker, one hopes, needs a few minutes to water his throat.
17. *Imagination permitted.* Although it may seem only your left brain is involved in listening, actually your whole brain is at work. Try to develop—or not to interfere with the spontaneous formation of—mental images of the information you are receiving.
18. *Hunt with your ears.* Ever notice with what undivided attention a cat stalks a bird or mouse or a dog cocks his ears to the wind? Bring this intensity of mental poise to your listening.
19. *It gets better when you practice.* Your listening skills can improve noticeably the more you practice and the more you believe it is possible for you to be a skilled listener.
20. *Hone your own talk.* Practice your communication skills to see how the other half lives in a typical conversation.

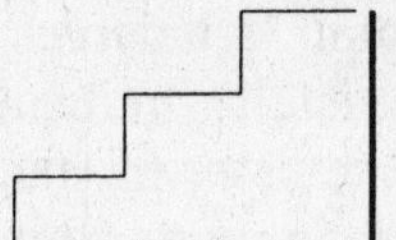

BRAIN-BUILDING SECRET #67

The AntiFrantic Hour—Take a Daily Sound Bath for Maximum Brain Relaxation

There is little argument that one of the prices you pay for the comforts, affluence, and technological amenities of American culture is a high level of stress. The sources of stress are innumerable: career, family, income, urban environments, health problems, commuting, work obligations. As you have learned already, stress is bad for your health and brain power.

REMOVING THE STRESS FROM YOUR LIFE WITH MUSIC

One of the reasons for this debilitating effect is that stress weakens your body's immune system, depressing its activities and leaving you more vulnerable to infections, colds, and other contagious illnesses.

Stress actually destroys brain cells and causes the brain itself to age, even atrophy, and to decline in vitality and efficiency, according to the latest brain research. Bearing in mind that brain scientists believe you have a fixed number of brain cells whose population steadily declines as you age, when too many brain cells die, your ability to concentrate, call up memories, compute, and learn new information is impaired.

Most of us have probably experienced the temporary decline in brain power that occurs when we must work under pressure for long periods or without enough sleep, food, or relaxation. While you cannot eliminate all stress from your life—in fact, psychologists suggest a small amount of stress is healthy for the nervous system—you can take steps to minimize its effect and its tendency to drain off your brain power.

Our brain-building secret is this: *You can use music to keep your brain cells alive and happy during periods of stress.*

Consider the calming effect of music. Musicologist, composer, and performer Steven Halpern recognized this problem of contemporary life some years ago and decided to write music that would specifically deal with our overstressed nervous systems. He called his musical approach AntiFrantic (or, alternatively, Inner Peace, Inner

Directed, and Music Rx). Music can be an Rx against brain cell depletion or loss due to stress. Halpern composes his music to induce relaxation and inner harmony as fast as possible in the listener. His idea is that people in general do not know how it feels to be relaxed and that his music (now available on about two dozen CDs and cassettes), because it is composed primarily with relaxation in mind, will quickly show us what it does feel like.

THE 3 STEPS FOR USING MUSIC TO MELT ALL YOUR BONES

Two examples of Halpern's music that I have personally used are *Radiance: Spirit in Sound* (Sound Rx, CD #7844, 1989), an hour-long anthology of Halpern's best from the past 15 years, and *Higher Ground* (Sound Rx, CD #7848, 1992), which provides a major relaxation response available as a foundation for meditative states. Here he creates a "sound environment" that quickly gets your brain waves into states of deep relaxation, ease, even euphoria—within about 15 minutes.

These two CDs were so richly relaxing, so luxuriously calming, that I felt as if my bones melted, as if my entire skeletal system sighed and dissolved.

1. Take a daily 15-minute "sound bath" with music deliberately composed and performed to be relaxing. This practice can work wonders in stress reduction.
2. Experiment with other widely available stress reduction, relaxation tapes and most New Age music, some of which combines music, natural sounds (waterfalls), with positive affirmations. For example: *The Rainbow Path*, Kay Gardner; *Birthing*, *Crystal Rainbows*, *Runes*, Don Campbell; *Dolphin Dreams*, Jonathan Goldman; *Music for Airports*, Brian Eno; *Ocean Dreams*, Dean Evenson; *Desert Moon Song*, Dean Evenson; *Sedona Suite*, Tom Barabas. (See the Resources for ordering information)
3. As a complement to this music-assisted relaxation, try the lavender bubble bath, described earlier. Spend at least 20 minutes fully immersed in the calming bubbles. Stay in the bubbles for the length of the CD. Your brain cells will thank you.

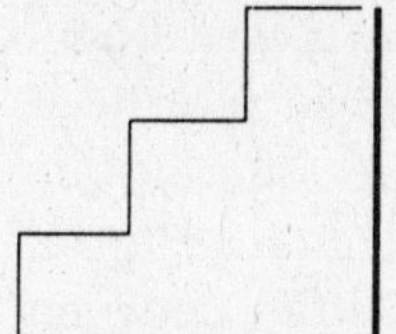

BRAIN-BUILDING SECRET #68

The Rhythms and Music of Accelerated Learning—How to *Suggest* More Brain Power

Back in 1956, Bulgarian research psychologist Georgi Lozanov made a breakthrough in how to promote rapid, thorough learning. The result was a radically innovative learning accelerated system now used in hundreds of schools in Europe and the United States. The Lozanov system is based on the power of positive suggestion coupled with appropriate visual and auditory cues.[3]

Lozanov drew from hypnosis, sleep-learning, music, parapsychology, and drama to put his approach together. Lozanov's idea turned on the power of suggestion, which is why he christened his approach, *suggestopedia*. Practitioners of the Lozanov method claim students can learn 1,200 new words of a foreign language in a single day.[4]

9 STEPS TO MAKE SUPERLEARNING WORK FOR YOUR BRAIN

1. *Desuggest*. You have to change your attitude about what is possible regarding mental abilities. You have to *desuggest* your preconceived ideas and remove your negative mental blocks against having more brain power; you replace these with positive suggestions.
2. *Relax*. Relaxation is central to the process of rapid and effective learning. Relaxation removes stress and regulates the breathing that makes information assimilation easy and recall long lasting.
3. *Mapping it out*. Create a mental map of the new information to be mastered. If this involves mastery of a new language, then you review the lesson in English first so you have an overview of the information terrain and a sense of context. Then you read the lesson through in the particular language you are studying.

4. *Active concert.* Next comes the active concert. Say you're studying French. You read (or hear read to you) the French text out loud in a dramatic manner while in the background Baroque classical music is playing, such as Bach, Telemann, Haydn, Albinoni, or Vivaldi, or other compositions written between 1700–1750. The reading voice follows the rhythms of the music as if the voice itself were a musical instrument.[5]
5. *Study the text.* While this is happening, you study a bilingual text, with English on one page, French on the other. You may be concentrating on the French, but your peripheral vision is also taking in the corresponding English words. Meanwhile, the music, with its precise rhythms, is stimulating your right-brain hemisphere. The combination of superliminal sound and subliminal visual stimuli work together to speed the entry of the new information into your memory.

   In other words, the sound and visual factors work at the high and low end of the threshold of your conscious awareness, enabling you to learn much more than if you went about the study in the "normal" academic way.
6. *Take a break.* Then you take a break. Researchers have proven that if you take regular study breaks, say, a 5-minute break every 30 minutes, your information recall later significantly rises. If, during this 5-minute lull between study, you practice deep breathing and relaxation exercises, the effects are enhanced.

   These factors help move information from short-term to long-term memory, which, by way of analogy, is a bit like moving loose papers from stacks on your desk to orderly hanging files in a file cabinet.
7. *Review.* Review your newly acquired information frequently. A woman who kept a diary for 4 years forgot 65 percent of the materials she never reviewed after initially writing it down. On the other hand, four reviews in one year's time could cut the level of forgetting down to 12 percent, which means these same four reviews can increase recall by 88 percent.

   For example, spend 5 minutes reviewing your study material after 10 minutes; after 1 day has elapsed, spend 5 minutes reviewing it again; after 1 week, spend 3 minutes; after a month, spend 3 minutes; and after 6 months, spend 3 minutes.

When you constantly boost your recall by active reviews in this manner, you can potentially improve your retention by as much as 400 percent, according to Lozanov practitioners. You begin to see the awesome possibility of correctly managed memory.

8. *Receptive concert.* Next comes the receptive concert. Here while it seems you are doing almost nothing, a great deal of mental activity is transpiring, as it were, behind the scenes. You relax in your chair, close your eyes, and listen to the music. Meanwhile, the French text is still being read out loud although you only hear it at the margins of your attention. Your subconscious mind, meanwhile, is taking in every word and remembering them.

   Your relaxation coupled with the music produces an ideal mental state to effortlessly absorb the new information, because the spoken language rides the rhythms of the Baroque music smoothly into your brain's "filing cabinets." Lozanov practitioners explain that this approach coordinates the activities of both brain hemispheres that in turn produces "a quantum leap in learning speeds and retention."

9. *Activations.* The class lasts 2 hours. After a night's sleep, you move into the phase called activations. Here you engage in certain games, puzzles, even plays that review the words studied yesterday; the environment is childlike, fun, and free of the usual stresses associated with intense learning.

   For example, the instructor tosses a ball to you while asking you a question in French (or the language you are studying). You have to answer spontaneously as you catch the ball. The correct words seem to pop out unexpectedly and correctly.

   The review session this day reinforces the new words assimilated the previous day. Each student gets a French name and character to master in a skit. If you make a mistake and fluff some lines, then you don't blame your English-speaking self, but your new French persona. Therefore, your emotional reaction to learning difficulties does not intrude with your actual study.

A SHOPPING LIST OF 8 MORE TECHNIQUES FOR SUPERLEARNING

Here is a shopping list for faster learning and more thorough recall based on Lozanov's superlearning approach.[6]

1. Relaxation is vital to creating the ideal conditions of receptivity and ease of gaining new information. It is also a brain state associated with alpha waves, which "consume" less energy and thus make more brain energy available for the learning task at hand.
2. New information enters your mind and is placed in short-term memory. To convert short term to long term, you need to review and rehearse the information immediately and frequently.
3. The key to registering new information is to bring it into your awareness through some form of strong encoding or association. This might be through emotions, bodily sensations, movement, or visual stimulation. The stronger, more pronounced the original encoding, the more likely you are to remember it later. Linking words with pictures makes information easier to recall. That's because, as the data presented above show, visual memory is almost perfect; recall of visual information is state of the art for memory skill.

   Therefore, when you improve your ability to visualize and to see visually and to encode informaiton with visual associations, you are guaranteeing that you will remember more.
4. More is better when it comes to learning and study, but a technique called distributed practice works even better. This means you rehearse or review new information immediately after you have learned it, then test yourself on recall; review again after the first hour, then again in the morning; then after a week, then after a month.
5. Make sure what you are learning has inherent meaning; that you understand its context and background and have a view of the overall map before you start; that you learn the principle involved first then the individual example; that you learn not by rote but by example.

6. Suggest to yourself frequently that you can learn this information quickly and thoroughly, despite whatever notions you may have formed in childhood or have heard from disparaging teachers.
7. Set up subconscious cues and reminders in your learning environment. Baroque classical music is one example. "Since possibly up to 90 percent of communication is at the subconscious level, the greater the number of subconscious stimuli that are orchestrated to aid learning, the faster and more effective is that learning," explains superlearning expert Colin Rose.
8. The key to accelerated learning is that positive, creative, supportive suggestion can produce a thriving educational environment. In such an environment, students of any age can learn quickly, with little conscious effort and with actual enjoyment. These approaches include:
   - presenting two texts side by side, so that your peripheral vision takes in one while your direct vision studies the other
   - playing games and acting out roles specific to the information or language
   - displaying posters and cards around the room with the same information you are studying
   - learning grammar and words through stories rather than lists
   - presenting the material in a way that engages your bodily, auditory, and visual senses

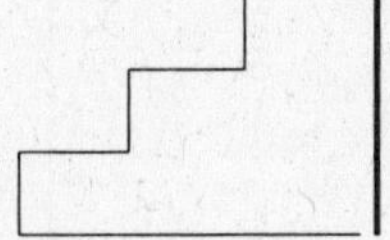

THE ANATOMY OF BRAIN POWER #12

Brain Waves—The Key to Redesigning Your Brain

Perhaps one of the most accurate statements we can make about the brain is that is runs on electricity. Each of your brain's 15 billion neurons (minus the 50,000 you lose every day) discharges a minute electrical current.

The overall electrical activity of your brain can be measured by various sensitive recording devices, including the electroencephalograph, or EEG. An EEG reading of your brain's electrical life gives a picture not of the individual firings of brain cells, but of the patterns of electrical activities for millions of brain cells working together. In a sense, the EEG gives you a brain weather map.

Another name for these patterns of electrical activity is *brain wave*, and when it comes to brain waves, neuroscientists divide them into four major categories according to frequency. The subject of brain waves gives you a key to understanding the relationship between the degree of electrical activity in your brain and certain typical states of mind and activities. (See Diagram 6-1.)

Think of a brain wave the way you picture a wave in the ocean. The brain wave represents the combined electrical pattern of the entire brain. Their frequency, or the rate at which new waves form, is measured in terms of *hertz* (Hz); 1 Hz is one cycle or wave per second, 60 Hz is 60 waves per second.

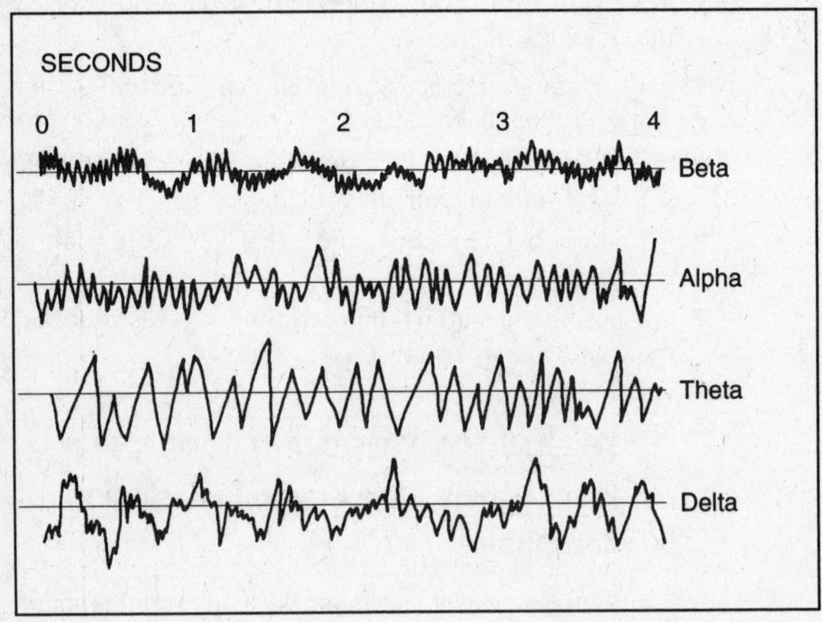

Diagram 6-1

THE 4 BRAIN WAVE STATES—YOUR KEY TO BRAIN POWER

1. *Beta waves*. These range from 14 Hz to 100 Hz and describe the electrical condition of your brain during a normal, everyday state of awareness. It is the brain pulse rate of ordinary consciousness, in which logical thought, analysis, and willed action take place.

   Your eyes are open, focused on the world and its affairs or you are working on a specific task, such as problem solving or talking. Your mind is alert, concentrated, focused, aware, and possibly a little anxious. People in the standard beta brain wave state sometimes report feelings of worry, anger, fear, frustration, tension, and excitement.

   Some neuroscientists make further distinctions about beta, classifying it as approximately 12–16 Hz. Then there are high beta (16–32 Hz), K-complex (33–35 Hz), and superhigh beta (35–150 Hz). In the *K-complex* state, which you may experience only in short bursts, you may find a "place" of high creativity and insight. In *superhigh beta*, you may find yourself having an out-of-body experience.

2. *Alpha waves*. When you close your eyes and start to relax into a more passive, unfocused, meditative state, your brain waves slow down to a range of 8–13 Hz. Alpha waves are calming and pleasant, a kind of neutral or idling state in which you're not particularly outwardly alert yet you're not entranced or asleep.

   People experiencing alpha brain waves report feelings of pleasure, tranquility, pleasantness, relaxation, and an increased awareness of their own thoughts and feelings.

   Alpha is an ideal state in which to master stress management. In other words, if you can lower your brain waves from beta to alpha, you will automatically enter a state of relaxation.

   This is also an optimum brain energy state for learning new languages and the fast assmilation of facts, partly because it removes the stress normally associated with mastering new subjects.

3. *Theta waves.* Here your sense of inner relaxation starts to shift into drowsiness, deep meditation, and reverie, as your brain waves slow to 4–8 Hz. This is the twilight state; you could drift off into sleep or you could have insights, intuitions, inner visions, memories, and dreamlike imagery.

   This is the state of mind you slip into just before falling to sleep; it is a highly suggestible brain state. Theta is ideal for various kinds of accelerated learning and self-programming approaches (using audio tapes or affirmations).

   In theta, while still awake, people often report sensations of problem solving, memory of problems, future planning, daydreaming, uncertainty, switching thoughts.

4. *Delta waves.* Here you are technically asleep as your brain waves break slowly in the range of 0.5–4 Hz. Yogis are able to fall asleep while staying awake in this theta state. Their bodies are asleep and a fair degree of their brain's activities are shut down, yet they are still aware of their environment and themselves and are able to think about things.

   For most everyone else, if your brain has enterd delta, you're probably unconscious. If your brain wave activity drops below 0.5 Hz, you are, technically, brain-dead.

SHIFTING BRAIN WAVE STATES—THE SECRET OF BRAIN-BUILDING

While these brain wave classifications make the brain appear to be something like an automobile's five-speed transmission, your brain rarely operates in a single brain wave frequency nor is it always in the same one. In fact, your brain has a unique brain wave signature. Were you to have a brain scan, it would reveal a unique *neuromap* of your precise brain wave patterns.

It may surprise you to know that you can fairly easily and deliberately change your brain wave state at will and to your best advantage. In this way you can speed up your brain power potential and become master of your brain states through such techniques as biofeedback, meditation, and inner imagery.[7]

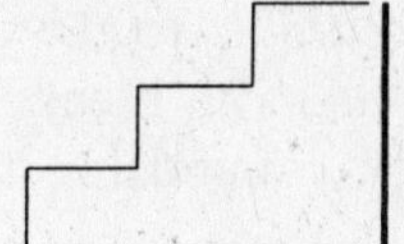

BRAIN-BUILDING SECRET #69
3 Superlearning Breathing Secrets to Unlock Your Brain Power

BREATHING FOR THE CHILD WITHIN YOU

This is a beginning breathing exercise suitable for using with schoolchildren or for the child within you.

- Place your hand over your heart. Feel your heart pumping; feel its rhythms. Know that with each heart beat, you are breathing. Breathe through your nose.
- Imagine that your chest is an accordion that opens and closes as you inhale and exhale. As you breathe in, the accordion expands; as you exhale, the accordion contracts. As you inhale, push your abdomen out; as you inhale, gently pull it back in.
- Place your hands on your abdomen so you can directly feel this accordion effect in your breathing rhythms.
- Follow your breathing, as if you were playing the accordion for 5 minutes.
- Do not be distracted. Give your complete attention to every inhale, as the chest accordion opens, and to every exhale, as the chest accordion closes again.
- Now let's add another element—the rhythm section. As you breathe in, count 1, 2, 3, 4, 5. As you exhale, count 1, 2, 3, 4, 5.
- Count silently to yourself. If you have a metronome, you might set it to tick at 60 beats a minute. Count your breaths in this way for 5 minutes.

CONCENTRATE ON YOUR BREATHING

When you breathe correctly, you reestablish the natural link between your mind and your body. You will also find it an excellent means to hone your concentration and focus and to put some energy into both through your natural breathing rhythms. According to the yoga tradition, from which it comes, breathing techniques can break up the cycle of worry and anxiety that too often plague our minds.

- You need to practice this exercise in a quiet room where you will not be disturbed by people or telephones.
- For this exercise, lie *face up* on the carpet or bed but with your head *facing north* so that you are aligned with the Earth's magnetic field.
- Move both your feet together. Position your hands against the sides of your body so that they are palms up.
- Breathing through your nose only, with your mouth closed, visualize that as you bring the air into your body, through the top of your head enters a warm, yellow-gold energy and light of the sun. This lovely golden light energy moves down through your head and permeates your body all the way to your toenails.
- As you exhale, visualize that at the same time you are drawing up through the soles of your feet a refreshingly cool, moist, blue energy from the moon. This cooling energy sweeps up through your body to the roots of the hairs on your head.
- For the next 15 minutes, without distraction, inhale golden Sun energy and exhale blue cooling moon energy.
- You might see these as two poles of an electric current running through your body in a regular rhythm. The yellow-gold comes in from your head and vibrates you all the way to your toes. The cooling blue comes in through your feet and vibrates you all the way to your head.
- Try to sustain this energizing sensation that with every in-and-out breath your body is being *electrically charged* by two different but healthy energies.

THE BEAT OF BREATHING

The idea of this practice is to learn how to control your breathing by making it rhythmical; this, in turn, will slow down and calm your body-mind rhythms.

- To do this exercise, sit comfortably in a chair, with your shoes (and glasses) off or lie on a soft carpet on the floor.
- Relax your entire body. Inhale deeply through your nose, as much air as you can without straining; then exhale very slowly, allowing only a little stream of air to pass through your lips.
- When you think you have fully exhaled, express a little more from your lungs. Repeat this several times.
- As you inhale, distend your abdomen. As you exhale, tuck in you abdomen. Hold your breath for a count of 3, then exhale slowly.
- Now inhale, counting to 4; hold your breath to the count of 4; then exhale, counting to 4 again, like this: inhale, 2, 3, 4; hold, 2, 3, 4; exhale, 2, 3, 4; pause, 2, 3, 4. Do this four times; then relax.
- Now repeat this sequence but count to 6. This means you must slow down your breathing even more to stretch it out for a count of 6.
- Follow the same pattern as explained in the previous bulleted step. Do the counting to 6 a total of four times, then relax.
- Now extend the cycle to the count of 8, following the same procedure, and do this four times.

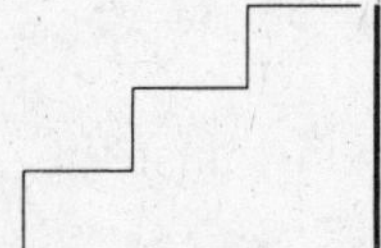

BRAIN-BUILDING SECRET #70
How to Relax Yourself, Psychologically, by the Numbers.

Not only does your physical body—with its muscles, tendons, and organs—need to feel relaxed for superlearning, but your mind and your psychological sense of yourself needs to chill out as well.

To do this exercise, sit comfortably in a chair, with your shoes (and glasses) off or lie on a soft carpet on the floor. You could have someone read this to you out loud, or you could record it on a tape cassette and then play it back when you're ready.

1. Close your eyes and do four inhales/exhales, slowly, deeply, without straining. Now pretend you are on the seventh floor of a building. The walls are vivid red.

   You walk down this red-lined hallway to a silver escalator going down. It makes no sound, is handsomely made, and inspires security in you when you contemplate it. You put your hands on the guide rails as the escalator noiselessly descends.

   You know you are descending, in safety and with calmness, to the inner, central part of this building. As you start to escalate downward, already you are feeling more relaxed.

2. As you glide down, visualize the digit 7, saying the number out loud several times and seeing it framed largely against the bright red hallway you have just left. Continue to breathe fully, with awareness.

3. Now you step off the escalator at the sixth floor, where you see the digit 6 framed against bright orange walls. After noting this, you get back on the escalator and resume your downward glide.

   Breathing deeply, recite the digit 6 out loud several times as you remember it against the orange walls.

   Notice that as you proceed farther down the escalator, you feel even more relaxed and laid back than you did just one floor above.

4. Now you reach the fifth floor, where the walls are a bright yellow-gold. You walk through these corridors of yellow-gold then reenter the escalator.

   As it descends, visualize the digit 5, framed against the yellow-gold walls, and recite it aloud several times. You are even more deeply relaxed and at ease than you were on the sixth floor.

   Allow your senses to revel in the colors you have witnessed.

5. Now you come to the fourth floor, where the walls are a lovely spring green. Again you stroll through the green corridors, then reenter the escalator.

   As you do, visualize the digit 4 framed against the spring green walls and recite the number out loud several times.

6. As the escalator brings you to the third floor, you feel yourself bathed in a peaceful, calming blue. The walls are all in this color. This reminds you of a serene lake or ocean or broad blue sky you have seen and loved.

   The blue also instills a sense of harmony and balance which is deeply relaxing. As you continue to breathe in and out with awareness, visualize the digit 3, and say it aloud several times.

7. Once more the escalator continues its downward journey. The walls of the second floor are painted royal purple, and you absorb this rich color as you wander through the hallways.

   Back on the escalator, you see the digit 2 against the purple walls and say this number out loud.

8. At last, you approach the first floor, which is awash in a radiant ultraviolet hue. You get off here, seeing the digit 1 framed against this violet background.

   You are almost unbelievably relaxed; you never suspected this degree of relaxation was possible. You also feel rested, alert, and focused, yet free of stress.

   If you wish, you can instantly revisit any of the previous six floors and enjoy the healing vibrations of their colors.

   When you are finished, count to 3, then open your eyes and enjoy your new state of relaxation.

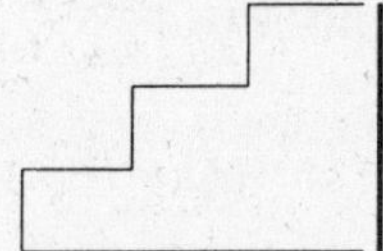

BRAIN-BUILDING SECRET #71
Achieving Supermemory by the Music

Use this exercise when you have a specific body of information you need to study and learn, such as a foreign language, material for an exam, or anything new and complex you wish to understand. For this exercise, you need to have somebody read the material out loud to you or you can prepare it in advance using your own voice speaking into a tape recorder.

Let's say you want to master more words of a foreign vocabulary or even to improve your working vocabulary of English.

THE SECRET OF SUPERMEMORY LIES IN THE NUMBER 4

- First, you learn how to synchronize your breathing to the rhythm of the spoken material.
- Review the steps explained in Brain-Building Secret #69.
- When you hear the material being read to you, hold your breath for a count of 4. The voice reads to you for 4 seconds—for example, *la maison*—house—*la maison*—house—*la maison*.
- As you hear the words, you are holding your breath to the count of 4. Then you exhale to the count of 2; then as you start the inhale cycle again, counting to 2 on the inhale, another 4 seconds of material is read to you.
- In other words, you start your breathing cycle in segments of 4, for inhale, holding, exhaling, pausing; then insert the study material in 4-second installments into this breathing rhythm. It goes like this: inhale 1, 2; hold 1, 2, 3, 4; exhale 1, 2. Then repeat.
- As someone reads the material to you (or you hear it on tape in your own voice) read through this same material silently, following the words on the page as you hear them spoken on the tape.
- Now add the 8-beat cycle of breathing: inhale 1, 2; hold 1, 2, 3, 4; exhale 1, 2. The speaking voice will read for 4 seconds, then pauses 4 seconds, then reads 4 seconds, until the material is finished.
- Remember to hold your breath during the 4 seconds the speaker is reading the material.
- Now go through the same material, continuing with the rhythmic breathing while listening to music in addition.[8]
- Not any music, but Baroque music, because its rhythms (60 beats per minute) are perfectly timed for this exercise.
- Continue your breathing rhythms like this: inhale 1, 2; hold 1, 2, 3, 4; exhale 1, 2. But also be aware of the music and its rhythms in the background as you hold your breath every 4 seconds to absorb the spoken material.

BAROQUE MUSIC FOR SUPERLEARNING—WHAT TO LISTEN TO

Here you might wish to prepare your own special superlearning tape cassette based on these selections from Baroque composers.

- *Johann Sebastian Bach*: Largo from Concerto G Minor for Flute and Strings; Aria to the Goldberg Variations; Largo from Solo Harpsichord Concerto in F Minor.
- *Antonio Corelli*: Sarabanda (largo) from Concerto No. 7 in D Minor; Preludio (largo) and Sarabanda (largo) from Concerto No. 5 in E Minor.
- *George Friedrich Handel*: Largo from Concerto No. 1 in F; Largo from Concerto No. 3 in D; Largo from Concerto No. 1 in B flat Major, Opus 3.
- *George Telemann*: Largo from Double Fantasia in G Major for Harpsichord; Largo from Concerto in G Major for Viola and String Orchestra.
- *Antonio Vivaldi*: Largo from "Winter" from The Four Seasons; Largo from Concerto D Major for Guitar and Strings; Largo from Concerto in C Major for Mandolin, Strings, and Harpsichord.

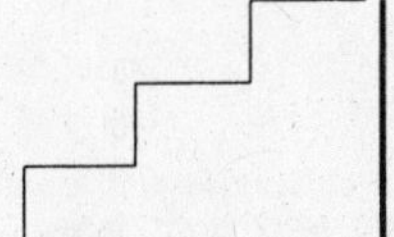

BRAIN-BUILDING SECRET #72
Music for the Brain—Recipes and Meal Planner

In Brain-Building Secret #68, we touched on the effective use of Baroque music to set the sound foundation for accelerated learning. There are other key applications of music, sound, and frequency that work equally well in boosting brain power.

CHANTING AS TOP-SHELF BRAIN FOOD

About 30 years ago, Dr. Alfred Tomatis, a French ear, nose, and throat specialist, discovered that sound is nourishment for the brain.

Tomatis found that the music of Gregorian chant actually *energizes the brain*. Somehow this musical style charges the brain with electrical potential—in fact, up to about 90 percent of the whole body's charge, Tomatis claimed.

After all, your brain needs about 3 billion stimuli a second for at least 4.5 hours a day just for you to stay awake, focused, dynamic, able to think and operate with vitality. Of these stimuli, approximately 60 percent come from sound and vibration, and they all must pass through your ears. Thus, your ears are a principal key to brain stimulation, providing they are in top working order. Many ears are not, said Tomatis.[9]

Our brain-building secret is straightforward: *Listen to Gregorian chants and related sound-nourishment music, sounds, or frequencies as often as possible as food for your brain, even as background music while you're working. If at all possible, learn how to sing along and get added benefits.*

For Gregorian chant and polyphony, listen to

- *Chant Grégorien*, Deller Consort, Harmonia Mundi, HMC 90234, 1987. A fine example of the high-energy Gregorian music, thematically featuring the entry of Christ into Jerusalem.
- *An English Ladymass*, Anonymous 4, Harmonia Mundi, HMU 907080, 1991. Lovely female voices doing thirteenth-century medieval chants and polyphony around the theme of the Virgin Mary.

EAR FORCE = BRAIN FORCE

The ear has functions that have been completely ignored by science, Tomatis added. The human ear is able to relay external stimuli (sounds) to the brain where they charge the "cortical battery." That's why he says *ear force = brain force*; ear force is the overlooked key to memory power.

The anatomy of the inner ear itself is the key to the mystery of ear force. Here you have, in the midst of the spirals of the snail-shaped cochlea of the inner ear, an estimated 24,600 sensory cells.

You might think of these, as Tomatis did, as brain batteries. Except it is not the brain and its metabolism that energizes these cells; it can be recharged only through external stimuli, such as special frequency sounds. These sounds then stimulate the Corti cells in the cochlea; then as sound is transformed into energy, your brain's cortex can then redistribute this energy throughout your body's nervous system. High-frequency sounds, especially around 8,000 Hz, are the master key to optimum brain energy

Gregorian chant is such excellent brain food because it contains all the frequencis of the human voice, from 70 cycles per second up to 9,000 cycles per second, but in a way that sounds different from what you hear in normal speech. Tomatis discovered that it's the high-frequency sounds, especially around 8,000 cycles per second, that are most beneficial. Whenever he has a long job to do or a complex mental task, Tomatis plays Gregorian chants in the background in his study "because it enables me to remain charged without difficulty." It also enables him to get by with only 4 hours sleep a day and to maintain a very productive schedule.

60 MINUTES A DAY OF GREGORIAN CHANT IS BRAIN ENERGY FOOD

Merely listening to properly recorded Gregorian chant for 30–60 minutes a day (as he did for years) can allow the sounds to work their brain-energizing magic, making them uniquely "a fantastic energy food." There is another brain tonic quality to Gregorian chant.

This is the fact it has rhythm but no tempo; listening to it, you have the sensation nobody ever pauses to breathe. But this becomes beneficial to the listener, working as a kind of "respiratory yoga," putting one into a state of tranquility with slow, calm breathing. In effect, listening to Gregorian chant trains your own breathing rhythms (and cardiac rates) to the calming, healing pace implicit in the music.[10]

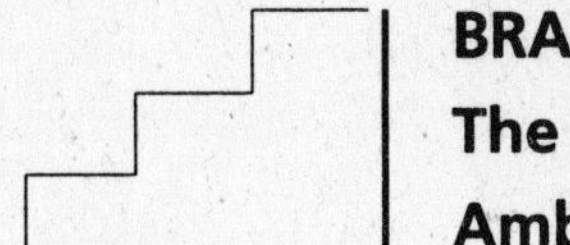

BRAIN-BUILDING SECRET #73
The Electronic Ear on Walkman—Ambrosia for Your Brain

In the 1980s, an innovative Canadian author, playwright, and broadcaster named Pat Joudry hit upon the idea of transferring Dr. Tomatis's Electronic Ear onto the Walkman.

Previously, Tomatis's system, though achieving excellent results with many health conditions, including building brain power, was simply too expensive for the average person. To get all the equipment, you needed about $20,000 or access to a Tomatis Center. Here you would listen to specially filtered electronic sounds, most often the music of Mozart with all the low notes and frequencies removed.

ENERGIZE YOUR BRAIN WITH ELECTRONICALLY FILTERED SOUNDS

The result didn't sound too much like *The Magic Flute* because what you—your inner ear, that is— mostly hears are frequencies in excess of 8,000 Hz. Lower-frequency bands below 2,000 Hz are suppressed, and the stereo dominance favors the right ear.

While this might displease the fastidious lover of classical music in its pure form, it produced astonishing results in the listeners, especially when Joudry put it all on simple cassettes for Walkmans.

After 100–200 hours of listening to filtered sounds in the 8,000–16,000 Hz range, it is like having a new, radically improved, unbelievably energized brain, according to the testimonials of hundreds of users.

One man was cured of his insomnia and so bubbled over with energy that he drove 2,500 miles in his car nonstop. A professor announced: "After three days [of listening] I was aware of an energy and mental clarity such as I had not experienced since before entering university many years earlier."

BENEFITS OF THE WALKMAN BRAIN-ENERGIZING SOUNDS

The range of other comments included praises for

- opening the door to creativity
- enabling users to sleep, think, and write better
- enabling a dyslexic child to show terrific improvement in writing
- greatly increasing energy, stamina, and endurance

- improving concentration
- improving the ability to focus the mind
- improving memory and learning ability
- providing a boundless supply of energy
- relieving chronic migraines
- helping autism
- relieving nausea
- relieving dizziness
- improving speech defects
- providing stress relief

LISTEN MORE, SLEEP LESS, AND CONCENTRATE BETTER

One typical result is a condition Joudry calls *hypersomnia*, or Supersleep: you sleep better with fewer hours. You get concentrated, time-efficient sleep because your system, especially the brain, has been so energized and recharged through Sound Therapy that it literally needs less time at night to refresh itself. Typically 2–3 hours of nightly sleep can be shaved off in this way.

Think of it this way: If you are now 40 and you start doing sound therapy, you could add 6 years of usable time to your life.

"First, improvement in memory, concentration, retention, and ease of learning is invariably reported by Sound Therapy listeners," says Joudry. Older people report they can retain information easier and that their minds are less like a sieve. "This is because Sound Therapy (among its other effects) unblocks neural pathways," Joudry adds. You should figure on listening 100–200 hours before you get significant results, Joudry advises. See the Resources for listings.

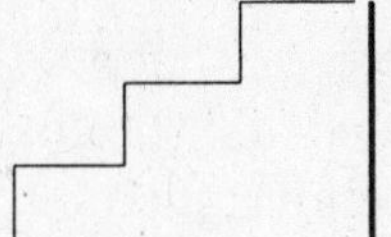

BRAIN-BUILDING SECRET #74
Overtoning the Brain—Use Your Own Voice to Feed Your Neurons

In Brain-Building Secret #72, it was noted that when you use your own voice to chant, you increase the energy charge delivered to your brain. In this discussion, we'll have a look at how to use your voice to feed your neurons.

Another form of music both quite different from Gregorian yet similar in its brain-energizing effect is an approach called *overtone chanting* or *vocal harmonics*. Again, this is sound nourishment that you can consume as a listener or player. Singers, or chanters, in this discipline are able to use their throat to project three different notes at the same time—upper and lower versions, or harmonics of the same note—creating what musicologists call "one-voice chords."[11]

When you listen to music that is rich in harmonics, this can energize your brain's cortex, lower your heart rate, slow down your breathing, reduce your brain wave activity, stimulate the flow of cerebrospinal fluid through the brain, and basically thoroughly relax you. It's not been proven yet, but some musicologists and sound therapists speculate that Gregorian chants and overtone harmonics may stimulate your brain cells to develop more connections at the synapses.[12]

8 STEPS TO MAKE VOWEL SOUNDS SERVE AS BRAIN FOOD

Here is an exercise that uses your voice and specific vowel sounds to stimulate your entire body, including your brain. It should take you perhaps 15 minutes and will be remarkably relaxing and energizing.

1. Find a quiet room in the house that is adequately lighted. Sit comfortably in a straight-backed chair with your feet flat on the floor and a couple of inches apart. Preferably, remove your shoes and socks; if you wear glasses, remove them. Rest your hands in your lap. You may close your eyes if you wish. Breathe naturally several times through your nose until you feel relaxed.
2. Now make your first sound. Pitching your voice as deep as possible, make the sound UH. Say it as you exhale. Make this sound at your normal speaking volume or quieter if you prefer. As you make the sound UH, place your attention in your groin.

   As you exhale, make the sound UH as if you were sitting at the base of your spine. You will feel the UH sound resonating in your throat of course, but imagine that it is vibrating the base of your spine. Make this sound with every exhale for perhaps 1 minute then stop and relax.

3. Now move your attention up the spine to the area of your pubic region or about 3 inches below the navel. Make the sound OOO on the exhale. Pitch this OOO sound a little higher than the way you sounded UH. As before, try to feel this sound vibrating in your pubic area. Do this for a minute then stop and relax.
4. Find the third energy center at your navel. This is called the solar plexus and occupies the region from the base of your sternum to the belly button. Focus your attention here as you make the sound OH on the exhale. Make the OH sound a little higher in pitch than you did for OOO; this would put it at about the middle range of your voice. Do this for a minute then stop and relax.
5. Now move your attention up to the heart. This is the chest area, essentially between the shoulder blades and the bottom of the rib cage. As you focus here, make the sound AH, pitched a little higher than you did for OH. Feel this sound resonating throughout your chest cavity. Do this for a minute then stop and relax.
6. Next, focus on your throat and neck. With your attention focused here, make the sound EYE at a pitch somewhat higher than you did for AH. Feel the sound EYE vibrating in your throat. Do this for a minute then stop and relax.
7. The next energy center is located between your eyebrows. Here you make the sound AAY on the exhale. Visualize that this sound AAY vibrates inside your brow. Do this for a minute then stop and relax.
8. Finally, make the sound EEE for the top of your head. Visualize that as you make the sound EEE it vibrates throughout the top of your head. Do this for a minute then stop and relax.

This completes the exercise for sounding your energy centers. You may feel slightly light-headed. This is natural and will pass in a few minutes. Continue breathing calmly through your nose. If you wish, you can reverse the exercise and proceed down through the centers, making the sounds again in reverse order. Or you may open your eyes, look around, and stand up.

8 STEPS TO MAKE OVERTONES SERVE AS BRAIN FOOD

Here are a few quick practices for overtoning as a way of stimulating your brain[13]:

1. Hum the sound MMM at a range that is comfortable for your voice. Allow your lips to vibrate strongly. Substitute different vowels, such as MMMUUU (moo), MMMOOO (go), MMMAAA (ma), MMMIII (my), MMMAYE (may), MMMEEE (me).

   Open your lips only slightly to let the sounds pass through softly yet with some force. You should be able to hear extra sounds at different ranges as you make these sounds.
2. Position your lips as if you are to whistle; then open your lips slightly, puckered. Make the sound MMMOOORRR (as in more). Make this sound at the bottom of your palate as you slowly exhale.
3. Place two fingers on either side of your nose and press lightly. As you exhale, make the sound NNNEEE (knee). See if you can make the sound vibration actually vibrate your fingers at your nose.
4. Now try making the sound NNNUUURRR (rhyming with her). First, let your nose vibrate with NNN; then add the UUU and RRR sounds. As you make the RRR sound, place your tongue about one-fourth inch behind your front teeth but barely touching the upper palate.
5. As you continue to make this sound, experiment with moving your tongue slowly from the back of your mouth to the front. There will be one particular spot where you hear a high-pitched whistle tone. When you find it, experiment with changing the shape of your mouth, which in turn will produce different sounds.
6. Now try the sound NNNNGONG. As you make the nasal sound NNN, say GONG; then do NNN again and add GUNG instead; then add GANG; then GING.

7. Finally, try putting them together. Start with MMMOOORRR; then go to NNNUUURRR and NNNNGONG.
8. Once you have the technique down, you might try practicing this for 10 minutes every day. Follow with listening to any of the discs listed here.

MUSICAL RESOURCES FOR OVERTONES AND HARMONICS AS BRAIN FOOD

- David Hykes, *True to the Times/How to Be*, New Albion Records, 1993, NA057CD. An exploration of the harmonic chant as a unified field; includes mode, text, and polyrhythm in a trio format (with accompanists).
- David Hykes, *Windhorse Riders*, with Djamchid Chemirani, New Albion Records, 1989, NA024CD. A study in the vibrant, subtle harmonics within the human voice as examples of harmonic polyrhythm.
- David Hykes, *The Harmonic Choir/Hearing Solar Winds*, Ocora (France), 1989, C. 558607, distributed by Harmonia Mundi, Los Angeles. A tour de force, an awesome harmonic parable of creation, incarnation, and transcendence.
- David Hykes, *Harmonic Meetings*, Celestial Harmonies, 14013-2, 1986. Hykes adds liturgical words to the harmonic chant as an experiment in singing pure vibrations.
- *From Ancient Worlds for Harmonic Piano*, Michael Harrison, New Albion Records, NA042CD, 1992. Harrison refitted a grand piano to Just Intonation, producing richly nuanced harmonics like ethereal voices and ringing bells.
- *Tibetan Tantric Choir*, The Gyuto Monks, Windham Hill Records, WD-2001, 1987. Aural prayer, not performance, demanding the listener's meditative participation.
- *Tantric Harmonies*, Gyume Tibetan Monks, Spirit Music, Inc. JSG-13007 (cassette), 1986. Similar sonic rituals, with Tibetans horns, bells, and cymbals, that induct the listener into the Tibetan cosmology.

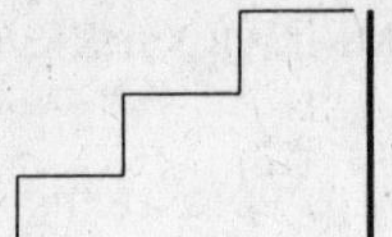

THE ANATOMY OF BRAIN POWER #13
What Really, at the End of the Day, Is Brain Power?

Considering the work and superlearning technique of Dr. Georgi Lozanov prompts a philosophical question. Is brain power, in the final analysis, simply a matter of more neurons with more dendrites and faster synaptic time? Or is there something even deeper at play?

MORE BRAIN POWER MEANS MORE CONSCIOUSNESS

I suggest that at the end of the day brain power is really about consciousness—more of it. I say this because in the case of Dr. Lozanov's work, the ancient spiritual practice of yoga, which aims at enhancing consciousness, and the modern opportunities of superlearning, which aim at fast intake and deep recall, converge in the same effort. More brain power is an aspect of more consciousness.

Think of all the categories of brain power we're trying to improve—we want more awareness, attention, concentration, focus, memory, range, flexibility, problem-solving ability, and creativity. Surely we can say of these that they are one and all to do with more consciousness, perhaps *unlimited* consciousness. This, after all, was the prime insight motivating Dr. Lozanov to develop suggestopedia.

TAPPING THE RESERVES OF THE MIND

Lozanov, after studying a special mental branch of yoga for 20 years, concluded that the human ability to remember and learn is virtually limitless. The technique is all about "tapping the reserves of the mind," coming, as it were, into a large legacy of unsuspected brain power.

Lozanov's is a truly holistic enterprise because the abilities of both right- and left-brain hemispheres are called into action, lending their support for the goal of superlearning. All of its programs are designed to remove your built-in psychological obstacles to learning, such as fear, self-blame, negative self-images, and negative conditioned responses or subsconscious suggestions that keep telling you that you cannot be any smarter or learn faster.

Lozanov found a uniquely successful way to apply altered states of mind, which have long been known to spiritual and parapsychological traditions, as a new foundation for learning, memory, and intuitive development.

For example, he writes that he once met Yogi Sha, a lawyer, at the Sri Yogendra Institute in Bombay, India. This yogi practiced yoga exercises daily for years after which he developed "supermemory." He could immediately recall 18-digit number columns, as well as the name and day of the week for any date in any century; he also had photographic memory.

Even more impressive, there were dozens more people in India like Yogi Sha who had also developed supermemory using yoga practices. These practices included visualization, concentration exercises, techniques to govern the mind, and special breathing routines.

Within the yoga tradition, these techniques, if taken far enough, lead to extraordinary powers such as a photographic memory, the ability to do instant calculations, the ability to control and subdue internal pain, and other paranormal abilities, including telepathy and ESP.

THE HUMAN MEMORY IS THOROUGH BEYOND BELIEF

All this convinced Lozanov that the "human mind remembers a colossal quantity of information, like the number of buttons on a suit, steps on a staircase, panes in a window, footsteps to the bus stop. These 'unknown perceptions' show the subconscious has startling powers."

It's as if you have a natural video recorder in your head. The Canadian surgeon Wilder Penfield once demonstrated this vividly. During brain operations on patients on low-level anesthesia, he used a weak electric current to stimulate certain areas of the brain. The patients would report detailed visual playbacks of old memories and life events, conversations, songs, jokes, birthday parties, and family outings.

All this information had been perfectly, accurately recorded and here it was, available to memory once again. All you have to do, Lozanov realized, is free the brain from everything that distracts or hampers its full natural range of abilities so that it can act like a sponge, absorbing and retaining vast amounts of information.

THERE IS NO OUTER LIMIT TO YOUR BRAIN'S POTENTIAL

The key is suggestion, the trained, directed use of thought and awareness coupled with a certain rhythm in the functions of body and mind to open the mind to greater awareness. Get the students into a calm state of mind, through breathing exercises, deep relaxation, and music; then present the information rhythmically, in short spurts and fragments.

They will remember almost everything, as thousands of Lozanov students have demonstrated in the last 30 years. Further, the supermemory sessions enhance awareness in all respects, even to the extent of cultivating heightened sensitivity, telepathy, and intuition.

Does your mind's potential have any outer limits or cutoff point? No, says Lozanov. Once you master the secret of opening your mind to superlearning, the capacity to remember seems almost boundless. And this capacity, Lozanov's work seems to imply, is really nothing other than the powers of human consciousness itself.

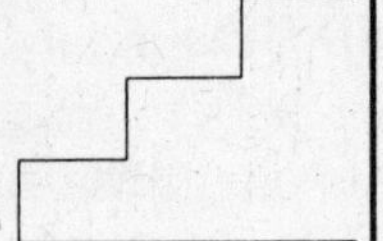

BRAIN-BUILDING SECRET #75
Getting in Sound Sync with the Hemispheres of Your Brain

Some of the most exciting research on how to sound the brain waves has come out of The Monroe Institute (MRI) in Faber, Virginia. There they have developed dozens of sound tapes that use sound to address everything from pain control, addiction release, physical coordination, insomnia relief, stress management, immune boosting, to self-transformation and psychic and intuitive development.

It's all based on former businessman Monroe's unique sound technology called Hemi-Sync™ which synchronizes the activities of both brain hemispheres.

Our brain-building secret here is this: *Try listening to some of these Mind Food sound tapes based on Hemi Sync and other approaches, given here, and see if they don't noticeably boost your brain power in a matter of a few weeks.*[14]

Monroe Institute sound engineers spent two decades figuring out the precise sounds to match those desired brain states until they found the right frequencies. They can now generate specific sound waves so accurately that they become subtle and powerful tools to change the state of your brain. Through a generous series of tapes, Hemi-Sync teaches listeners how to use their own brain resources at their maximum capability. They can even make a unique map of the way the brain responds to these different frequencies.[15]

HEMI-SYNC IMPROVES BRAIN POWER IN THE CLASSROOM

Some of the claims for MRI's Hemi-Sync are being born out by independent research, particularly its use in the field of accelerated learning. A study conducted by the U.S. Army found that students using Hemi-Sync showed a 77.8 percent improvement in mental and motor skills, plus stress reduction, enhancements in self-control, performance, and motivation.

An educator at Tacoma Community College in Washington State tested Hemi-Sync with his college students in areas involving focused attention. He used Hemi-Sync in a variety of class settings, including creative writing, drawing, psychology, speech, philosophy, and foreign languages. The experimental group heard the standard lectures while Hemi-Sync played in the background. The Hemi-Sync group outscored the non–Hemi-Sync group in all test categories by an average of 10.9 percent, which, to the teacher, was a letter grade higher.

A SHOPPER'S SAMPLING OF BRAIN POWER TAPES

Monroe Hemi-Sync Tapes

- ▼ *Practical Application Mind Food Tapes*, for specific applications, including focused attention, accelerated learning, stress and tension reduction, recharging and refreshing.
- ▼ *Awake & Alert*, uses Hemi-Sync signals to keep you awake and focused for brief periods of time.
- ▼ *Concentration*, strengthens your focus and attention for studying, reviewing visual information.

- *Retain-Recall-Release*, contains sound-encoding cues to help you remember information.
- *Nostalgia*, uses Hemi-Sync to guide you into remembering your personal history.
- *Progressive Accelerated Learning*, PAL *Album Series*, trains you in gaining focused attention by getting both brain hemispheres to work together.[16]

Megabrain Zones

Six tape cassettes that focus on peak performance, relaxation, focus, flow, exploration, and awakening, based on the science of audio psychotechnology, including music plus "psychoactive sounds." $74.95, developed by Michael Hutchison, noted author, educator, and demonstrator in this field.[17]

Mind Gymnastiks. A Program to Boost Brain Function and Performance

Six audio tapes for body-mind reeducation to stimulate creativity, clarity in thought and perception, and information-processing speed.[18]

High Coherence: Ascend to Higher Levels

Sound waves that move your mind, according to its producer Kelly Howell, in a 60-minute tape combining music with precisely-engineered sound waves to keep your mind alert.[19]

Mind Flow—Enhance Cognition

Using music and the sound of chanting monks, these two cassettes deliver theta and beta frequencies associated with higher cognitive functions, memory formation, visual acuity, and concentration.[20]

Ataraxia, A State of Peace

One of a series of specially sound-engineered tapes based on the concept of brain hemisphere synchronization from Brother Charles, this set of two 30-minute tapes for "environmental listening and contemporary contemplation."[21]

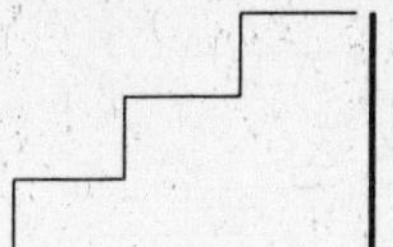

BRAIN-BUILDING SECRET #76

The Megabrain—Neurotechnology Will Get You There

Not only can music and sounds heighten your brain power, but a rapidly growing field called neurotechnology—technologies for the brain—may get you there by way of manipulating frequencies, the real music your neurons listen to anyway. There is now a rich assortment of new, personalized consumer microelectronic devices to make this happen.

The whole idea is to make practical use of what is known about the relationship between brain waves and brain states and then to do a little manipulation of both to get the desired results. The manipulation is done via the mind machines, which are based on minicomputers and hand-held controls.

GET YOURSELF A DESIGNER MIND AND BRAIN POWER BY THE VOLT

Designer minds, brain wave manipulated attitudes, positive feelings instantly—that's the kind of promises neurotechnology is making. The field of portable, affordable "mind machines," as they're popularly called (using precise frequencies of light and sound chaneled through the eyes and ears into the brain), is burgeoning.

And if industry spokespeople can be trusted, mind machines may put accelerated learning, heightened creativity, and even the sublimities of meditation in your hands, virtually at the touch of a minicomputer button. Neurotechnology promises you more than a map or even access to your brain; it offers transportation through the *megabrain*.[22]

The claims that manufacturers make for their brain machines are rather considerable. They include

- ▼ relaxing stress
- ▼ improving IQ
- ▼ stimulating memory
- ▼ solving problems holistically

- ▼ alternating in space/time perception
- ▼ enhancing self-esteem
- ▼ correcting breathing patterns
- ▼ reducing critical logical blocks
- ▼ heightening creativity
- ▼ concentrating deeply
- ▼ thinking with the whole brain
- ▼ improving vision
- ▼ accelerating learning
- ▼ balancing brain hemispheres
- ▼ removing acne
- ▼ normalizing blood pressure
- ▼ reducing pain
- ▼ eliminating addictions
- ▼ boosting self-assertiveness
- ▼ stabilizing emotions
- ▼ increasing intuitive abilities
- ▼ augmenting energy
- ▼ lifting your mood

A QUICK REVIEW OF MIND MACHINES

The cranial electric stimulation, (CES) device, not much larger than an electric pencil sharpener, sends a minute electrical current (less than 1 milliampere) into the brain at a regular pulse rate of 0.5 Hz, and up, according to your adjustment.

Electrodes are attached to your ears or temples through which the minute electrical currents pass directly into your brain. Once inside your brain hemispheres, the electrical stimulation produces various brain states, including heightened relaxation, deepened awareness, calm alertness, a sense of well-being, even euphoria.

The CES was originally developed as a way of controlling and reducing pain—by the person in pain. More recent studies have shown CES highly useful in cases of treating drug addiction withdrawal, depression, anxiety, and insomnia. CES is also used successfully in treating patients with learning disabilities, including "attention-to-task deficits" resulting from head injury.

After three weeks of daily CES work, many aspects of brain power had been restored, including concentration, speed, and perception. In other cases involving amnesia and short-term memory disorder from head injuries, CES also racked up considerable success.

Brain machine technology, like computers, changes fast. Here are a few samples of CES-type brain machines, available through stores or catalogs, at fairly reasonable prices, usually $400–$1,000. See Resources for a listing of brain machine catalogs.

1. The *Brain Tuner-6*, invented by Robert Beck in 1983 and modified five times since, uses direct CES applied at each ear through clip-on electrodes. Clinical research shows that BT-6's minute current stimulates the brain's hypothalamus and boosts (or restores) neurotransmitter activity within 40 minutes of application.

   The clinical use of CES has a long and successful medical history in the West, particularly with the treatment of drug dependency and methadone withdrawal, depression, insomnia, and headaches. "We have new technology for enhancing consciousness rapidly, safely, right now, with no side effects," declares Beck. The BT-6 contains 256 preset frequencies, including the 7.83-Hz Earth resonance, fits in a coat pocket, and may have restorative effects on the immune system after only a month's use.
2. The *AlphaPacer III Plus* addresses psychotechnology's three worlds, combining electrical current, pulsed magnetic field, and light/sound stimulation.

   This triply synchronized input makes sense, says AlphaPacer's inventor Keith Simons, because "the more of the sensory channels you make an impact on in one device, the more likely you are to produce entrainment and the more deeply. It's like meditation, only we're using a more technical method to slow down the brain waves more quickly. All kinds of effects *may* be possible, but we can't claim any of these until all the research is done."

3. The *Alpha-Stim* CS, released in 1981 and by 1992, reportedly used worldwide by more than 1 million people, combines TENS and CES techniques to speed pain relief, eliminate migraines, improve memory, and accelerate healing.
4. The German-made *Mind Man* produces CES frequencies from 0.5–510 Hz and 13 preset frequency harmonic mixes.
5. *Nustar* uses a biofeedback principle and electrode headband to teach users how to produce desired frequency states within their brain in as little as ten 40-minute sessions.

7 EXERCISE YOUR BRAIN

▼▼▼▼▼▼▼▼▼▼▼▼▼▼▼▼▼▼▼▼▼▼▼▼▼▼▼

How to Exercise Your Brain Power "Muscles" to *Smarten Up* Your Neurons

Exercise your brain. Finally, here is the cart of brain power, now that you have put the "horse" in its rightful place. Brain-building exercises can get much better traction and results when you do them in a prepared environment. Creating this environment is what the brain-building secrets of Chapters 1–6 are all about; now even a little practice with some of the exercises in this section will give you far better results than if you had tried them first.

Now we arrive at the real mental gymnastics, the time when you can start pumping ions and building IQ fitness. You have laid the proper foundation through the first brain-building secrets introduced in Chapters 1–6. Now you can enjoy the rewards for your hard effort. The benefits of practicing the brain-building secrets in this chapter will be multiplied many times over because you have prepared the organic foundation for your brain power through the previous 76 brain-building secrets.

Now you can work on building memory; expanding your mental abilities for words and numbers; developing your visual abilities, which many believe are the key to memory; and get busy with a variety of brain power calisthenics.

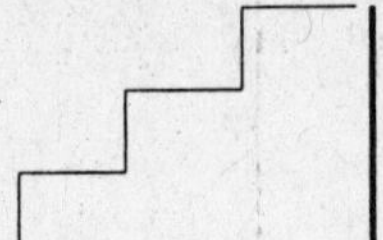

BRAIN-BUILDING SECRET #77
There's Brain Power in Your Eyes and How to See It

Generally speaking, the way your eyes move and how you track objects in space is an aspect of how your brain works as a whole. That's why, if you practice certain eye movements, you can actually stimulate your brain and build brain power at the same time. If you have difficulty in using your eyes to track objects, this, in turn, suggests there are blockages in your brain's processing centers that interfere with your natural brain power. (See Diagram 7-1.)

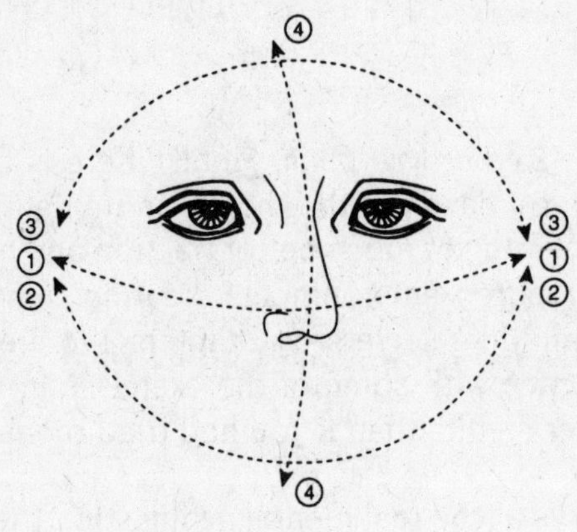

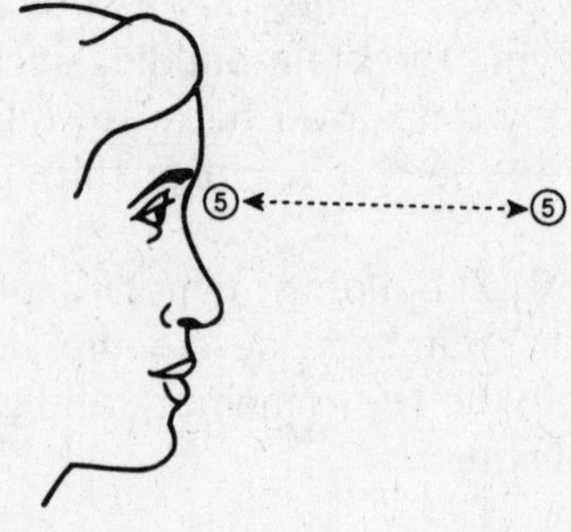

Diagram 7-1

One way to tell for yourself if your eyes are draining off valuable brain power is the following exercise.

- Take a pencil flashlight or a nightlight and turn it on in a darkened room or closet.
- First, look at the light; then move your eyes away from it slowly either to the left or right. If the after-image is a smooth and straight track, then no problem, but if it is wobbly and uneven, then you can benefit from the exercises to follow.
- Next, suspend the pencil light from a hook.
- Look at the light; then move your eyes across the wall behind the light, making arcing curves upward from right to left; then downward arcing curves from left to right; then straight lines, from right to left; then straight lines from top to bottom, then at close range; then at far range.
- Close your eyes. Examine the after-image track.
- Are the lines straight and smooth or wobbly and interrupted?

BETTER EYE TRACKING CAN MEAN BETTER SCHOOL PERFORMANCE

The quality of the after-image tracked by your eyes is the key to your eye-brain fitness. If your eyes cannot easily and smoothly track a moving target, such as the lighted tip of a pencil flashlight, then your brain itself may be having difficulties in its activities. Brain power expert Win Wenger reports that he once worked with a 6-year-old girl who was having troubles learning how to read. He tested her eyes by having her track the tip of a pencil eraser as he moved it across her field of vision.

At first her eyes had difficulty tracking the moving target, but after a few minutes her eyes were getting the trick and tracking the movements more smoothly. He spent 10 minutes in two 5-minute sessions retraining the girl's eyes in this manner; immediately afterward she was able to read at the level of a third-grade student. While he admits the shift in eye tracking rarely happens that fast, generally it takes only a few hours of eye tracking to register dramatic improvements.[1]

Here's how to take immediate steps to improve your eyes' tracking ability and thus the part of your brain involved in this vital activity.

- You'll need a partner for this exercise.
- Take a ball-point pen with the point retracted. Focus on this end.
- Your partner should hold the pen 18–36 inches away from your eyes then move the pen according to the five tracking directions mentioned earlier.
- Up and down; straight across, left to right; near and far; sweeping upward arc; sweeping downward arc.
- Your partner should vary the speed with which the pen is moved. Meanwhile, hold your head still and track the moving pen only with your eyes.
- Notice in which of the five tracking arcs your eyes wobble, blink, jump, or have difficulties, then practice this specific tracking direction until your eye tracking goes more smoothly.
- Practice this for no more than 3–5 minutes at a time.

2 MORE EYE EXERCISES THAT ENHANCE BRAIN POWER

1. *Palming*. Finish this exercise with a relaxing technique from the field of optometry. Developed many years ago by William Bates, it's called *palming*. If you wear glasses, remove them.

   Cup your palms over your eyes, close your eyes, and hold your palms gently in position for 5 minutes. Tune into the gentle relaxing depth of the blackness which you can see and feel with your eyes closed.

2. *Flick gazing*. This neurological exercise also works with your eyes.[2] This exercise will engage about 80 percent of your brain to process visual information at a rate approximately 100 times its normal speed—or at least, that much faster than the speed you are accustomed to.

   You can do this anywhere—in your house, outside, in a shop, art gallery, bookstore, restaurant, supermarket. Flick your gaze around the room, pausing on individual objects for no more than one-half second.

- Every half-second, move your gaze to something new.
- Do this for 3 minutes; repeat two more times each day for 2 weeks.
- Every half second your brain is interpreting new visual data and providing the results to your awareness: chair, toaster, red hair, blue shoes, calendar, and so on.
- Your neurons can get quite nimble on this kind of exercise program.

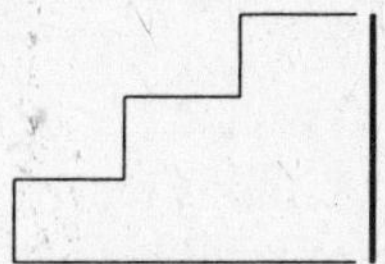

BRAIN-BUILDING SECRET #78
Why a Slap on Your Face Is the Best Memory Tool You'll Ever Get

There is a memorable scene in the movie *Beaches* in which Bette Midler slaps her husband on the face just as they are pronounced husband and wife. Naturally, he asks why she whacked him on the face. "This is the happiest day of my life and don't you forget it," she replies.

There is much wisdom in this simple strategy. If you register each moment with heightened attention, which is exactly what a quick hand across your cheek will do, you will remember it.

THE SNAPSHOT TECHNIQUE OF REMEMBERING THINGS

A variation on this approach is the snapshot method. Regardless of whether you are competent with a camera, you walk through your days as if you were taking photographs of the key events every 15 minutes. You willfully commit each moment, each scenario, each little family drama to memory by taking a mental picture of it. As you take the picture, you say to yourself: "Here I am committing this scene to memory and here I am aware that I am committing it to memory."

THE EMOTIONAL FIX TECHNIQUE OF REMEMBERING

There are other similar approaches to the face slap approach to memory. Correlate your information with sensory or visual associations.

Give the information a context; that is, assign an emotional quality or weight to it. Note what is distinctive, different, or outstanding in the information. See if it has anything to do with your personal survival, sense of personal importance, or personal association. Repeat it several times to yourself, to reinforce the impressions. Do this first and last in any memory-building sessions. In other words, if it is an important item of information, go over it at the beginning of a study session, then reiterate it just before you finish.

FINDING THE SECRET REASONS WHY YOU DON'T WANT TO REMEMBER

Admittedly, brain-building secrets will give you many techniques to improving your memory, but I wish to tell you frankly that in my opinion a great deal of the worry given to memory and memory loss is entirely overrated.

By the time you get to this brain-building section on memory, you will already have taken many steps that will naturally improve your ability to commit information to memory and to recall it.

As you learned in earlier chapters, many aspects of the way you probably live interfere with the natural vitality and range of your memory. Remove these, add a few health-promoting practices and substances, and you are already in a new memory league.

Bear in mind that there are a number of factors that can interfere with your natural memory ability. Most of these we have already touched on in the book, but I will quickly review them again. Obviously, if you have Alzheimer's, any form of senile dementia, or multi-infarct dementia, your memory will not be working like the good old days.

Other organic problems interfering with memory include syphilis, encephalitis, meningitis, metabolic problems and biochemical imbalances in your body, congestive heart failure, chronic illness such as cardiovascular disease, colds, flu, ear infections, or bronchitis.

You should know by now that many conventional medications, both over-the-counter and prescription drugs, can interrupt your memory processes. It's imporant to note, too, that if you have undiagnosed vision problems (such as presbyopia, which is middle-aged nearsightedness) or hearing deficits, this may significantly get in the way of your processing information and committing it to memory.

Other memory-inhibiting factors include fatigue, lack of exercise, alcohol, and smoking.

YOU'VE GOT AN ATTITUDE—THAT'S WHY YOU AREN'T REMEMBERING

There are psychological factors that can interfere with your ability to remember. One is highly obvious yet often overlooked. Your attitude or self-concept. If you believe you cannot remember an item or subject, this belief becomes self-fulfilling and you forget it.

If you think your memory is poor, *your attitude itself* keeps weakening what might otherwise be a strong memory power. Depression, stress, and anxiety also put blocks on your natural memory abilities.

Throughout this book, I have encouraged you to first *remove the obstacles* to your natural brain power and then to add brain power enhancing practices. Many memory books put the cart before the horse. They give you numerous tips for improving your memory but never show you how to remove all the hidden obstacles that make your memory less than perfect in the first place.

WHY THE BEST MEMORY DEVICE IS A POCKET NOTEBOOK

Let me share a secret. My memory is reasonably good and usually doesn't let me down. I can remember the names and faces of obscure movie actors who appear in numerous different films—from the 1940s or the 1990s. This seems to impress friends. I can usually remember what I need to do on errands or shopping expeditions or if I'm having a meeting or giving a seminar.

What's my technique?

First: I *pay attention* as the information is presented to me.

Second: I make *lists*.

Third: I write myself a copious amount of *notes*.

Fourth: I keep a *running journal* of important events, interesting thoughts, or people encountered.

Fifth: I keep an *active* Rolodex of names and addreses, birthdates, anniversaries.

Sixth: I enter appointments and tasks in a *daily desk diary* that opens out to two pages.

Technically, I don't have to remember that much with these systems in place; I only have to remember to consult them. What's the difference, anyway, whether I commit the information as short-term memory in my mind or if I remember to write myself notes and keep lists, Rolodexes, diaries, and journals?

BE THERE IN THE FIRST PLACE TO REMEMBER IT WHILE IT HAPPENS

Give yourself a break. And be honest with yourself: sometimes there are emotional reasons why you do not wish to remember an item, face, or person. Find out if this is the case with you; otherwise, you will be pushing the boulder uphill.

If you can't remember things, write yourself a lot of notes. And next time something interesting comes before you, *pay more attention*, take a mental snapshot of it, slap yourself on the face, do a voice-over as if you're a TV journalist—*be there in the first place* to be able to remember it later.

If you are about to commit something important to memory, calm yourself, pay attention to your breathing, take 5 minutes to chill out. Practice Brain-Building Secrets #12, 13, 40, and 42 to develop inner calm and outer attentiveness. Biologists call this *state-dependent learning* and behavior.

If you are calm and focused when you study a subject or commit an item to memory, you need only return to this same state of mind to be able to easily recall it later. In other words, probably the smartest thing you can do to improve your memory is to prepare the best state of mind and body for brain power. Your *calm breathing and focused attention* will be your most reliable memory tools.

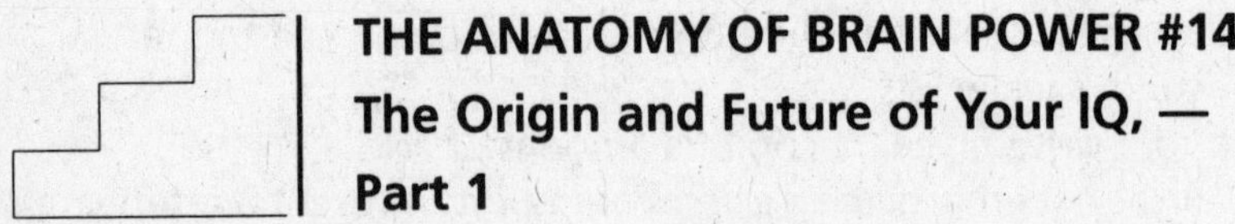

THE ANATOMY OF BRAIN POWER #14

The Origin and Future of Your IQ, — Part 1

So much of the way you think about your brain power is measured in terms of IQ, or intelligence quotient. But where does this measurement come from, how does it work, and does it really say anything accurate about how smart you might be?

Technically, IQ is a comparative score or number that indicates how intelligent a person is relative to that person's age in comparison with other people of that age or societal group. According to the child psychologists who originally devised it, you take a person's mental age, divide it by his chronological age (calculated at less than age 14), then multiply this by 100 to eliminate decimal points.

The most well-known intelligence test is called the Stanford-Binet and was developed and first used in France in 1905. At that time, the French government asked two psychologists, Theodore Simon and Alfred Binet, to devise a test that would distinguish slow-learning children from "normally" learning ones. The idea was to figure out a standard learning rate for children at different mental ages. The IQ test, after some improvements, included 129 categories.

Over the years the test was further revised, with an important addition being contributed by Lewis Terman of Stanford University in 1960—hence, the present name, Stanford-Binet. It tested children age 2 up to young adults, age 23, in areas such as vocabulary, arithmetic, ingenuity, sentence memory, understanding opposite analogies, sentence building, orientation, reversing digits, reconciling opposites, perceiving basic differences, and other mostly verbal or logical subjects.

Now, more than 90 years after it was first devised, psychologists rely on the Stanford-Binet test to tell them about the IQ of "normal," "retarded," gifted, and superintelligent children.

In 1949, another IQ test came along, called the Wechsler Intelligence Scale for Children. Originally, the test was very limited in scope, based on the exclusively Caucasian children drawn from families whose fathers worked in nine specified fields. Eventually, the test, renamed Wechsler Adult Intelligence Scale, or WAIS, was broadened to reflect the IQs of children from other social groups and family backgrounds.

Even so, both WAIS and Stanford-Binet are still criticized for being misleading and not completely reliable gauges of IQ. In fact, psychologists have shown that the IQ results of a single child can vary by 20–30 points a day or a week, depending on psychological and health conditions of the child. So who can say if your 8-year-old boy's IQ is 110 or 140? It depends on how he feels when the test is given.

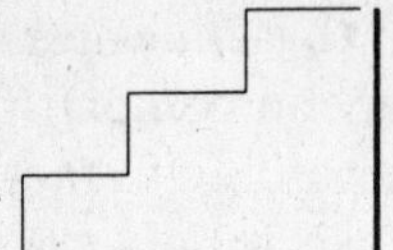

BRAIN-BUILDING SECRET #79
Talk to Both Sides of Your Brain and Unite the Hemispheres

The great nineteenth-century American jurist and author Oliver Wendell Holmes, known as "the autocrat of the breakfast table," once suggested that an excellent way to increase brain power is to think 10 "impossible thoughts" before breakfast. In our own time, the popular humanist educator Jean Houston has adapted Dr. Holmes's breakfast advice by often having her workshop participants start the day off by telling one another "three outrageous lies."

The idea, of course, is to stretch the brain by reinventing reality.[3] The idea behind the exercise is to integrate many brain functions of the left- and right-brain hemispheres, such as words and images, senses and emotions, numbers and holistic perception.

This brain-awakening exercise will take you about 25 minutes. It will work best for you if you read these instructions into a tape recorder so you can listen to the tape without interruptions and with your eyes closed.

VISITING YOUR BRAIN FROM THE INSIDE, FROM LEFT TO RIGHT

- Sit comfortably in a chair with your back straight, both feet on the floor. Take your shoes and glasses off; close your eyes.
- Breathe calmly and slowly; pay attention to your breathing, watch it rise and fall, inhale and exhale until you feel relaxed and attentive.
- Focus on the left side of your brain and then your left eye, still closed. Keeping your eye closed, look down, then up, then left, then right, then rotate it clockwise, then rotate it counterclockwise.
- Focus on the right side of your brain and then your right eye, still closed.
- Keeping your eye closed, look down, then up, then left, then right, then rotate it clockwise, then rotate it counterclockwise.

- Then relax, keep your eyes closed, and place your palms over them to ease the relaxation for 3 minutes.
- Keep your eyes closed. Place your attention in the left side of your brain for 10 seconds, then shift to the right side and hold it for 10 seconds.
- Repeat. Do you notice any differences in feeling, content, or concentration as you shift back and forth between your brain hemispheres? Is one easier to focus on than the other?
- Keep your eyes closed and visualize or imagine the following items on alternating sides of your brain: left brain/number 1; right brain, letter A; left side, number 2; right side, letter B; left side, number 3; right side, letter C.
- Continue with this all the way through the alphabet and up to the number 26.
- Rest for 3 minutes, then reverse the process. Right brain/number 1, then left brain, letter A; right side, number 2, left side, letter B; and all the way up to Z and 26.

Now go through this series of imaginings, alternating from your left brain to your right. After each image, let it dissolve before doing the next:

- right, a couple getting married
- left, nuns walking in pairs through a church
- right, a hurricane flooding a coastal town
- left, an atom
- right, a galaxy of stars
- left, an apple tree with white blossoms
- right, tree branches covered with snow
- left, a sunrise
- right, a sunset
- left, a tropical jungle
- right, a snow-covered mountain peak
- left, a three-ring circus

IMAGINARY ACTIVITIES—IT'S ALL HAPPENING INSIDE YOUR HEAD

Now shift to images that require you to imagine the sensation involved, moving from the left to the right sides of your brain:

- right, feeling a thick fog on your face
- left, climbing rocks and breathing vigorously
- right, caressing a baby's skin
- left, putting your hands into warm mud
- right, making snowballs with your bare hands
- left, pulling taffy
- right, punching a pillow
- left, hearing the sound of a fire engine
- right, hearing summer crickets
- left, hearing a car ignition turned on
- right, hearing a person singing in a high voice
- left, hearing waves breaking on a beach
- right, hearing your stomach growling
- left, smelling the aroma of a pine forest
- right, smelling fresh brewed dark roast coffee
- left, smelling gasoline fumes
- right, smelling the aroma of bread baking
- left, tasting a crisp, juicy apple

CROSSING THE BRIDGE BETWEEN THE HEMISPHERES

- Keeping your eyes closed, use your left eye to look "into" your left brain, as if you are exploring it with a searchlight.
- Do the same with your right eye and right brain.
- Use your left eye to trace triangles inside your left brain; then do rectangles, then stars. Do the same with your right eye in your right brain.
- Make a series of circles that overlap one another in your left brain; imagine that these circular lines give off healing light to this hemisphere.

- Do the same in your right brain.
- Now use both eyes, still closed, to make circles in the center of your forehead and head, in the corpus callosum that bridges both brain hemsipheres.
- From this point, widen the circles of light to include all of your brain. Then, make very wide circles in your brain and slowly make them smaller and smaller until the circle has become a point in between your eyes.
- Keep your attention and breathing focused on this single point in your brain.

IMAGINARY TREES, HARPS, AND EAGLES IN YOUR BRAIN

- Imagine there is a large tree growing in the center of your forehead, from out of this single point.
- Now imagine there is a golden harp in your left brain and a drum in your right.
- Dissolve these pictures and imagine an eagle in the left side, a canary on the right. See them both at once then let the image go.
- Focus your attention on your left brain and try to imagine what it looks like, with its folds of gray matter. Do the same for your right brain.
- Now sense both sides at once, your whole brain. Be aware of the billions of brain cells talking to one another, sending messages, electrical sparks, and brain chemicals.
- Sense that your very concentration in this moment has made possible this huge amount of neuronal activity.
- Link your breathing with your whole brain. As you inhale, your brain expands; as you exhale, it contracts. With every breath, your brain is enriched with oxygen and brain power.

ORDERING UP NEW BRAIN CELLS AT THE NEURONAL PHARMACY

- Now it's time to talk directly to your brain. Tell it you want it to make more brain cells available to you, to grow more dendrites connecting the cells, that as a result, you will have more brain power, faster thinking, and greater mental abilities.

- Give your brain a chance to respond in whatever way it chooses.
- Meanwhile, you might take your palms and place them a few inches from your head and caress the energy field of your brain power. Try this for 3 to 5 minutes.
- Relax and continue breathing quietly for a few minutes, then open your eyes.
- Quite likely you'll feel relaxed and alert, and you may have a brand-new attitude about the 3 1/2-pound universe you've been carrying on top of your shoulders all these years.

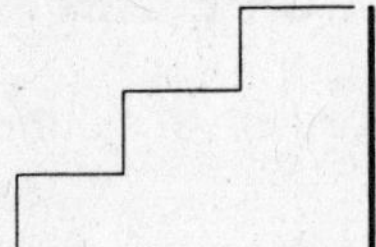

THE ANATOMY OF BRAIN POWER #15
How the Two Halves Live Inside Your One Brain

Right-brained, left-brained—how many brains do you have? We hear quite often that a person is too *left*-brained or completely *right*-brained, and in either case most often the person saying this means it critically. Of course you have only *one whole* brain, but according to brain scientists, different mental functions appear to be localized in different sections of the brain.

Scientists call this the *lateralization* of brain function, meaning that different mental abilities are parceled out laterally, to either the left or right hemisphere. It is also well known by now that your brain's two hemispheres are not biologically equal; they are, in fact, asymmetrical, naturally, in terms of shape and function.

Your left hemisphere has more gray matter, a greater specific gravity, and a wider occiptal lobe; your right hemisphere is heavier, has a wider frontal lobe, and shows a larger internal skull size. That is why *brain asymmetry* is a natural feature of your brain.[4]

For example, studies of brain waves (EEGs) of subjects performing different tasks showed this difference of function between the hemispheres quite clearly. While the subjects were working on a task requiring visual and spatial integration, the brain waves showed that the left hemisphere was idling in a kind of relaxed electrical state. Then when the subjects changed activities and started to write letters, the brain waves of their right brain were idle.

AN ANATOMY OF BRAIN POWER SECRET

Certain key qualities of brain function, such as visual-spatial orientation and verbal-analytical activity, also appear to be localized in either of the brain's two hemispheres.

Left hemisphere. In your brain's *left hemisphere* occur the activities of reading, writing, arithmetic and number skills, calculation, spoken language and language skills, scientific skills, reasoning, linear, logical processing, and right-hand control. In the left hemisphere you have your brain's basic language center, which is basically a linear information-processing activity.

Right hemisphere. In your brain's *right hemisphere* you have music awareness, spatial construction and artistic intelligence, holistic thinking, imagination, insight, intuition, three-dimensional and pattern perception, and left-hand control. In the right brain, you have the center for geometry, rotating shapes in your mind, mental map-making, and all aspects of spatial perception.

The bridge between the two. Your two brain hemispheres are linked by the *corpus callosum*. This is a thick bundle of 200 million nerve fibers that is white in appearance and 4–6 centimeters in length. The corpus callosum is both an instant communication bridge between the hemispheres and a kind of inhibitor that prevents too much electrical stimulation from jumping across the hemispheres and upsetting brain function. Each of the 200 million nerve fibers in the corpus callosum originates in one hemisphere and goes directly to the opposite.[5]

20 MILLION MORE NERVE FIBERS IN THE WOMAN'S BRAIN

Biologists have determined that there are distinct differences between the corpus callosum of a male and female brain. The corpus callosum on the average is 10 percent larger in females and it matures up to 3 years sooner in women than in males, usually between the ages of 9–12. This difference in size implies that the female corpus callosum may contain 20 million more axon nerve fibers than in the male brain.

Further, brain impulses travel 5–10 percent faster in the female corpus callosum than through the male's, which means that women can potentially process information and generate solutions to mental problems faster than the average man.

BRAIN-BUILDING SECRET #80

A Meeting of the Hemispheres—In Your Brain

Here is an exercise for getting acquainted with your brain hemispheres and for seeing into which of the two now-famous brain camps you belong.

Is your preference left brained (verbal/analytical/rational) or right brained (visual-spatial/intuitive)? Check one answer for each question.[6]

1. In your opinion, is *daydreaming* (a) a waste of time, (b) an amusing way to relax, (c) helpful in solving problems and thinking creatively, (d) a good way to plan your future?
2. What's your attitude about *hunches*? (a) Your hunches are strong and you follow them. (b) You are not aware of following any hunches that come to mind. (c) You may have hunches but you don't trust them. (d) You'd have to be crazy to base a decision on a mere hunch.
3. When it comes to *problem solving*, do you (a) get contemplative, thinking it over on a walk, with friends; (b) make a list of alternatives, determine priorities among them, and take the one at the top; (c) consult the past, by remembering how you handled something similar to this situation before; (d) watch television, hoping the problem will go away?
4. Take a moment to relax, put this book down, close your eyes, and put your hands in your lap, one on top of the other. Which hand is on top? (a) Your right hand; (b) your left hand; (c) neither, because they are parallel?
5. Are you goal oriented? (a) True; (b) False.

6. When you were in school, you preferred algebra to geometry? (a) True; (b) False.
7. Generally speaking, you are a *very organized* type of person, for whom everything has its proper place and there is a system for doing anything. (a) True; (b) False.
8. When it comes to speaking or writing or expressing yourself with words, you do pretty well? (a) True; (b) False.
9. When you're at a party, do you find yourself more natural at listening rather than talking? (a) True; (b) False.
10. You don't need to check your watch to accurately tell how much time has passed. (a) True; (b) False.
11. When it comes to athletics, somehow you perform even better than what you should expect from the amount of training or natural abilities you have. (a) True; (b) False.
12. If it's a matter of work, you much prefer going solo to working by committee. (a) True; (b) False.
13. You have a near photographic memory for faces. (a) True; (b) False.
14. If you had your way, you would redecorate your home often, take trips frequently, and change your environment as much as possible. (a) Yes; (b) No.
15. You are a regular James Bond when it comes to taking risks. (a) Yes; (b) No.

Here's how to score yourself: **1.** (a) 1; (b) 5; (c) 7; (d) 9. **2.** (a) 9; (b) 7; (c) 3; (d) 1. **3.** (a) 7; (b) 1; (c) 3; (d) 9. **4.** (a) 1; (b) 9); (c) 5. **5.** (a) 1; (b) 9. **6.** (a) 1; (b) 9. **7.** (a) 1; (b) 9. **8.** (a) 1; (b) 7. **9.** (a) 6; (b) 3. **10.** (a) 1; (b) 9. **11.** (a) 9; (b) 1. **12.** (a) 3; (b) 7. **13.** (a) 7; (b) 1. **14.** (a) 9; (b) 1. **15.** (a) 7; (b) 3.

After you total your points, divide this by 15 for your hemisphere score. The lower your number, the more left-brained you are; the higher the count, the more right-brained. For example, if your score is 1, by this measure you are a first-class professional left-brained person; on the other hand, if your score is 8, you are intuition incarnate, exceptionally right-brained; a score of 5 means your corpus callosum is intact, and there is regular traffic between your two brain hemispheres.

ENTRAINMENT OF THE HEMISPHERES IS A KEY TO BRAIN POWER

Let's add one more item of interest about your brain hemispheres. Neuroscientists have demonstrated that each of your brain's two hemispheres has its own characteristic brain wave pattern. On a practical level, this means the EEG frequency of your left hemisphere isn't always in phase or coherent with that of its neighbor on the right. Your brain hemispheres are like ships passing in the night.

The brain does not ordinarily show a high degree of hemispheric coherence, but when it does, under special circumstances, wonderful things result: heightened creativity, insight, rapid learning, enhanced well-being, inner peace, meditative states. When the brain waves of both hemispheres lock into a common, integrated step, that's called *entrainment* (some call it whole brain "synchrony")—two waves beating together, as electronics people say.

Entrainment apparently heightens the release of specific brain chemicals called neurotransmitters—most well known of which is the mind's chief opiate, beta-endorphin—which enhance mental, emotional, and physiologic function and often produce euphoria.

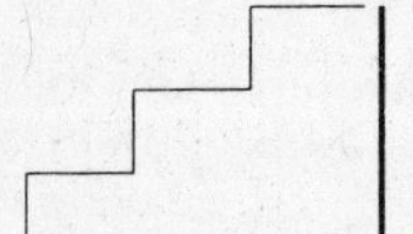

BRAIN-BUILDING SECRET #81

2 Ways to Get Neurologically Friendly with What You're Studying

According to brain power expert Win Wenger, if you want to learn better, you must increase your *neurological contact* with the material you are trying to learn. To do this, Wenger teaches a method he calls *freenoting*. Say you're attending a lecture; pay no attention to what the speaker is saying.

FREENOTING

With perhaps just one ear cocked to hear the general drift of the speaker's argument, devote the rest of your attention to writing down at a "furious" pace and without pausing all the thoughts that come to mind relative to the topic.

Do this for 5–15 minutes, without repeating yourself but keeping your writing at least tangential to the lecture topic. The goal of this unusual exercise is not to insult the speaker by outdoing him or ignoring him, but to see what untapped treasures of insight you might have available within you.

In fact, Wenger invites readers of his books to freenote him while they read, even to write "furiously" in the margins and inside covers in response to what they encounter in the text.

The exercise gets you into direct, even intimate, neurological contact with the material you are studying. Your commentary, critique, and independent brainstorming inspired by the book actually brings your mind in close, working relationship with the book material. That in itself is both stimulating and an aid for memory.[7]

The more you express out loud or in spontaneous writing of what you perceive, the more you actually are able to perceive. Similarly, you will learn far more when it comes as feedback from your own activities; in this case, your freenoting commentary on somebody else's information.

TAKING NOTES PLUS WISECRACKS

This is a variation on freenoting. Say you are at that same lecture, or perhaps it's after the break and you've just sat down again for part two of the talk.

- Divide your notebook pages into a two-third column on the left and a one-third column on the right.
- In the left column, write down the substance of the talk or study information, the facts, figures, quotes, reasons, problems.
- In the right column, write down your thoughts, feelings, impressions, daydreams, attitudes, reactions, commentary, questions, disagreements, and concerns with the same material.
- This column is a stream-of-consciousness running commentary on the material you are summarizing in the left-hand column.

What happens here is that your conscious and subconscious mind are simultaneously engaged in purposefully reporting and responding to the same set of mental events and information. It's like having two reporters, not one, covering the event.

Or you might see it as having one reporter on hand to report the facts, while the other handles the gossip. Feel free to use symbols, cartoons, balloons, arrows, exclamation marks, happy faces, stars, crosses, or other unusual symbols to concentrate your impressions.

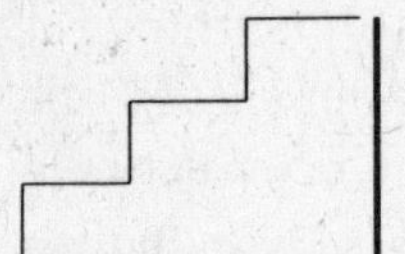

BRAIN-BUILDING SECRET #82

2 Ways to Map Your Mind and Herd Your Ideas into Clusters

The Holographic Mind Map

Yet another variation on this idea is based on a technique brain power researcher Tony Buzan developed in the 1970s, called MindMapping™ which numerous brain power teachers have been working with ever since.

Making a map of the mind is a whole-brain approach that takes advantage of how your brain actually organizes information and relates one idea to the next. It is not linear or sequential by any means, but holographic. That means everything is connected to everything else and each part contains information about the whole.

Linear, logical, rational thinking is not the original way your mind processes information. It is the outcome of a great many simultaneous and complex mental processes by which your brain orders, selects, searches, sorts, links, formulates, organizes, and makes sense of pictures, symbols, feelings, sounds, and images, so that it can put it all together into words and sentences that somebody else can comprehend.

In other words, in the beginning—as far as the secret inner life of your brain is concerned—all is diverse, random, even chaotic impressions and thoughts that need to be organized into logic-based expressions.

So why not take this fact and make it the centerpiece of a brain-building exercise? The Mind Map calls on your whole brain to generate a visual pattern of connected ideas. The result is a kind of interactive mirror of how your mind goes about making connections, seeing relationships, generating ideas, and making plans.

You can use this approach to take notes at a lecture, summarize information from a textbook, to register impressions and thoughts while interviewing somebody for a post, or to plan a speech or paper.

- You start with a large blank piece of paper and several colored pens.
- Determine what your main idea or theme is, then print this in the center of the page and enclose it in a circle or square.
- Think of several key related points and add these to the page, as if they are branches extending out from the central square.
- Connect them to the center with single lines. You might use a different color to make each branching point.
- Write a descriptive word on each branch as a kind of guide to the contents of the point.
- Add pictures, symbols, or illustrations as you feel inspired. Underline words, write them in bold or capital letters as you feel necessary to make your idea map personal.
- Let the Mind Map grow organically as your thought processes kick into high creative gear.
- The end result may well resemble a road map to a complex neighborhood, except in this case it's your thinking on a single idea.

HERDING YOUR THOUGHTS INTO A CLUSTER

The idea here is to make a clustering of ideas on paper in such a way that they mirror how your mind processes and sorts information in a creative way. You quickly sort through a jumble of ideas and put them down on paper without judging or editing them.

In this way you actually trace the path your brain takes in developing a concept out of a mass of raw unsorted information. Like making Mind Maps, clustering shows you how to see and make connections between ideas and how to expand on these concepts.

All thoughts are given equal rank, which sets up a chain reaction of associations and relations—a cluster of ideas.

- Start with a large blank piece of paper.

- Select a key idea, a big term or word, such as *freedom*, *vacation*, *work*, or with opposites such as *men/women*, *love/hate*, *single/married*.
- Circle this word.
- Now think of all the associated ideas or concepts that relate to this key word.
- Write these down in circles and connect the secondary circles to the primary one at the center of the page.
- Keep the process going in a lively, spontaneous, unedited way, until you have generated a page of clustered ideas.

The value of this exercise is that it shows you how to work creatively and productively with a host (a cluster) of ideas without pulling in the reins, without editing them. Because you are not censoring associations as they come up, your brain is inspired to keep generating more connections.

Eventually, you might find a nugget of gold amid all the circled words. It keeps your thinking flexible and it may well help you to write more easily, even if it's only a letter to a friend.

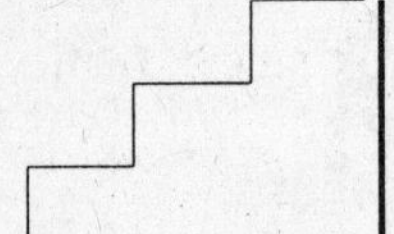

THE ANATOMY OF BRAIN POWER #16
The Origin and Future of Your IQ—Part 2

Now there's a new IQ test being tried out by child psychologists in Canada. There are no questions, no written test, nothing to do with what a child may have learned in school. Instead, this unusual IQ test is based on looking at a light.

The child wears electrodes on his head to pick up brain waves, and this information goes to a computer that displays them using a special device called an oscilloscope. This, in turn, flashes a light every second for 2 minutes. The idea is to see how quickly the brain respond to the flashing light.

According to the test's inventors, this will show, objectively, how capable the child is at learning, how *quickly* the child can understand what is required, and whether these results are appropriate to the child's age.

According to the psychologists, this is the basis of IQ. Of course, there is a problem here. Suppose your child is slow on the draw in terms of figuring out connections between words and objects, actions and results, problems and solutions. Yet your child is a mechanical genius or has great ability, at age 6, on the piano. Is she smart or dumb? The standard IQ test may give you a wrong impression, and it may set you off on a disappointing track for years.

Since standard IQ tests do not accurately measure all the aspects of brain power, your child—or perhaps yourself—may spend years and decades with a serious *underestimation* of your real brain power.

Creativity studies have shown that people with high IQs may still have gaps in their whole brain abilities. They may be unable to think independently, lack a sense of humor, be unreasonable, be unappreciative of beauty, be unable to deal with complexity or novelty, be original, fluent, flexible, or asture.

Be careful with the IQ numbers. They are at best relative indicators of a few aspects of your potential brain power but not the whole "cerebral" ball game by any means.

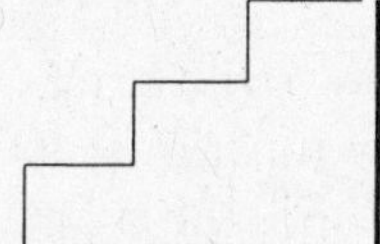

BRAIN BULDING SECRET #83
Say It Out Loud to Amplify Your Intelligence

This exercise is based on an idea called *image streaming*. The goal is to take the impressions that your right brain gathers and translate them into spoken words. This exercise focuses your (left-brained) attention on the (right-brained) stream of *spontaneous* mental imagery.[8]

You describe your inner experiences and impressions by speaking them out loud. In this way, your two brain hemispheres are encouraged to work together. When you make the effort to describe out loud the sensory impressions, fantasies, and inner images happening in your nonverbal right-brain hemisphere, this linkage strengthens your brain and its overall abilities.

Remarkably, this act alone helps increase your IQ and language ability; it will also improve your ability to be alert, attentive, observant, and mindful, which, as you saw earlier in the book, are important foundations for brain power. In this case, you're watching your mind at work.

YOU ARE A JOURNALIST COVERING THE ACTS OF YOUR OWN PERCEPTION

The exercise is easy and entertaining. Here are the steps:

- Select some music that you know helps you relax, tune inward, and generate images and impressions, and play this at a low volume. (See Brain-Building Secrets #67, 68, 71, 72, and 73 for suggestions on brain power enhancing music and mind-training tapes. See the Resources for ordering information.) You can do this exercise without music if you wish.
- Sit comfortably in a chair in a room where you won't be disturbed, take off your shoes and glasses, relax, close your eyes.
- For maximum benefit from this *left-brain enhancing* exercise, check your nasal cycle to see which nostril is dominant.
- If your left nostril is clogged, this means your left brain is active and the appropriate brain hemisphere for this exercise is dominant.
- If your right nostril is blocked, this means your right hemisphere (regulating nonverbal, spatial, intuitive functions) is dominant. You can either wait 90–120 minutes until the brain hemispheres shift naturally, or you can apply Brain-Building Secret #33 and voluntarily shift your nasal cycle and brain hemisphere dominance now.
- Breathe calmly and slowly; pay attention to your breathing, watch it rise and fall, inhale and exhale until you feel relaxed and attentive.
- Pretend that you are holding the microphone for a tape recorder in your hands. You are going to interview yourself.
- Now observe what is happening in your mind. Are there images, pictures, dream fragments, thoughts, memories, emotions, or physical sensations?
- Note what is happening right now and start to describe it, as if you were a journalist objectively describing an important event to a live radio or television audience.

- Be thorough; emphasize the details, such as color, shape, texture, sound, movement. Make it interesting; try to convey what you are seeing or sensing in vivid, exciting language.

THE MOST IMPORTANT THING IS TO *SAY IT OUT LOUD*

- Don't worry if what you are saying seems to make no sense; saying it out loud is what is most important.
- Try to continue this oral description for 15–20 minutes. You needn't worry about your mind running out of material; your mind is unbelievably creative, and unless you have spent a very long time meditating, it will never cease to generate new impressions and sensations.
- If you are unable to generate a spontaneous stream of images in your first attempt, there are some alternate strategies to get things started.
- Try remembering a recent dream and start narrating the details of one of its most dramatic scenes. If you can't think of a dream, bring to mind a beautiful scene you have recently visited or seen, such as a park, beach, waterfall, mountain vista, or view from an airplane.
- Describe this out loud. If this doesn't work, stare directly at a light bulb for about 30–45 seconds then look away and close your eyes.
- Examine the after-image this bright light has left on your retina, and start describing what you see. Even if you are a remarkably nonvisual person, after 3–6 tries with this approach, images will start streaming.
- The goal is to have new images spontaneously arising even as you are describing them.

LYING ON YOUR BACK AND WATCH THE IMAGES STREAM DOWN YOUR LEGS

After you've tried image streaming, do it again, adding this new factor.

- Lie flat on your back on the floor, without a pillow, and put your feet up on a chair so that they are about 12 inches off the floor and higher than your head.
- Bend your knees comfortably so that your legs can rest on the chair without falling asleep.
- Take several deep and relaxing breaths, exhaling through your nose.
- Then do image streaming again in this position.
- When you are finished, lower your legs and sit up slowly, remaining in this position for a few moments until your circulation stabilizes again.[9]

AN EXERCISE THAT CAPITALIZES ON THE WAY YOUR BRAIN WORKS

This exercise is based on taking advantage of certain facts about the physiology of your brain. Your right brain (associated with spatial, intuitive, and artistic functions) apparently works 10,000 *times faster* than your left brain (which deals with language, analytical, linear activities).

Your left brain moves at the speed of language, which is quite slow; your right hemisphere processes at something approaching light speed, at least metaphorically speaking. In practical terms, your mental activity is many times faster in your right brain (and in effect unconscious or beyond your consciousness) than anything that your conscious left brain can handle.

Add to this the fact that for one consciously registered thought or impression (in your left brain), your right brain is picking up probably 100 more peripheral impressions—"seeing out of the corner of your eye," as the popular expression has it.

In some miraculous way, all these right-brain sensory impressions are still stored somewhere in your memory, even though you were barely aware of them in the first place. They remain available as a kind of superbrain resource; in moments of insight or spontaneous intuition (or dreams) they become available to your conscious mind.

You have in effect a vast data bank of information that normally you do not call upon. Image streaming, or "focused describing," starts to call up this data and make it available to your conscious mind.

It may strike you as both odd and hard to believe, yet several independent studies on this technique have shown that it can increase IQ factors, such as your ability to solve problems and your ability to use languages by approximately 1 point for every 80 minutes of practicing the exercise.[10]

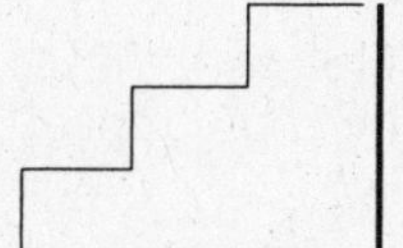

THE ANATOMY OF BRAIN POWER #17 Profiles of the Great Rememberers and Their Feats of Memory

History is rich with anecdotes of men and women with outstanding memory abilities, people we shall call GRs.

GR. Cardinal Mezzofani spoke 60 languages, most of them fluently.

GR. Dario Donatelli, still living, broke the world's speed memorization record when he accurately recalled a list of 73 numbers only 48 seconds after he first heard the number series. The previous world record had been, since 1911, a series of 18 digits.

GR. A Bombay yogi named Shaa could after only one hearing or reading repeat 1,000 phrases from memory. The legend has it that he could master any poem, in any language, after one hearing.

GR. Antonio de Marco Magliabechi, an Italian born in 1633, had an awesomely accurate photographic memory coupled with a mastery of speed reading. He could write out the entire contents of a book after one reading. He gained a reputation for being able to speed read books and memorize their entire contents—a walking, talking encyclopedia.

GR. There are Hindu students who have committed the entire text of the Rig Veda, one of India's sacred texts, to memory. This text includes 153,826 words.

GR. The twentieth-century Russian newspaperman Solomon Veniaminoff had one of the most astounding memories ever studied by scientists. Upon hearing a list of 70 numbers once, Veniaminoff could recite them back at once, forward or backward, with complete accuracy. He could be shown a list of 13 number pairs, with 4 numbers per pair; he would study it for 3 minutes, put the list away, then accurately call out the numbers in order or different combinations, even diagonally.

The scientist studying him—the famous psychologist Alksandr Luria, who studied him for 30 years—admitted his feats put him in a state of confusion. "I simply had to admit that the capacity of his memory had *no distinct limits.*"

GR. Christian Friedrich Hernaker, the infant genius of Lübeck, Germany, was born in 1721. By the age of 10 months he could repeat every word spoken to him; by age 1 year, he knew every event described in the first five books of the Old Testament; by age 3, he could speak Latin and French and had a comprehensive knowledge of geography, world history, and all the facts of biblical history. He even predicted his own death, at little over 4 years old.

GR. A Turk named Mehmed Ali Halici accurately quoted 6,500 verses from the Koran in 6 hours.

GR. An Edinburgh University professor could correctly remember the first 1,000 decimal places in the mathematical function called π (pi). A Japanese prodigy supposedly could recall the first 10,000 places of π.

GR. George Parker Bidder, born in 1806 in England, was known as the child prodigy of calculation. He could perform complex math calculations instantly in his head, without paper or hesitation. His photographic memory was such that he apparently could see the long rows and columns of numbers visually in his mind.

GR. Maori Chief Kaumatana from New Zealand could recite the entire history of his tribe, spanning 45 generations and 1,000 years; it would take him 3 days and he never used any notes.

GR. Paul Charles Morphy, an American born in 1837, was one of the greatest chess players of all time. More impressive yet was his ability to play chess blindfolded, which requires perfect recall of all previous moves, without the aid of having ever seen them.

Even more astonishing, he could play several chess games at the same time, blindfolded. Morphy claimed that he could remember every chess move he had ever made in all the chess games he had ever played in his long career, even the ones in which he had been blindfolded.

GR. Dan Mikels, a memory instructor at SuperCamp, an educational environment for "Quantum Learning" devised by Bobbi DePorter, memorized the entire contents—names, addresses, and phone numbers—of the Los Angeles telephone directory and went on national television to prove it.

GR. History and folklore is rich with tales of clever idiots, or idiot savants. This strange phenomenon is exemplified in the recent movie, *Rain Man*, in which Dustin Hoffman plays a man whose brain power is focused solely into a remarkable ability with number calculations; otherwise, he is technically, severely retarded.

GR. Jacques Inaudi was a French "clever idiot" who at 13 could not read or write yet could calculate the cube root of 9-digit numbers and the fifth root of 12-digit numbers—in his head in seconds. He completed a complex calculation in 20 minutes that would have taken the ordinary intelligent person 15 days to figure.

GR. An American named Truman Safford was able to calculate the square of an 18-digit number in 1 minute. According to observers, his technique—or the way his body cavorted while his mind was performing the calculations—was rather striking: "He flew round the room like a top, pulled his pantaloons over the top of his boots, bit his hand, rolled his eyes in their sockets, sometimes smiling and talking and then, seeming to be in an agony, in not more than one minute replied."[11]

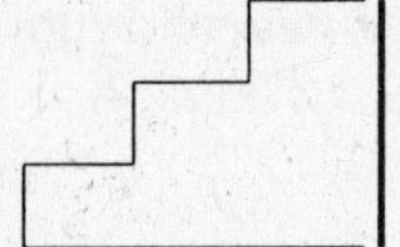

BRAIN-BUILDING SECRET #84
Play It Again, Sam, and Meet Your Brainier Half in the Future

This exercise is both similar to and different from Brain-Building Secret #83 which deals with image streaming. Now you will describe out loud a stream of *directed* images, pictures, and memories that you deliberately set into motion and then observe like a TV journalist reporting live from the scene.[12] The idea is that you build brain power by actively describing and attentively observing a remembered event.

REPORTING LIVE, FROM YOUR PAST

- Search through your memory banks for a pleasurable memory of an experience, location, or encounter that you would like to revisit to mine for yet more enjoyment. This could be
- the day you got married (or divorced)
- a high school or college graduation
- an awards ceremony
- a surprise meeting with a long-lost acquaintance
- an unexpected but deserved raise or promotion at work
- Close your eyes; then narrate the details of this event, out loud, as you remember them, and speak into your tape recorder. If you prefer, tell it to an impartial listener. The idea is to expand your perception within the given framework of a single event, retrieved from your memory.
- Describe this remembered scene in as much detail as possible. Pretend that you are there again, in person, in that time, experiencing the event for the first time.
- Narrate it with this in mind, emphasizing as much of the sensory detail as possible, what the weather is like, what the air smells like, what clothes you are wearing, how you feel, what the environment around you is like.
- Act as if you are a live anchorperson for a television news station covering an important event live for an interested viewing audience. *Make sure you speak of it out loud and in the present tense; act as if it is happening right now.*
- Try to remember another 4–6 events from your past and run them through this *Play It Again, Sam*, describe out loud technique.

OUR SPECIAL GUEST, THE SUPERMASTER BRAIN POWER EXPERT—YOU

With this practice established, you are ready for the next level of directing your imagery. In this case, you will be imagining yourself as a person in the future who has already mastered all the brain-building secrets outlined in this book and who now embodies the highest in brain power possibilities.

- You are about to meet the brainier part of yourself, as you could be (and probably would like to be) in the future. Or if you want to think in terms of science fiction, you will meet yourself as you are now in an alternate or parallel reality as a brain power master.
- Start by picturing yourself standing in a lush, sensory-rich setting, perhaps on a beach, under the bright sun, by a waterfall, in a tropical garden, in an apple orchard in blossom, on a mountain top.
- Describe out loud how you appear to yourself. Remember, this new version of yourself is a brain power master, the possessor of everything you ever hoped to gain in terms of mental abilities, memory, information-processing speed, creativity, and intuition.
- Describe out loud into your tape recorder how this alternate you is—how you look, feel, what impression you give.
- Now step into this alternate you and become your brainier self. As you do so, try to remember the process of becoming this brain power master, how you mastered all the brain-building secrets, all the exercises you mastered, the techniques you practiced, and the amazing gains in brain power you achieved.
- Recite your impressions and "memories" out loud in complete detail.
- Return to your "old" less smart self and take stock of your impressions of how this feels, after having been, at least momentarily, a near genius disguised as your humble self.
- Remember to describe all your impressions out loud into your tape recorder, just as if you were an impartial TV journalist covering a fast-breaking news development.
- Return to being your brainier self. Describe any new sensations, thoughts, or impressions.

ANY COMMENTS FROM YOUR BRAINIER HALF?

- How does it feel to be *this smart*, at last?
- Does It feel differently being in this body of your brainier self? Are your perceptions sharper, do you hear and see and smell more keenly?

- Now, see if you can think up a phrase, single sentence, or even one word that summarizes the novel experience of being your brainier self. For example, you might say
- "exalted intellect"
- "formidable mind"
- "all-encompassing, competent beyond belief"
- "He (she) is able to think anything."
- Finally, returning to your "old" self, use this word, sentence, or phrase as a way of summoning up the experience of being your brainier self.
- When you say the phrase *exalted intellect*, for example, you immediately move into the state of mind—and the brain power—that is your brainier self. *Believe it until it's real.*

This is like pulling yourself up by your own bootstraps or a kind of *brain power petard*: you are self-launched into a brainier state. When you can feel the mind qualities of this brainier self, you have in effect claimed them already for your own.

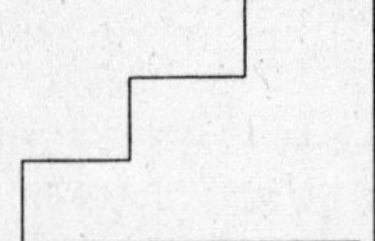

BRAIN-BUILDING SECRET #85
Seeing the Picture with Your Mind's Eye—And Describing It

This exercise involves some of the principles and techniques of Brain-Building Secret #84 but works in the reverse direction. Here you will study an actual picture, describe its features out loud, then memorize it and recreate it inside your mind.

This exercise will train your mind to be better at *visualizing*, that is, recreating complete images in your imagination based on your memory of them when your eyes were open and looking at them. The exercise will also strengthen your *memory and recall* mind muscles.[13]

It's all *subliminal* impressions from here on in. This shows why, when you work with the visual response part of your brain function, you may get remarkable results. That is the part that is already awake and active; this means, stimulating your brain's visual response is a doorway into a larger untapped part of your brain power.

HANGING YOUR FAVORITE PAINTING INSIDE YOUR BRAIN

- Select some music that you know helps you relax, tune inward, and generate images and impressions, and play this at a low volume. (See Brain-Building Secret #72 for suggestions on brain power enhancing music and mind-training tapes. See the Resources for ordering information.) You can do this exercise without music if you wish.
- You will need a color picture or photograph that is both rich in detail and personally fascinating to you. This can be a painting, an advertisement, or even a photograph, provided it has lots of detail, perspective, and complexity. You don't want to make things too easy on your brain, after all.
- Sit comfortably in a chair in a room where you won't be disturbed, take off your shoes and glasses, and relax.
- For maximum benefit from this right-brain enhancing exercise, check your nasal cycle to see which nostril is dominant.
- If your right nostril is clogged, this means your right brain is active and the appropriate brain hemisphere (regulating nonverbal, spatial, intuitive functions) for this exercise is dominant.
- If your right nostril is open, this means your left hemisphere (governing verbal, analytical, speech skills) is dominant, which will hinder your exercise.
- You can either wait 90–120 minutes until the brain hemispheres shift naturally, or you can shift your nasal cycle and brain hemisphere dominance now.
- Put the picture directly in front of you. Pretend there is a blind person with you who wants to know what this picture represents.
- You will be a journalist now and describe in as much detail as possible all the features of the picture, including overall theme, design, color, color contrast, perspective, individual objects, and shapes.
- Be thorough; spend 5 minutes if necessary.

HOW TO BE AN ASTUTE ART CRITIC, WITH YOUR EYES CLOSED

- When you feel your blind companion has the picture in mind, close your own eyes and become the blind person yourself.
- Bring the picture to mind in color in all its details before your inner mind's eye.
- Go through the process of description again. Now there are two blind people in the room, yourself and your blind companion.
- Try to bring all of the picture to mind and describe everything in it that you see. Probably you will not recall all of it. If so, go back to your first oral description of it and go through this again.
- If you can't remember anything, open your eyes and repeat the previous step of describing the picture out loud while you look at it.
- Once you have been able to visualize most of the picture with your mind's eye and after you have been able to describe most of it out loud with your eyes closed, then start seeing it in three dimensions.
- Give the picture depth and perspective. Pretend you can see around and behind objects in the picture.
- Now take it one step further. Imagine you are walking into this picture and now walking through it, seeing everything in three dimensions, just the way you normally see the physical world around you.
- What does it feel like to be in the picture? Do objects look differently when they are part of a new three-dimensional landscape that is nonetheless "all in your mind"?

HOW TO SPIN A FRUIT BOWL 360° WITHOUT USING YOUR HANDS

- Select an object in your picture, such as a statue, vase, or fruit bowl.
- Try to rotate it slowly so that you can see it from 360 degrees.

- Make the object turn around in a circle while you remain stationary.
- Now try rotating yourself, turning slowly around in a complete circle.
- Keep your eyes on the three-dimensional picture as you turn around within it.

These last two steps, admittedly, are difficult, and may take you a lot of practice to master. On the other hand, you may surprise yourself to discover that you are a very accomplished right-brain visualizer.

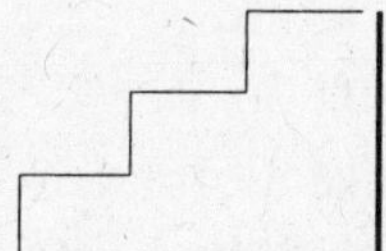

BRAIN-BUILDING SECRET #86
Brain Aerobics: Easy Calisthenics for Your Neurons

In the mid-1980s, the French government established the National Institute for Research on the Prevention of Cerebral Aging. There was concern about the declining mental status of their elderly citizens, and some of the more progressive bureaucrats saw the writing on the wall for the future as well. An aging, mentally incompetent population would cost a great deal in social services and would produce a population that was mentally unfit and probably unhealthy, too.

Brain fitness expert Monique Le Poncin was engaged as director. She developed a 4-week brain fitness program based on a series of graduated exercises that would train people to develop speed and diversification in their mental abilities.

That is, they would learn how to respond to a wide range of questions and situations quickly involving such key aspects of brain power as verbal activity, perception, visual-spatial (being able to quickly estimate distances, areas, volumes, and proportions of objects in space), structuralization (building logical wholes from different elements), and logical activity (reasoning, strategizing).

Her key assumption was that neuronal function could be molded, expanded, and quickened. Le Poncin believed that brain cells that were not specialized for any particular mental ability could be activated and in a sense converted to new brain power functions. She was able to test and measure her assumptions. Using advanced brain scan imaging equipment, she prepared a series of *brainprints* that showed the energy patterns in brains according to different mental activities, according to age, neuronal health, or disease, such as Alzheimer's.[14]

It's only a metaphor, but you might try thinking of your brain as a muscle. The more you use it, the more developed, nimble, flexible, and supple it becomes. That's where brain aerobics come in. The following are simple brain calisthenics to trim your brain power "muscles" and give them new fitness.

HOW TO WRITE A COMPLETE SENTENCE WHILE IN A HURRY

Study these words for 15 seconds, Then try to make a complete sentence out of them in less than 60 seconds. (See note 15 for answer.)

---

believed evening
in her cup
had that
drinking feel tea
relaxed of
she made
always a the
more

HOW TO GO SHOPPING WITH ONLY A LIST AND NO SUPERMARKET

Each of these 2-letter pairs starts a word, and all the words they start represent items you can find in a typical supermarket. Study these letter pairs for 20 seconds, then find the words they begin in less than 2 minutes. (See note 16 for answer.)

	TO		BE	
OR		SQ		
	PL	CE		
ST		BA		TU
			ON	

AFTERWORD

Congratulations. By now, you have completed all 140 Brain Builders! recommendations contained in this book. You have, I hope, sampled many of the Brain Builders! Workouts, perused the Anatomies of Brain Power, and probably tried out a fair number of the Brain-Building Secrets. You may even have considered a new way of looking at intelligence and the mind and the important role your health, attitude, and lifestyle play in the full expression of your brain power.

I hope some of these Brain-Builders Secrets were new ideas for you. That, after all, is the purpose of a book; but more than that, many books on self-development and building brain power often do not consider the entire picture, or to use the popular term, they are not *holistic*. In other words, intelligence depends on more than the speed of neurons and synapses in your brain, or whatever so-called IQ you were born with, as if it's a tangible part of your physical brain.

As you learned in the early chapters of this book, your attitude and life-style—even your living environment—can actually detract from your brain power by creating obstacles. When you remove these obstacles, you automatically gain brain power points. Here you learned, first, to *believe your brain*, then second, to *free your brain*. Those two tasks accomplished, you learned how to *get in rhythm with your brain*, to use your body and brain's natural rhythms and energy cycles to best advantage in your quest for more brain power.

From here, you started to move into the positive steps you could take to build brain power. You learned how to *feed your brain*, how important nutrition is in the healthy life of your brain. Then you saw the value of *moving your brain*, which means exercise, physical movement, even special breathing techniques to build brain power. But it didn't stop here. Your sixth Brain Builders! Secret was to sound your brain, to use music, sounds, even electronic frequencies, to stimulate your brain cells to greater efficiency.

Finally, you got into what most brain power books (mistakenly) give you first; namely exercises, tricks, puzzles, and workouts to *exercise your brain*. Because you got to these valuable exercises last, on the basis of a strong, carefully built foundation of the six previous Brain-Building Secrets, you received the maximum benefit from these mental gymnastics. By carefully following the seven steps to better brain power, you have no doubt gained the most from the 140 techniques presented in this book. In fact, if you take away nothing else from this book other than the 7 major brain-building points, you would have done your intelligence a big favor. So, once again, congratulations on your new brain power, "built" by you, at home, because you believe in your brain (and yourself) to be better.

NOTES

CHAPTER 1

[1]A study of 1,000 schools—which included interviews with 27,000 teachers, students, and parents in 1984 by a University of California educator—revealed similarly disturbing findings. Barely 3 percent of classroom time goes to praise, expressions of joy or humor, or even spontaneous outbursts of delight. Less than 1 percent of a typical day is devoted to students sharing their opinions or openly reasoning on a topic. Teachers run the classrooms virtually like tyrants; the creative input of the students is not solicited or expected.

About 70 percent of school time is taken up with a teacher *talking* to the students—in effect, cramming them full of facts and figures. Students spend the better part of their time waiting for teachers to hand out materials or give them instructions; even so, barely half the kids questioned ever feel they understand what is expected of them. Almost no time is spent in innovative activities such as group learning, role playing, and creative problem solving; almost all classroom teaching is from books, and precious little of the average 13,000 school hours from kindergarten to high school graduation have anything to do with real-life activities or challenges.

"Shared laughter, over-enthusiasm, or angry outbursts are rarely observed," the researcher noted. And it only gets worse the older the students become. As they move through the school system, their interest in all academic subjects noticeably drops from elementary to high school—whereas 56 percent of elementary students said they liked math, that number dropped to only 27 percent of senior high school students.

[2]That's the idea behind an exciting book on brain power written by Adam Robinson (*What Smart Students Know*) who as a student back in 1980 developed a revolutionary new way for preparing for the standard college tests like SAT and GRE. More than a decade later, Robinson interviewed hundreds of successful students to find out their secrets for superlearning—how to get maximum grades, achieve optimum learning, and spend a minimum of time doing it.

[3]These, and the previous 12 steps, are adapted from Robinson's survey *What Smart Students Know*.

[4]This idea comes from Thomas Armstrong, a brain power educator and director of Armstrong Creative Training Service, who teaches the theory and practical uses of Gardner's multiple intelligences.

[5]Gardner's theory has another implication for our idea of what makes intelligence, says Armstrong. Standards of high ability in the areas of memory, attention, perception, and problem solving—what psychologists call "cognitive processing"—may vary according to the kind of intelligence involved. For example, if your intelligence is musical, you may have a flair for remembering melodies but you may forget faces, names, and addresses. The theory of multiple intelligences, says Armstrong, is already being proven by psychological tests and experimental research. "It constitutes the most up-to-date synthesis of research on the topic of intelligence currently available."

[6]This is adapted from Thomas Armstrong's "Multiple Intelligences Checklist" in his book, *7 Kinds of Smart*.

[7]Many of these suggestions have been adapted and expanded from Thomas Armstrong's excellent material.

[8]Brain cells of elderly individuals when photographed reveal a thinning of the dendritic branches between brain cells. Quite often the brains of the elderly have some swollen neurons and fewer neurotransmitters; in fact, Alzheimer's patients may be missing 60–90 percent of the enzymes needed to make acetylcholine, a brain chemical necessary for memory and a 90 percent depletion of cells in a tiny brain segment called the *nucleus basalis of Meynert* that releases acetylcholine.

Your *locus ceruleus*, a brain region associated with the cycles of sleep and wakefulness, emotion, and memory, will probably lose 40 percent of its cells as you age; and the *hippocampal cortex*, involved with memory, shows a decline in nerve cells after the age of 60. All of this can mean fewer messages will be sent through the brain, resulting in a general slowing down in mental processing. But that's the wonder of the human brain. Aging *does not* have to mean this.

[9]In a sense, your brain is equipped with such an astonishing *surplus* because it is destined to lose a lot of them, but for the most part, the brain cells you lose in the natural course of aging are probably *redundant*, and their loss shouldn't affect your brain power at all. The current thinking is that during your mental life, you actually sculpt the neuronal form of your brain; you don't add new materials (brain cells) but shape (and discard) the original raw materials into a smoothly working, intelligent organ. When you were born, you had far more brain cells than you would ever need, so to lose 50,000 a day is no big deal.

[10]A healthy neuron has a "dentritic tree" whose branches are connected with a network of several hundred thousands of other dendrites. When your brain loses dendrites and their richly connected system, this slows down the communication network and makes learning harder and slower. Contrarily, when your brain gains more dendrite branches, learning can happen faster and more efficiently.

[11]A brain scan of the brains of individuals aged 21 to 83 showed that the healthy *aged* brain can be just as active and efficient as the healthy *young* brain. A neuroscientist analyzed brain tissues from 20 brains and found a definite relationship between the degree of education the person had received and the length of their neuronal dendrites. In other words, stimulate your brain more, and your dendrites grow more connections; it is a proven fact.

[12]This exercise comes out of the application of Neuro-Linguistic Programming to the field of education.

[13]Richard Bandler calls this *The Swish*. He claims to have succeeded in getting a woman to quit smoking in 11 minutes—after she had tried unsuccessfully to drop cigarettes for 11 years.

[14]A woman, age 63, lived in a house insulated with urea formaldehyde foam insulation (UFFI). Each year her house was upgraded with new carpets, furniture, tile floors, or other construction. Four years after the insulation, she developed severe episodes of arrhythmia, chest pain, light-headedness, arthralgias, and muscle weakness. She consulted a series of specialists, yet none were able to prescribe anything. Two years later she was unable to enter a shop-

ping mall unless supported with a cane or her husband's arm; once outside again in fresh air, her symptoms would start to clear up.

A test of her room showed that the walls were foam insulated, her mattress was foam filled, and the bed had a particle board headboard, all of which raised the level of formic acid in her body to dangerously toxic levels. Merely by changing her sleeping arrangements so that she slept on an old cot in a different room reduced her formic acid levels by 50 percent; when she had the new carpeting and brand-new furniture removed from her home, her symptoms disappeared.

[15]A 10-year-old excelling student started to get failing grades, was disruptive in class, and was judged to be unteachable. Tests showed that he was hypersensitive to a chemical family called phenol; exposure to this synthetic substance alone would send him into a frenzy of screaming and aggravation, such that he would lay on the floor and kick the walls.

CHAPTER 2

[1]A now-famous medical study from 1982 used CAT scans to examine the brains of men age 24–39 who had been tortured as political prisoners.

The scans showed that their brains had physically aged and even started to deteriorate, at the level of tissue and neurons, as a result of the prolonged stress from being unjustly held as prisoners. They had unusual difficulty in concentrating and remembering; they suffered headaches, depression, anxiety, numbness, and disturbances in sleeping. In a general sense, the high level of stress hormones released had literally damaged their brains.

Another study of how 100 men and women age 45–64 cope with the ordinary small stresses of life—such as being late or stuck in traffic, missing appointments—had a stronger influence on their overall psychological health (and brain power) than the more traumatic and dramatic events.

[2]An estimated 350,000 Americans experience and survive a stroke every year, and about 2.7 million people have thickening of the arteries in their brain, which is a predisposing factor in strokes. Even short of having a stroke, hypertension (or high blood pressure), compounded with chronic stress, can weaken your mental functions. A

study of 1,700 men and women with hypertension showed that having high blood pressure negatively affected their ability to retain information and use short-term memory.

[3]For example, a "normal" blood pressure is 140 (systolic) over 85 (diastolic) or lower for either type. When you get 90–104 for the diastolic reading, you're into mild hypertension; 115 and above and you have severe hypertension. For the lower pole, the systolic reading, borderline hypertension starts at readings of 140–159.

[4]One of the standard items from the field of natural health is called flower remedies. This is a gentle approach first formulated in the 1930s by an English physician named Dr. Edward Bach, who discovered a direct healing connection between the blossoms of certain plants and trees and specific human emotions.

[5]The Bach remedies gently move the deeply set emotion into your awareness, then help to change its energy and diffuse its strength in a process poetically akin to melting, boiling, and, finally, evaporating ice. As an adjunct to taking a flower remedy—it's preferable to try one at a time—you might consider keeping a daily journal in which you record thoughts, emotional reactions to people and situations, dreams, and daydreams.

In addition to the 38 remedies in the Bach system, there are several other prominent collections now available in the United States. All these flower remedy systems greatly increase the varieties of emotions and mental states that we might wish to change through this simple, nonchemical, noninvasive approach.

[6]Technically, a healthy person has a blood sugar content between 70 and 110 milligrams per deciliter of blood, but someone with hypoglycemia may be as low as 50 mg/dl. Generally, if your blood sugar level is at this level or lower, you will feel symptoms of depression, fatigue, nervousness, and experience sleep disturbances. Further, if you are seriously depressed, whether from hypoglycemia or from other dietary factors, it is quite likely your system is lacking at least two key amino acids, L-tryptophan and tyrosine.

L-tryptophan helps make the neurotransmittter serotonin, while tyrosine is needed to make dopamine and norepinephrine, also key brain chemicals. When your brain is low in serotonin and dopamine, most likely you're depressed to some degree. The important point to consider is that excess sugar intake may interfere with your brain's supply of serotonin and dopamine by affecting the two key amino acids needed to make them.

[7]They were developed by the diet's inventor, Larry Christensen, author of *The Food-Mind Connection. Eating Your Way to Happiness*; Pro-Health Publications, College Station, TX, 1991.

[8]A medical study of 12 depressed women who had attempted suicide revealed they all had low intakes of vitamin C compared to another group of 12 women who were not depressed or suicidal; in fact, the difference in vitamin C levels was the *only* difference the study found.

[9]There are now about 3,000 practitioners of behavioral optometry (out of 24,000 licensed optometrists; see the Resources) now practicing in the United States, showing clients the direct relationships between how you see and how you behave—and how to improve both.

[10]Behavioral optometrists conduct much longer eye examinations that check the visual system for other criteria besides the standard ones and then prescribe lenses that are not compensating, which is the norm for glasses, but that are remedial, developmental, and preventive. It's a way of retraining and supporting your eyes to see correctly so that your brain can process the information appropriately.

[11]Today Alzheimer's disease affects between 3 and 5 million Americans, producing 100,000–200,000 deaths every year, making it the fourth or fifth most deadly disease in the country. Worldwide, the statistics are similar. In Great Britain, 2 million have it and in Australia it's 1 out of 6; it almost seems that the longer you live, the more likely you are to develop some of the signs of Alzheimer's.

[12]However, a study of 648 elderly individuals divided the patients into seven different groups based on the amount of brain lesions each had. In the three groups that had the highest amount of plaques and tangles, fully 100 percent showed signs of amnesia, in age groups 67–76. In the three groups with a lesser amount of brain lesions, amnesia affected 72–87 percent of the individuals; and in the final group that had no brain lesions, only 30 percent showed any signs of amnesia.

The doctors concluded that the brain lesions were directly related to memory loss and most of the mental changes found with Alzheimer's.

[13]Scientific studies have shown that alcoholics who have good nutritional standards and who abstained from drinking during the test period still tested markedly below average in learning abilities that required strong recent-memory function. Long-term alcohol use definitely influences progressive loss of memory.

Incidentally, about 10 percent of those who use alcohol are considered abusers or alcoholics. But this is misleading because some people, depending on their body weight and physiology, can get seriously drunk on the most minute quantity of alcohol. And people with brain injuries, stroke, tumor, or a history of epilepsy can have dangerous reactions from one or two drinks alone.

In fact, statistics show that suicide is 30 times more prevalent among alcohol-abusers, more than 50 percent of drivers in fatal car crashes have alcohol-poisoned brains, two thirds of drowning victims and half of those who burn to death or die from falls have high levels of blood alcohol, and brain poisoning by alcohol is involved in a high number of incidents of domestic violence. As much as 10 percent of annual deaths in American can be attributed in part to alcohol. However, from your brain's viewpoint, it gets even worse.

[14]"Long-term alcohol use, we thus concluded, even by well-nourished individuals, produces structural changes in the brain," declares Vernon H. Mark, a neurosurgeon and medical researcher at Massachusetts General Hospital in Boston, a recognized expert on brain power and memory loss, and the physician who treated the epileptic alcoholic. "Your brain is the most precious organ in your body. It needs the utmost protection—especially from brain poisons. My own view is that for optimal brain function the intake of alcohol should be zero."

[15]Caffeine seems to affect the brain chemical called adenosine; when this neurotransmitter is given to animals, it sedates them and lowers their blood pressure and body temperature. Perhaps you have had the queer experience of having a second cup of coffee on a morning when you're not quite in sailing shape and it actually makes you drowsy. A recent study of 1,500 college students proved that moderate to high coffee use was linked to low grades in academic perfor-

mance. Another study of college students suggested that caffeine may impair short-term memory and word recall ability by as much as 20 percent.

[16]In one study 23 smokers were divided into two groups. One group smoked nicotine-based cigarettes while the others smoked nonnicotine cigarettes. Then they all took a memory test involving the recall of 75 items. After three tests, the subjects who had smoked the nonnicotine cigarettes scored 24 percent higher in memory recall than those with nicotine cigarettes. In another experiment, 37 smokers and 37 nonsmokers were tested on their recall of a list of 10 names. After 10 minutes, the nonsmokers impressively outscored the smokers in their recall of the names.

[17]Consider how frequently you encounter consumer advertisements on television and in mainstream magazines for drugs either for constipation or diarrhea. Consider the alarming statistics: colon cancer will kill somewhere between 57,000 and 100,000 Americans each year, second as a cancer threat only to lung cancer; many more Americans will contract colon cancer without dying from it; an estimated 70 million Americans have bowel problems of some kind; and still more will have frequent or virtually permanent constipation.

[18]According to Dr. Bernard Jensen, one of the country's foremost natural health educator's and authors, an autopsy of one person's colon revealed that while it was 9 inches in diameter, it had a usable passage of a pencil width. The rest of it was thoroughly caked and clogged with old matter. In another autopsy, a stagnant colon was weighed in at 40 pounds; here was a person carrying around 40 pounds of accumulated fecal matter as part of his body weight, some of which had the consistency of truck tire rubber. Further, Dr. Jensen estimates that worldwide some 200 million people have harmful intestinal parasites, which can range from single-celled organisms to tapeworms 20 feet long.

[19]The symptoms of "cerebral vascular deficiency" include ringing in the ears, dizziness, headaches, depression, short-term memory loss, and general impairment of your mental abilities—all of which are now commonly found in the elderly as the supposedly "unavoidable" symptoms of aging.

[20]According to Michael Hutchison, author of *Mega Brain Power*, "Many young and middle-age people today are suffering from dam-

age and deterioration of their basic intelligence and ability to think, of their powers of memory, and of their capacity to learn." Millions of supposedly healthy people are actually "victims of premature senility," Hutchison says.

[21]These recommendations come from Melvyn Werbach, M.D., a member of the American College of Nutrition, a clinical professor at the UCLA School of Medicine, and the author of two influential books on nutrition and illness.

[22]For example, a prolonged vitamin deficiency compounded with alcohol abuse (which depletes your system of B vitamins) can lead to memory loss. A 62-year-old woman drank too much white wine on a regular basis and tended to forget to eat proper meals in between her drinks. Eventually she paid the price of this neglect; one day friends found her confused and irrational and making strange eye movements.

She had lost a huge portion of her recent memory and was functionally amnesiac. She received various technical diagnoses from psychiatrists to account for her state, but what truly helped her was the nutritional prescription by her physician. He suspected she might be deficient in vitamin B1 as well as B5 (pantothenic acid) and B6 (pyridoxine). He gave her massive doses of these three B vitamins and had favorable results. Most of her symptoms went away and almost all of her memory returned.

[23]In another case, a 23-year-old college student maintained a healthy vegetarian diet, avoiding alchohol and other dietary poisons. Even so, she started developing fatigue and memory loss, which interfered with her studies. A nutritional evaluation showed she was deficient in B12, although it was only in the low to normal range. Her B12 intake was too low to give her brain enough "lift" to function properly. Fortunately, her condition was easily corrected with B12 supplements, which reversed her symptoms, ended her depression, and improved her memory.

[24]Medical studies in the last two decades have shown that even supposedly healthy men and women eating balanced, nutritious diets are low in magnesium; those on nutritionally inferior diets were dangerously low in magnesium. A 1988 study showed that the average American diet supplies only 40 percent of the adult recommend-

ed daily allowance (RDA) for magnesium; one noted nutrition expert estimated that as much as 80 percent of Americans have a hidden (undiagnosed) magnesium defiency.

As nutrition expert Sheldon Saul Hendler, notes, "It is becoming increasingly evident that marginal magnesium deficiency is very common." In his view certain groups are especially vulnerable to this widespread problem: the elderly, diabetics, people on low-calorie diets, people taking drugs that are diuretics or based on digitalis, people who drink alcohol, pregnant women, and men and women who exercise regularly and strenuously. All these factors can reduce your magnesium levels.

[25]"We have an epidemic in disguise," writes Sherry Rogers, a prominent physician and author in the field of environmental medicine. "For here we have a group of people who are seriously ill and are often barely able to function. Their major target organ is the brain, and so they are not only depressed and irritable, but they cannot think well."

[26]For example, a study of 803 New York City public schools showed dramatically the effects of dietary change on academic work. During a period of four years, the schools changed the foods they served at lunch. They eliminated all the synthetic additives and preservatives and the sugar content in the meals. After a short time on these dietary changes, the students, who had normally tested out average on a national level, now scored 16 *percent higher*.

[27]One medical study of 144 students, from kindergarten to college, proved that the average IQ of students on larger doses of vitamin C was higher than those on lower amounts. The study also showed that when the group on the lower dose of vitamin C started taking a glass of orange juice (high in vitamin C) every day for 6 months, their IQs showed a greater increase than the group of students already receiving a higher daily dose of vitamin C.

[28]A medical study showed that 28 children who had difficulties in learning had higher than average levels of aluminum in their blood. Another study proved that higher than normal levels of aluminum were found in the hair of students known to be dyslexic or learning disabled.

[29]In our modern industrial and urban environment, lead is far more common than it was for our great-grandparents. It's in the air,

the soil, soldered metal cans, drinking water, household or street dust, and our blood. Children are far more susceptible to lead toxicity than adults, as they absorb five times more—and the target organ for lead in the body is the brain. Estimates made in the early 1980s suggested that most people were absorbing 300 micrograms of lead a day from polluted air, water, and food and that each year another 400,000 children have increased blood levels of lead, of which 16,000 need treatment for toxicity.

[30]These suggestions come from Sherry Rogers, M.D., author of *Tired or Toxic? A Blueprint for Health*, Prestige Publishing, Syracuse, NY, 1990; and *The E.I. Syndrome: An Rx for Environmental Illness*, Prestige Publishing, Syracuse, NY, 1986.

[31]These suggestions come from Julian Whitaker, M.D., as part of the Whitaker Wellness Program, in *Dr. Whitaker's Guide to Natural Healing*, Prima Publishing, Rocklin, CA, 1995.

CHAPTER 3

[1]A woman suffered from extreme tension due to overwork and pressure; she had aches and muscle pains in her lower back from too much bending at work, plus she had congestion in her lungs from excessive smoking. Her aromatherapist gave her a mixture of juniper, lavender, and sandalwood for topical massage, inhalation through burners, and for dispersion baths.

After one treatment she reported that it felt as if a great weight had been removed from her shoulders and head, in addition to feeling exceptionally rested and relaxed. Further hand massage with these oils on her back, knees, and hands brought more deep relief. In general, she found afterwards that her well-being and sense of relaxation was greatly enhanced by the aromatherapy treatment.

[2]You may find it interesting that this spot is next door to two important endocrine glands located in your brain, namely, the pituitary and hypothalamus. Presumably, this exercise stimulates their activities. According to brain power expert Tom Kenyon, who teaches this exercise often in his "Brain States" workshops, a woman once came to him saying she had not had a period for one year and always had painful cramps during menstruation. Kenyon recommended she practice the

one-inch gate meditation for several weeks. She reported back that her period had suddenly returned; months later, her menstrual cycle was regular and far less painful. Evidently, the exercise had helped rebalance her endocrine system working through the master glands in the head. Kenyon also recommends this exercise for inducing deep states of rest, such as after a long airplane journey across time zones.

[3]The purpose of the last five steps in this exercise is to close an energy circuit in your body, to lock it into place so no energy can leak out. According to the Taoists, your basic mind-body energy, life force, or chi normally circulates up your spine, through your brain, and then down the front of your body to your perineum.

When your tongue is locked against the roof of your mouth, this actually locks the energy in like a switch. When you relax your tongue, this opens the circuit again; when you press it against your upper palate, this closes the energy circuit.

[4]Called "noise removal breathing," it was developed by the noted brain power authority Win Wenger, author of numerous popular books on intelligence, genius, and creativity.

[5]This is according to psychobiologist Ernest Lawrence Rossi, who has studied human biological rhythms and their effect on mind-body health and functioning.

[6]Scientists call this the rhythm of brain hemispheric dominance, and your key to charting it is your own nasal cycle, the flow of air through each nostril. In the next 24 hours, you will breathe about 21,600 times or about 13-15 times a minute; in effect, for 12 hours your breathing will primarily flow through your right nostril, then for 12 hours, it will move through your left nostril.

During this naturally occurring rhythm, your body will shift between the two poles of your autonomic nervous system, between the sympathetic and the parasympathetic branches. The blood vessels and mucosal glands in your nostril will either constrict or expand, allowing more or less air to pass through them as you breathe.

[7]A study by two Boston physicians in the late 1970s of nursing homes in that area revealed that about 90 percent of all patients in nursing homes had lost some of their brain power, 40 percent presumably had Alzheimer's, and 20 percent were suffering the results of a stroke.

However, the physicians estimated that 20 percent of the patients they studied had known numerous causes underlying their symptoms of mental decline and that all of these would have been treatable had the doctors diagnosed them properly much earlier. Another 20 percent had symptoms that were a mixture of treatable and untreatable. The researchers were amazed by their findings.

"For the first time it struck me that tens of thousands of people were being put away prematurely in nursing homes when, in fact, they could have been leading productive lives," comments one of the study's doctors, Vernon H. Mark. Senility is not the natural result of aging, argues Dr. Mark. "If someone's brain isn't working properly, it is because of brain disease or injury." In a study of postmortems on patients who had been diagnosed with Alzheimer's, fully 14 percent did not have the classic symptoms and in fact had something else.

[8]Jean Houston, psychologist, author, and director of the Foundation for Mind Research in Pomona, New York, took Cicero's advice to heart and developed this memory-building exercise, adapted here. Houston's approach is to help people reclaim memories from childhood as a way of strengthening the "memory muscles" in general.

[9]Back in 1975, Harvard Medical School scientist Herbert Benson, described the "relaxation response." As Benson saw it, this is a technique to relieve inner tensions, deal effectively with stress, lower blood pressure, and improve your emotional health. Benson drew equally upon Eastern meditation techniques and Western scientific information about the nervous system and the brain, which he then put in terms familiar to Americans. The *relaxation response* is a way to let the brain rest, naturally, while you are awake.

[10]The idea comes from Charles T. Tart, an internationally recognized authority on psychology, meditation, and mindfulness.

[11]The idea comes out of Buddhism and is advocated by the popular Vietnamese Buddhist teacher, Thich Nhat Hanh.

[12]This mindfulness affirmation (and the others that follow) is courtesy of Thich Nhat Hanh.

[13]The body scan was developed by Jon Kabat-Zinn, a Zen Buddhist teacher and director of the Stress Reduction Clinic at the

University of Massachusetts Medical Center. Here he teaches hospital patients with chronic pain how to use their minds constructively to alter their experience of discomfort.

CHAPTER 4

[1]In a study, 40 men between the ages of 18 and 28 had a large serving of turkey for lunch and then were asked to perform complicated mental tasks. Another day these same men had, instead, an almost completely carbohydrate lunch and then sat down to do the same mental work. The result was that their brain power was "significantly impaired" following the high-carbohydrate meal, but not following the protein lunch.

Another study showed that the sleep-producing effects of carbohydrates are even stronger in people over 40. In a study of 184 men and women, one half were fed a high-protein lunch, the others a dish of sherbet, which is almost pure carbohydrate. Those eating the sherbet uniformly felt spaced out and mentally asleep, but those over 40 in this group had twice the difficulties in mustering up concentration, recall, and ability to perform mental tasks. Yet another study placed this drop in brain power, among women tested, at 46.7 percent—not the kind of dip in brain power that makes for a productive afternoon on the job.

[2]In a U.S. Army study with two-dozen soldiers about to make a stressful military maneuver, half received tyrosine, the others a placebo. The maneuver was performed and then the soldiers got another dosage of the amino acid, except that those who had first received the placebo got the tyrosine and those who had tyrosine before, this time had the placebo. During the course of the two drills, all the soldiers were evaluated for their performance under stressful conditions.

The researchers found that for those soldiers who normally felt stressed and even depressed such that these conditions would affect their performance and thinking (plus producing headaches, fatigue, and "clouded" brain function), the tyrosine dramatically improved everything.

[3]Western scientists have studied ginkgo's brain-building properties in recent decades. In fact, since 1975, 34 clinical studies have shown that ginkgo increases blood flow in the brain and body at large.

[4]In one study, healthy volunteers were given one dose of *Ginkgo biloba*, five times greater than a normal dosage. An hour later when they took a battery of tests to gauge memory, the group showed a significant increase in short-term memory. Ginkgo alters brain wave patterns and thereby increases general alertness.

An EEG study with the elderly who were showing signs of mental decline showed that ginkgo changed the dominant brain wave pattern to mostly alpha waves, which are more favorable for learning and alertness; at the same time, ginkgo reduced the number of theta waves, which are associated with drowsiness, an unfocused state of mind, and poor attention. These results were noticeable after 3 weeks.

Other studies have shown that ginkgo is especially helpful if used by elderly who are showing the early signs of mental decline, dementia, or Alzheimer's; in these cases, it apparently delayed the progression of poorer mental function. Ginkgo is particularly helpful in reversing mental decline if the problem stems from depression or a restriction in the flow of oxygen to the brain.

Most recently, 20 patients with diagnosed Alzheimer's took 80 mg of *Ginkgo biloba* extract three times daily for 3 months. They were tested for memory and attention at the beginning of the experiment, then in the middle, and at the end. Memory and attention improved significantly after only 1 month on ginkgo, and continued so for the next 2 months as well. The patients also showed improvement in other areas of mental and bodily function as a result of taking the herb.

[5]Ginseng's ability to boost energy and to reduce fatigue has been demonstrated in clinical trials with mice. In an experiment, mice were required to swim in cold water and run up a very long rope. Mice given ginseng extract were able to endure the otherwise cruel test 183 percent longer than mice without ginseng. Experiments testing ginseng's antifatigue ability have been tested on humans as well. Nurses switched from day to night duty were first tested for their performance in mental and physical tasks; after taking ginseng, they scored much higher on the same tests.

In another study of telegraph operators, after taking ginseng for 30 days, all personnel showed heightened coordination of physical with mental reflexes, improved endurance, fewer mistakes, and stronger, more sustained concentration.

[6]"*Rasayana* substances rebuild the body-mind, prevent decay, and postpone aging; they may even reverse the aging process," comments Ayurvedic scholar David Frawley. According to Frawley, the ancient Ayurvedic practice of *rasayana* aimed at mutating the brain, which means so changing its physical nature and way of operating that higher consciousness, more awareness, and heightened mind function could be experienced.

In this system, what we call more brain power is an aspect of what the Ayurvedic physicians think of as heightened, clarified consciousness in general. Ayurveda considers the "old brain" to be habitual conditions of fear, anxiety, sluggish awareness, desire, even excessive egotism; *rasayana* aims to develop a "new brain" marked by more awareness, less selfishness, greater clarity of mind, and expanded consciousness.

[7]To order Ayurvedic herbs and products and to receive a free catalog, contact Maharishi Ayur-Ved Products International, P.O. Box 49667, Colorado Springs, CO 80949; telephone: (800)-255-8332.

[8]This list was compiled by Robert Haas, nationally recognized nutrition and fitness expert, as presented in his book *Eat Smart, Think Smart.*

[9]This information comes from herbalist Daniel B. Mowrey in his book *Scientific Validation of Herbal Medicine.*

[10]In a study of geriatric patients who were suffering mental confusion on account of a vitamin C deficiency, when vitamin C supplements were added to their diet, remarkable brain power improvements resulted. In another case, students who increased their vitamin C intake, scored, on average, 5 points higher on IQ tests compared to students with lower vitamin C levels. However, when this group was given vitamin C supplements for 6 months, their IQ scores climbed by 3.5 points.

[11]A study showed that subjects who took oral choline did much better in a short-term memory test; their ability to remember abstract words (such as "truth") also increased. Choline levels in Alzheimer's patients of course are quite low, yet in an experimental study with 11 Alzheimer's patients who took lecithin, 7 experienced a 50–200 percent improvement in long-term memory.

[12]College students who took 3 gm of choline daily during the semester did much better on word recall tests; in fact, an improvement in memory usually becomes evident in only a few days after beginning a choline supplementation program.

[13]The way scientists discovered that niacin in high dosages could reverse memory loss is a fascinating story in itself.

Back in 1953, when psychiatrists were (mistakenly) using electroconvulsive shock therapy (strong electrical jolts applied to the brain, abbreviated as ECT) to treat schizophrenia, they found in some cases this violent procedure severely damaged the memory of patients, almost to the point of not functioning. Following ECT, patients would experience significant amnesia.

One physician experimented with giving his patient 3 gm of niacin every day for a month; after 30 days, the patient's memory had returned and all signs of mental damage and amnesia had disappeared. In further trials with several hundred other patients, the physician found that niacin relieved most of the residual memory defects following ECT. Even discontinuing niacin after the return of memory did not then bring back the amnesia.

[14]In a study of 40 patients with depression, they all took phenylalanine supplements every day for up to 6 months in doses that grew from 500 mgs to 3–4 gm daily. They also took 100–200 mg of vitamin B6 to increase the working effect of the amino acid. After 6 months, 31 of the depressed patients reported that they felt they had benefited noticeably, and 10 said their depression had completely disappeared.

[15]EQ 02 is available from Design for Health, 6306 215th Street SW, Mountlake Terrace, WA 98043; telephone: (206)-771-6248.

[16]In this study, children on the special nutrient program, involving higher than average dose of vitamins and minerals, gained 7 IQ points. Students who received 100 percent of the recommended daily allowance for the 23 nutrients scored 3.7 points higher in the nonverbal IQ tests; students who received 50 percent and 200 percent of the RDA showed smaller increases of 1.2 and 1.5 points, respectively.

Not only did this study prove that nutrient fortification can improve school performance (as measured by IQ), but there is actually an ideal dosage range in which to get the best results. There is a provocative moral in this anecdote, as the study director commented. "The IQ difference between an average American and a doctor, lawyer, or professor is only about 11 points. The gain observed in one out of three [study participants] is the same as might be required for an average American to aspire to be a doctor, lawyer, or professor."

[17]In their recent book, *Smart Drugs II: The Next Generation*, researchers Ward Dean, John Morgenthaler, and Steven Fowkes publish a great many letters from readers of their previous book and newsletter, who have written reports of their positive experiences with using brain power building nutrients.

[18]In clinical studies with Alzheimer's patients, average age 67, Piracetam has fared quite well. These patients were given 2.4 gm daily of Piracetam for 8 weeks and then tested for a series of brain power abilities. The results were remarkable: 45 percent reduction in memory disturbances, 49 percent improvement in alertness, 42 percent reduction in perception disturbances, 37 percent improvement in sleep, and 32 percent reduction in depressive states. Healthy students who took 4.8 gm daily of Piracetam for 2 weeks had much improved memory for verbal information. Students, aged 7–12, with learning disabilities and dyslexia who were put on Piracetam for 36 weeks showed strong improvements in reading skills, verbal memory, short-term memory, and the equivalent of a 6-month's gain in reading scores.

[19]This is a sampling of the testimonials by Piracetam users, as quoted by Ward Dean and John Morgenthaler in *Smart Drugs & Nutrients* (1990).

[20]An American study of 148 healthy elderly people taking Hydergine over a 3-year period showed many positive results, including improvements in brain wave measurements, a decrease in negative subjective sensations such as dizziness, ringing in the ears, visual disturbances, an increase in heart rate, and normalization of blood pressure. All this led researchers to conclude that the smart drug slows down the aging process.

[21]It seemed especially capable of helping to lower hyperactivity in children, with increasing their attention span, reducing irritability, correcting learning disabilities, enabling them to perform better in schoolwork, and even, in some cases, increasing their IQ. During a 6-week trial, 17 subjects took DMAE daily in gradually increasing dosages. After the 6-week period, they demonstrated an increased ability to concentrate; they also had better muscle tone and needed less sleep and slept better; they had more energy, greater attentiveness, and worried less before school exams.

[22]For example, a 47-year-old woman suffered from lifelong learning problems and disturbances in her memory; a variety of therapies had failed to change this condition. It turned out, through blood tests, that her DHEA levels were far lower than average. When she was put on a DHEA supplementation program, all her brain power functions improved.

In a study of Alzheimer's patients, researchers found that their DHEA levels were lowering (by 48 percent) their body's ability to respond normally to outside stimulation.

CHAPTER 5

[1]Experts in "brain gym," Dennison's popular name for the approach, teach a long series of simple, quick exercises in schools around the world, including the United States. One group of learning-disabled elementary school students improved their reading skills by the equivalent of 1.5 years after practicing the brain gym routines for about 30 minutes a day in 5-minute sessions for one school year. The formal name for Dennison's complete system of exercises and principles, from which we have adapted the following exercises, is educational kinesthetics, which means "learning through movement."

[2]The circulating blood of a 20-year-old man will absorb about 4 liters of oxygen a minute, while that of a 75-year-old man take in only 1.5 liters. Oxygen deprivation in your brain can have a negative effect on the vitality and quantity of some of the key neurotransmitters, such as dopamine, norepinephrine, and serotonin. Bear in mind that the natural supplies of these brain chemicals declines with age, so if your oxygen intake is down on account of your age and lack of exercise, you can easily guess the consequences for your brain power.

[3]A study with 25 university students evaluated the effect of 4 month's worth of qigong practice on their performance in 10 test areas, such as recall ability, response speed, and accuracy. This group was compared to another equivalent group of students before beginning qigong; they differed in only 1 item out of 10. But after 4 months of qigong practice, that difference widened to 7 categories, due entirely to the exercises. The study also showed the positive effect of only 1 hour's qigong practice on various intelligence tests, including memory.

[4]Thanks to Sheila Ostrander and Lynn Schroeder for their translations from Lozanov's original texts, in *Superlearning*.

[5]This the way noted megabrain authority Michael Hutchison sees it: "What the rotation is really doing is 'exercising' the brain—altering and increasing the flow of neuroelectricity and neurochemicals to large areas of the brain. The first thing this kind of vestibular stimulation does is bring a dramatic increase in your motor and learning capabilities."

[6]If you ask the Sufis how the spinning benefits them physically, they might tell you that it stimulates a series of subtle energy centers located near the spine. These in turn feed the brain with refreshing vital force. If you ask a Western scientist the same question, you will learn that brain wave studies show that spinning has a highly positive effect on a factor called *neuroefficiency quotient*, or NEQ. This is a measurement that tells you how fast your brain's neurons can transmit electrical signals from one brain region to another; fast rates of transmission are connected with high IQs.

Some researchers in the field of body motion and NEQ have found that when you can increase NEQ you can sometimes get a corresponding IQ hike of up to 30 points. There are also changes in brain wave activity, such as a down-shifting from the more frenetic beta to alpha, the relaxation wave length; in addition, there is often an increase in brain wave coherence, which is a pleasurable and productive brain condition in which the otherwise different brain waves from different brain regions start to vibrate in harmony.

[7]There are devices that will twirl your entire body for you or simulate the same effect through sound conveyed through all your tissues and muscles. These devices include the Graham Potentializer, Symmetron, Somatron Chair, and Discovery Sound Table. Read about these and others in the catalog from Tools for Exploration, 4460 Redwood Highway, Suite 2, San Rafael, CA 94903; telephone: (415)-499-9050.

CHAPTER 6

[1]This quiz was developed by Tony Buzan, author of *Make the Most of Your Mind* (1988) and *Use Both Sides of Your Brain* (1989).

[2]The 20 steps are adapted from Tony Buzan.

[3]Dr. Lozanov got the idea after studying a variety of mental prodigies, such as a Russian who could out calculate a computer in multiplying 4-figure numbers or an Indian mystic who could remember 10,000 verses perfectly. Mikhail Keuni, a Russian artist, dazzled mathematicians during an experiment. They drew numerous interconnecting circles on a blackboard, so many that the board was nearly entirely white.Then, looking at it for the first time, Keuni told them in 2 seconds how many intersections the circles made.

It took the top mathematicians in the room 5 minutes to verify Keuni's correct answer. Lozanov saw no reason why such remarkable brain power should not be the possession of everyone. He brought to his system what he had learned after studying a form of mental yoga called *raja* for 20 years and other fields.

[4]The superlearning technique is now used widely around the world, including the United States. When tested at the University of Iowa, researchers found that this Baroque brain booster increased learning by 24 percent and enhanced memory by 26 percent. Other scientific studies in the past three decades have substantiated Lozanov's claim that this music-based approach could move listeners into a definite state of *alert relaxation*, which is the perfect state of mind for learning.

Clinical studies of students using this program back up Lozanov's claims for actual physiological changes during listening. Alpha brain waves increase by about 6 percent while beta waves decrase by 6 percent; the pulse rate slows by an average of 5 beats per minute; and blood pressure drops slightly but measurably.

[5]Lozanov discovered that most Baroque music is set to a standard rhythm of 60 beats per second, which corresponds to the average resting heart rate. This music synchronizes mind and body, outer environment with inner physiology; blood pressure, pulse rate, and brain waves slow down and your muscles relax.

[6]Brain power researcher Colin Rose, author of *Accelerated Learning*, spent 4 years researching the Lozanov method and related memory-building techniques and developed this shopping list. Lozanov method students typically master a new language in 30 days, which is about 7 times the norm, and they typically retained 90 percent of what they learned. There are Lozanov statistics from the 1960s

showing that some students mastered 1,000 words in a single day; in 1974, that figure jumped to 1,800 words; and by 1977, some students could absorb 3,000 new words daily.

[7]As Barbara Brown, one of the foremost biofeedback innovators in the 1970s, once remarked, "Watching brain waves gives me the feeling of suddenly having discovered where halos come from." She would often stand before the EEG machine "entranced" as the brain wave squiggles were recorded on the graph paper. It spoke of the mysteries of the mind. "Just to ponder the fact that living brains ceaselessly pour forth electrical activity gives one a profound sense of awe . . . and is an experience that never fails to excite."

[8]According to Lozanov, in 15 minutes of this coordinated breathing and listening, you should be able to remember as many as 80–100 new items of information, but even if you do 40–50, that's considered excellent.

[9]Using the ears as a conduit for brain stimulation was in fact the idea behind Gregorian chant as developed by Pope Gregory in the seventh century A.D. Here they use the human voice as a way of energizing the brains of the monks—as brain food made from sound, or as aural coffee to keep them awake for long periods to complete their devotional practices. And the fact that they, themselves, did the chanting, added an extra dimension to this sonic nourishment.

Tomatis discovered the link when he visited a Benedictine monastery in France that had discontinued its practice of chanting 6–8 hours daily. The abbot couldn't figure out why all his monks started getting tired and easily exhausted; doctors brought in as consultants could not get to the bottom of the mysterious fatigue either.

Finally, Tomatis was called in to consult. "I found that 70 of the 90 monks were slumping in their cells like wet dishrags." His remedy: He got them chanting again, "giving them back their sounds, their stimuli." Within several months, they were energized again. The secret here was that the sound of their own chanting literally energized them, enabling them to get by comfortably with only 4–6 hours of sleep.

[10]In passing, you should know that the Tomatis method, a unique listening-retraining system developed by Dr. Tomatis, now used in centers around the United States, has been successful in reversing numerous brain power-related problems in literally tens of

thousands of patients. Using a unique device Tomatis calls the electronic ear, which in his words is like a "fitness center for the middle ear," his approach has brought cures to conditions of dyslexia, autism, attention deficit disorders, and other learning disabilities.

[11]Tibetan monks at particular monasteries have the remarkable ability (captured in sound recordings) of singing whole chords by themselves, such as D, F#, and A, simultaneously. For example, the Gyuto monks of Tibet can chant a bass note two octaves below middle C, where it vibrates at 75.5 cycles per second (hertz, Hz). To put this in perspective, the lowest typical range of an opera singer is 150 Hz.

[12]Jonathan Goldman, a well-known sound educator, author, teacher, and advocate of sound therapy, once worked with a physician who used a device to measure heat emissions from the skin. The physician wanted to show, scientifically, the relationship of music on relaxation by registering differences in temperature on the skin of the listener.

Goldman, who teaches people how to make vocal harmonics, went through some of his routines while the physician's gauges were hooked up to his skin, especially his scalp, because he was deliberately projecting the sounds into his brain. The resulting photographs, says Goldman, "showed incredibly rapid changes in color on my forehead and the top portion of my skull. There were changes in the activation of skin temperature which matched the portion of my head where I had been projecting the vocal harmonics."

[13]Both exercises are adapted from Joanathan Goldman, *Healing Sounds. The Power of Harmonics*, Element Books, Rockport, MA, 1992.

[14]Hemi-Sync is a technology based on two fundamental facts about sound and hearing. The first, called frequency following response (FFR), is about *entrainment*. When as a listener your sound environment is dominated by specific sound frequencies, your physiology tends to reproduce them, and you can further become entrained to the state of awareness produced by those sounds and even learn to reproduce them at will.

The second fact is the *binaural* ("two ears") *beat*. Let's say your right ear hears a 100-Hz pulsed tone while your left ear gets 104 Hz; your brain will bridge the gap and perceive a new, third frequency of 4 Hz, which is the difference between the two sounds. Binaural beat generation feeds your brain with sound frequencies usually below the threshold of conscious hearing. There they stimulate "interhemispheric synchronization," which means both brain hemispheres work together as a single brain. This in turn guides you as the user into certain desirable, and preprogrammed states of mind, explains Monroe.

[15]Using a Neuromapper NRS-24, which is a computerized 20-channel EEG scanner that cross-references and analyzes brain wave patterns, MRI scientists can make a brain map in color showing the tangible effects of a Hemi-Sync session on the theta brain waves (4–8 Hz). To demonstrate the reality of hemispheric synchronization, MRI published two maps, a before and after shot of the same brain.

The differences are indisputable: the "before" brain wave pattern is imbalanced and disorganized; the "after" is stunningly symmetrical and focused. Hemi-Sync sound technology is also used successfully with brain injury recovery, psychotherapy, post-viral fatigue syndrome, quadriplegia, multiple sclerosis, dentistry, chemical dependency, cranioscaral therapy, among other problems.

[16]Available from The Monroe Institute (for Hemi-Sync tapes), Route 1, Box 175, Faber, VA 22938; telephone: (804)-361-1252.

[17]Available from Megabrain, P.O. Box 65676, Los Angeles, CA 90065; telephone: (800)-475-6463.

[18]Developed by Acoustic Brain Research/Quantum Link, 8665 East Miami River Road, Cincinnati, OH 45247; telephone: (800)-531-9283.

[19]Developed by Brain Sync Corporation, 235 Bayview Street, San Rafael, CA 94901; telephone: (800)-866-7707.

[20]Developed by Brain Sync Corporation, 235 Bayview Street, San Rafael, CA 94901; telephone: (800)-866-7707.

[21]From M.S.H. Association, Route 1, Box 192-B, Faber, VA 22938; telephone: (800)-962-2033.

[22]"The development of brain-exploring technology has become a hotbed of scientific activity, a hot spot of brain research," according to Michael Hutchison, author of two key books on the burgeoning field of consumer psychotronics, *Megabrain* and *Megabrain Power*. These electronically driven tools can be used like body building tools for cerebral

mental fitness, training wheels for the brain for "spicing up the brain soup" and triggering mind expansion, learning, memory, and creativity. According to Hutchison, mind machines are selling by the thousands in mainstream consumer catalogs and the manufacturers show no signs of letting up the pace of technological innovation.

CHAPTER 7

[1]According to Dr. Win Wenger, these tracking exercises reveal highly interesting and specific information about the state of mind of the tracker. His studies reveal that, for example, how well you can track the light making downward curving arcs indicates the degree to which you're in touch with your *feelings*. How well you can follow the light making the upward arc from left to right and to track carefully into the diagonal corners says a lot about your *memory* capabilities.

Tracking straight up and down is related to your ease at working with *abstractions* and details. If you have trouble tracking the light first close then far, this tends to correlate with problems in personal *relationships*, says Dr. Wenger. The important point is that your eye tracking movements reveal a lot about the degree to which your brain power is at your fingertips.

[2]This exercise was developed by Win Wenger, author of *How to Increase Your Intelligence*, D.O.K. Publishers, East Aurora, NY, 1987, and *Beyond Teaching & Learning*, Project Renaissance, Gaithersburg, MD, 1992.

[3]As a result, Dr. Houston uses a powerful brain-building exercise in her seminars, developed originally by her psychologist husband Robert Masters, "This kind of brain exercise is designed to increase the capacity of the brain to consider multiple possibilities, however outrageous," without the logical part of the mind voicing its opposition.

[4]Incidentally, brain size, which can vary, is no measure in itself of IQ. While the average brain weighs 1,349 grams (2.97 pounds), two famous writers, the English Jonathan Swift and the Russian Ivan Turgenev, had brains weighing 2,000 grams, or 4.4. pounds. On the other hand, the French novelist Anatole France had a brain that weighed only 1,017 grams (2.24 pounds), while the largest brain on record (2,049 grams, or 4.51) belonged to an idiot.

[5]Although this connecting link is found in the brains of other primates and animals, it has achieved its state of the art in the human brain in terms of its volume of nerve fibers in relation to other brain structures such as brain stem fibers. In the horse it is 0.70; in the dolphin, 0.93; in the elephant, 1.11; in the chimpanzee, 1.79; but in the human brain, it is 3.12.

[6]This exercise is adapted from Mark Bricklin, Mark Golin, Deborah Grandinetti, and Alexis Lieberman. *Positive Living and Health: The Complete Guide to Brain/Body Healing & Mental Empowerment*, Rodale Press, Emmaus, PA, 1990.

[7]"What is expressed *by* the learner is 100 times more productive of learning than what is expressed *to* the learner," says Wenger. As Wenger explains it, this exercise frees up the "traffic jam in your articulariae," which are tiny structures in several key parts of your brain believed to be active during speech, reading, or word processing.

[8]This ingenious exercise was developed by noted brain power expert Win Wenger. founder of Project Renaissance, an educational effort dedicated to finding new ways to improve brain power.

[9]Dr. Wenger recommends practicing this exercise for at least 10 minutes for 10 days in a row. After this time, you may expect impressive results in your brain power. "If you can persist 10 or more minutes per day of image streaming for 21 straight days, the improvements in your life become not only more profound but permanent."

[10]If these studies are to be believed, this means that if you practice image streaming for 23 minutes a day for 1 week your IQ may climb by 2 points. In fact, studies in 1989 at Southwestern State University in Marshall, Minnesota, tested out the assumptions in this exercise and found them to be accurate. Students actually gained 0.8 of an IQ point for each hour of practice, or about 20 IQ points for 25 hours practice, according to formal measurements. Remedial students gained 1.8 IQ points per hour of practice.

[11]Perhaps you don't have to be a genius to have powerful memory, especially if it involves visual images. Students at the University of Rochester were shown a series of 2,500 photographs, 1 every 10 seconds for 7 hours, spread out over 3 days. Then they were shown 300 pairs of photographs, 1 of which they had already seen among

the 2,500, the other new. When tested, they correctly recognized 85–95 percent of the original pictures. In another test, subjects were shown 600 pictures and then immediately quizzed; they scored 98 percent correct identification.

[12]Its originator, Win Wenger, calls it *instant replay*.

[13]Certain facts of brain physiology explain why visualization exercises can have a powerful brain-building effect. Studies based on EEG readings show that 80 percent of your brain power goes into visual response, in responding to visual information. Further, it's estimated that only 1 percent, at best, of your brain cells (or less than 5 percent of brain surface area) is involved with registering conscious experience, or under our ordinary control; the rest operates on automatic pilot or is, technically, unconscious as far as your attention is concerned.

[14]Even more impressive, in a test of 357 men and women who took the 4-week brain fitness program, she showed actual improvement in four brain power categories. In mental alertness, scores increased from 15.8 to 18.2; in visuospatial memory, they climbed from 4.8 to 7.1; in verbal memory, from 12.6 to 13.2; and in associative memory, from 5.1 to 5.3. Here was indisputable proof that brain fitness exercises could raise IQ in a short time period.

[15]ANSWER: She had always believed that drinking a cup of tea in the evening made her feel more relaxed.

[16]ANSWER: Tomatoes, beans, oranges, squash, plums, celery, strawberries, bananas, turnips, onions.

RESOURCES

BOOKS

Armstrong, Thomas. *7 Kinds of Smart. Identifying and Developing Your Many Intelligences*. Plume/Penguin Books, New York, 1993.

Bandler, Richard. *Using Your Brain for a Change*. Real People Press, Moab, UT, 1985.

Beaver, Diana. *Lazy Learning. Making the Most of the Brains You Were Born With*. Element Books, Rockport, MA, 1994.

Berwick, Ann. *Holistic Aromatherapy. Balance the Body and the Soul with Essential Oils*. Llewellyn Publications, St. Paul, MN, 1994.

Bourre, Jean-Marie. *Brainfood. A Provocative Exploration of the Connection Between What You Eat and How You Think*. Little, Brown, Boston, 1993.

Bricklin, Mark, Mark Golin, Deborah Grandinetti, and Alexis Lieberman, *Positive Living and Health: The Complete Guide to Brain/Body Healing & Mental Empowerment*. Rodale Press, Emmaus, PA, 1990.

Brown, Barbara B. *New Mind, New Body. Bio-Feedback: New Directions for the Mind*. Harper & Row, New York, 1974.

Buttram, Harold E. "Volatile Organic Compounds: Contributory Causes of Learning Disabilities and Behavioral Problems in Children." *Townsend Letter for Doctors*, May 1994, pp. 472–474.

Buzan, Tony. *Make the Most of Your Mind*. Fireside/Simon & Schuster, New York, 1988.

—. *Use Both Sides of Your Brain*. Plume/Penguin Group, New York, 1989.

Campbell, Don, ed. *Music, Physician for Times to Come*. Quest Books, Wheaton, IL, 1991.

Carper, Jean. *The Food Pharmacy. Dramatic New Evidence That Food Is Your Best Medicine*. Bantam Books, New York, 1988.

Carter, Philip J., and Ken A. Russell. *The IQ Challenge*. Barnes & Noble, New York, 1993.

Casdorph, H. Richard, and Morton Walker. *Toxic Metal Syndrome: How Metal Poisonings Can Affect Your Brain*. Avery Publishing Group, Garden City, NY, 1994.

Castaneda, Carlos. *The Art of Dreaming*, HarperCollins, New York, 1993.

Castorri, B. Alexis, and Jane Heller. *Mental Aerobics, Exercises for a Stronger, Healthier Mind*. Citadel Press/Carol Publishing, New York, 1992.

Chaitow, Leon. *Clear Body, Clear Mind. How to Detoxify Yourself Through Self-Help Techniques*. Greenhouse/Penguin Books Australia, Victoria, 1990.

Challem, Jack. "Keeping Your Marbles," *Natural Health*. January/February 1995.

Chang, Stephen T., with Richard C. Miller. *The Book of Internal Exercises*. Strawberry Hill Press, San Francisco, 1978.

Chisti, Hakim. *The Traditional Healer's Handbook. A Classic Guide to the Medicine of Avicenna*. Healing Arts Press, Rochester, VT, 1991.

Christensen, Larry B. *The Food-Mind Connection. Eating Your Way to Happiness*. Pro-Health Publications, College Station, TX, 1991.

Connor, Danny, with Michael Tse. *Qigong. Chinese Movement & Meditation for Health*. Samuel Weiser, York Beach, ME, 1992.

Csikszentmihalyi, Mihaly. *Flow. The Psychology of Optimal Experience*. HarperCollins Perennial, New York, 1991.

Davis, Patricia. *Aromatherapy*, An A–Z. C. W. Daniel Company, Saffron Walden, UK, 1988.

Dawkins, Hazel Richmond, Ellis Edelman, and Constantine Forkiotis. *Suddenly Successful—How Behavioral Optometry Helps You Overcome Learning, Health, and Behavior Problems*. Optometric Extension Program Foundation, Santa Ana, CA, 1991.

Dean, Ward, and John Morgenthaler. *Smart Drugs & Nutrients. How to Improve Your Memory and Increase Your Intelligence Using the Latest Discoveries in Neuroscience*. B & J Publications, Santa Cruz, CA, 1990.

—. and Steven Wm. Fowkes. *Smart Drugs* II. *The Next Generation.* Health Freedom Publications, Menlo Park, CA, 1993.

Dennison, Gail E., Paul E. Dennison, and Jerry V. Teplitz. *Brain Gym for Business. Instant Brain Boosters for On-the-Job Success.* Educational Kinesiology Foundation, Ventura, CA, 1994.

Dennison, Paul E., and Gail E. Hargrove. *Personalized Whole Brain Integration.* Educational Kinesiology Foundation, Ventura, CA, 1985.

DePorter, Bobbi, with Mike Hernacki. *Quantum Learning: Unleashing the Genius in You.* Dell, New York, 1992.

Devananda, Swami Vishnu. *The Sivananda Companion to Yoga.* Fireside/ Simon & Schuster, New York, 1983.

Epstein, Seymour, with Archie Brodsky. *You're Smarter Than You Think. How to Develop Your Practical Intelligence for Success in Living.* Simon & Schuster, New York, 1993.

Faelten, Sharon. *The Complete Book of Minerals for Health.* Rodale Press, Emmaus, PA, 1981.

Ferry, Georgina. "Alzheimer's Disease: A New Age." *New Scientist,* November 12, 1988.

Flaws, Bob. *Imperial Secrets of Health and Longevity.* Blue Poppy Press, Boulder, CO, 1994.

Franklin, Jon. *Molecules of the Mind. The Brave New Science of Molecular Psychology.* Atheneum, New York, 1987.

Frawley, David. *Ayurvedic Healing. A Comprehensive Guide.* Passage Press, Salt Lake City, UT, 1989.

—. and Vasant Lad. *The Yoga of Herbs. An Ayurvedic Guide to Herbal Medicine.* Lotus Press, Santa Fe, NM, 1986.

Gardner, Howard. *Frames of Mind: The Theory of Multiple Intelligences,* 10th ed., Basic Books, New York, 1993.

Golden, Daniel. "Building a Better Brain," *Life,* July 1994.

Goldman, Jonathan. *Healing Sounds. The Power of Harmonics.* Element Books, Rockport, MA, 1992.

Goleman, Daniel. "Mental Decline in Aging Need Not Be Inevitable." *The New York Times*, April 26, 1994.

—. "High Blood Pressure Tied to Memory Decline." *The New York Times*, April 26, 1994.

Haas, Robert. *Eat Smart, Think Smart. How to Use Nutrients and Supplements to Achieve Maximum Mental and Physical Performance.* HarperCollins, New York, 1994.

Hanh, Thich Nhat. *The Miracle of Mindfulness. A Manual on Meditation.* Beacon Press, Boston, 1975.

—. *Present Moment, Wonderful Moment. Mindfulness Verses for Daily Living.* Parallax Press, Berkeley, CA, 1990.

Harman, Willis, and Howard Rheingold. *Higher Creativity. Liberating the Unconscious for Breakthrough Insights.* Jeremy P. Tarcher, Los Angeles, 1984.

Hendler, Sheldon Saul. *The Doctor's Vitamin and Mineral Encyclopedia.* Simon & Schuster, New York, 1990.

Henig, Robin Marantz. *The Myth of Senility. The Truth About the Brain and Aging.* American Association of Retired Persons, Washington, D.C. 1985.

Herrmann, Ned. *The Creative Brain.* The Ned Herrmann Group, Lake Lure, NC, 1993.

Heyn, Birgit. *Ayurveda. The Indian Art of Natural Medicine & Life Extension.* Healing Arts Press, Rochester, VT, 1990.

Hoffer, Dr. Abram, and Dr. Morton Walker. *Smart Nutrients. A Guide to Nutrients That Can Prevent and Reverse Senility.* Avery Publishing Group, Garden City, NY, 1994.

Hooper, Judith, and Dick Teresi. *The 3-Pound Universe.* Jeremy P. Tarcher, Los Angeles, 1986.

Houston, Jean. *The Possible Human. A Course in Enhancing Your Physical, Mental, and Creative Abilities.* Jeremy P. Tarcher, Los Angeles, 1982.

Hutchison, Michael. *Mega Brain Power. Transform Your Life with Mind Machines and Brain Nutrients.* Hyperion, New York, 1994.

—. *Megabrain. New Tools and Techniques for Brain Growth and Mind Expansion.* rev. ed. Ballantine Books, New York, 1991.

Hyman, Tom. *Jupiter's Daughter*. Viking Penguin Group, New York, 1994.

Jensen, Bernard, with Sylvia Bell. *Tissue Cleansing Through Bowel Management, From the Simple to the Ultimate*. Bernard Jensen, Escondido, CA, 1981.

Johari, Harish. *Breath, Mind and Consciousness*. Destiny Books, Rochester, VT, 1989.

Kabat-Zinn, Jon. *Full Catastrophe Living, Using the Wisdom of Your Body and Mind to Face Stress, Pain, and Illness*. Delacorte Press, New York, 1990.

Kaminski, Patricia, and Richard Katz. *Flower Essence Repertory*. A *Comprehensive Guide to North American and English Flower Essences for Emotional and Spiritual Well-Being*. The Flower Essence Society, Nevada City, CA, 1994.

Kavner, Richard S. *Your Child's Vision*. A *Parent's Guide to Seeing, Growing, and Developing*. Fireside/Simon & Schuster, New York, 1985.

—. and Lorraine Dusky. *Total Vision*. Kavner Books, New York, 1978.

Kenyon, Tom. *Brain States*. United States Publishing, Naples, FL, 1994.

Laborde, Genie Z. *Fine Tune Your Brain. When Everything's Going Right and What to Do When It Isn't*. Syntony Publishing, Palo Alto, CA, 1988.

Lad, Dr. Vasant. Ayurveda. *The Science of Self-Healing*—A *Practical Guide*. Lotus Press, Santa Fe, NM, 1984.

Le Poncin, Monique. *Brain Fitness*, trans. by Lowell Blair. Fawcett Columbine, New York, 1990.

Mandell, Marshall, and Lynne Waller Scanlon. Dr. *Mandell's 5-Day Allergy Relief System*. Thomas Y. Crowell, New York, 1979.

Mark, Vernon H., with Jeffrey P. Mark. *Reversing Memory Loss. Proven Methods for Regaining, Strengthening, and Preserving Your Memory*. Houghton Mifflin Company, Boston, 1992.

—. *Brain Power*. A *Neurosurgeon's Complete Program to Maintain and Enhance Brain Fitness Throughout Your Life*. Houghton Mifflin, Boston, 1989.

Masters, Robert. *Neurospeak. Transforms Your Body, While You Read.* Quest Books, Wheaton, IL, 1994.

Minninger, Joan. *Total Recall. How to Maximize Your Memory Power.* MJF Books/Fine Communications, New York, 1984.

Morgan, Brian, and Roberta Morgan. *Brainfood. Nutrition and Your Brain.* The Body Press, Tucson, AZ, 1987.

Mowrey, Daniel B. *Scientific Validation of Herbal Medicine.* Cormorant Books, Lehi, UT, 1986.

Nagel, C. Van, Edward J. Reese, Maryann Reese, and Robert Siudzinski. *Mega-Teaching and Learning. Neurolinguistic Programming Applied to Education.* Metamorphous Press, Portland, OR, 1985.

Null, Gary. *The Egg Project. Gary Null's Complete Guide to Good Eating.* Four Walls, Eight Windows, New York, 1987.

Ornstein, Robert, and David Sobel. *The Healing Brain. Breakthrough Discoveries About How the Brain Keeps Us Healthy.* Simon & Schuster, New York, 1987.

Ostrander, Sheila, and Lynn Schroeder. *Superlearning.* Delta/The Confucian Press, Dell, New York, 1979.

—. *Supermemory. The Revolution.* Carroll & Graf, New York, 1991.

Payne, Mark. *Superhealth in a Toxic World. The Complete Environmental Medicine Health Plan.* Thorsons/HarperCollins, London, 1992.

Pearson, Durk, and Sandy Shaw. *Life Extension. A Practical Scientific Approach.* Warner Books, New York, 1982.

Pelletier, Kenneth R. *Mind as Healer, Mind as Slayer. A Holistic Approach to Preventing Stress Disorders.* Delacorte Press/Seymour Lawrence, New York, 1977.

Pelton, Ross, with Taffy Clarke Pelton. *Mind Food & Smart Pills. A Sourcebook for the Vitamins, Herbs & Drugs That Can Increase Intelligence, Improve Memory, & Prevent Brain Aging.* Doubleday, New York, 1989.

Pitchford, Paul. *Healing with Whole Foods. Oriental Traditions and Modern Nutrition.* North Atlantic Books, Berkeley, CA, 1994.

Potter, Beverly, and Sebastian Orfali. *Brain Boosters. Foods and Drugs That Make You Smarter.* Ronin, Berkeley, CA, 1993.

Price, Shirley. *Practical Aromatherapy, How to Use Essential Oils to Restore Vitality*. Thorsons/HarperCollins, London, 1987.

Rama, Swami, Rudolph Ballentine, and Alan Hymes. *Science of Breath. A Practical Guide*. The Himalayan International Institute, Honesdale, PA, 1979.

Randolph, Theron G., and Ralph W. Moss. *An Alternative Approach to Allergies. The New Field of Clinical Ecology Unravels the Environmental Causes of Mental and Physical Ills*. Harper & Row, New York, 1990.

Reid, Daniel. *The Complete Book of Chinese Health and Healing*. Shambhala, Boston, 1994.

Restak, Richard M. *The Mind*. Bantam Books, New York, 1988.

—. *The Brain: The Last Frontier—An Exploration of the Human Mind and Our Future*. Doubleday, New York, 1979.

—. *The Brain Has a Mind of Its Own. Insights from a Practicing Neurologist*. Crown Trade Paperbacks, New York, 1991.

Rick, Stephanie. *The Reflexology Workout. Hand & Foot Massage for Super Health & Rejuvenation*. Harmony Books/Crown Publishers, New York, 1986.

Rico, Gabriele Lusser. *Writing the Natural Way*. Jeremy P. Tarcher, Los Angeles, 1983.

Robinson, Adam. *What Smart Students Know. Maximum Grades, Optimum Learning, Minimum Time*. Crown Trade Paperbacks, New York, 1993.

Rogers, Sherry A. *Tired or Toxic? A Blueprint for Health*. Prestige Publishing, Syracuse, NY, 1990.

—. *The E.I. Syndrome: An Rx for Environmental Illness*. Prestige Publishing, Syracuse, NY, 1986.

—. *You Are What You Ate: An Rx for the Resistant Diseases of the 21st Century*. Prestige Publishing, Syracuse, NY, 1988.

Rose, Colin. *Accelerated Learning*. Dell, New York, 1985.

Rose, Steven. *The Conscious Brain*. Vintage Books, New York, 1976.

Rossi, Ernest Lawrence. *The 20-Minute Break: Reduce Stress, Maximize Performance, and Improve Health and Emotional Well-Being Using the New Science of Ultradian Rhythms*. Jeremy P. Tarcher, Los Angeles, 1991.

Ryman, Danielle. *Aromatherapy. The Complete Guide to Plant and Flower Essences for Health and Beauty*. Bantam Books, New York, 1991.

Sacks, Oliver. *Awakenings*. Harper Perennial/HarperCollins, New York, 1990.

vos Savant, Marilyn, and Leonore Fleischer. *Brain Building in Just 12 Weeks*. Bantam Books, New York, 1990.

Shih, T.K. "Qigong Elicits Latent Energy & Promotes Intelligence." *Qi—The Journal of Traditional Eastern Health & Fitness*, Autumn 1994, pp. 10–13.

Tart, Charles T. *Living the Mindful Life. A Handbook for Living in the Present Moment*. Shambhala, Boston, 1994.

Taylor, Gordon Rattray. *The Natural History of the Mind*. E. P. Dutton, New York, 1979.

Temple, Christine. *The Brain. An Introduction to the Psychology of the Human Brain and Behaviour*. Penguin Books, New York, 1994.

Tisserand, Robert B. *The Art of Aromatherapy. The Healing and Beautifying Properties of the Essential Oils of Flowers and Herbs*. Healing Arts Press, Rochester, VT, 1977.

Wade, Carlson. *Natural Energy Boosters*. Parker, West Nyack, NY, 1993.

Walker, Morton. "Excessive Tissue Manganese as a Cause of Antisocial Behavior." *Townsend Letter for Doctors*, December 1994.

Walker, Norman W. *Colon Health: The Key to a Vibrant Life*. O'Sullivan Woodside, Phoenix, AZ, 1979.

Warren, Tom. *Beating Alzheimer's. A Step Towards Unlocking the Mysteries of Brain Diseases*. Avery, Garden City, New York, 1991.

Wenger, Win. *How to Increase Your Intelligence*. D.O.K. Publishers, East Aurora, NY, 1987.

—. *Beyond Teaching & Learning*. Project Renaissance, Gaithersburg, MD, 1992.

Werbach, Melvyn. *Healing Through Nutrition. A Natural Approach to Treating 50 Common Illnesses with Diet and Nutrients*. HarperCollins, New York, 1993.

West, Robin. *Memory Fitness over 40*. Triad, Gainesville, FL, 1985.

Whitaker, Julian. Dr. *Whitaker's Guide to Natural Healing*. Prima, Rocklin, CA, 1995.

Wills, Christopher. *The Runaway Brain. The Evolution of Human Uniqueness*. Basic Books, New York, 1993.

Winter, Arthur. and Ruth Winter. *Build Your Brain Power. The Latest Techniques to Preserve, Restore, and Improve Your Brain's Potential*. St. Martin's Press, New York, 1986.

Wujec, Tom. *Pumping Ions. Games and Exercises to Flex Your Mind*. Doubleday, New York, 1988.

Wycoff, Joyce. *Mindmapping. Your Personal Guide to Exploring Creativity and Problem Solving*. Berkley Books, New York, 1991.

Yates, Francis A. *The Art of Memory*. The University of Chicago Press, Chicago, 1966.

Yepsen, Roger, B. *How to Boost Your Brain Power. Achieving Peak Intelligence, Memory, and Creativity*. Wings Books, New York, 1987.

Ziff, Sam. *The Toxic Time Bomb. Can the Mercury in Your Dental Fillings Poison You?* Aurora Press, Santa Fe, NM, 1984.

PRODUCTS AND SERVICES

Healing. Relaxing , Brain Food Music

Soundings of the Planet, P.O. Box 43512, Tucson, AZ 85733; telephone: (602)-792-9888. For Dean Evenson, Tom Barabas, and others.

Sound Rx, 1221 Andersen Drive, Suite H, San Rafael, CA 94915; telephone: (800)-726-39243. For Steven Halpern music and others.

Sound Therapy, Electronic Ear on Walkman: For tapes (set of 4 90-minute cassettes in ascending frequencies, $275 U.S., includes shipping), books (*Sound Therapy for the Walkman*, Pat Joudry, $10), and information: Sound Therapy, Steele & Steele, P.O. Box 617, Dalmeny, Saskatchewan, Canada, S0K 1E0; telephone: (306)-931-2522.

For Lozanov Superlearning materials: Superlearning, Inc., 450 Seventh Avenue, Suite #500, New York, NY 10123; telephone: (212)-279-8450. Catalog of tapes, books.

For Tomatis training and materials: Tomatis Centre, Inc., Ron Minson, Director, 55 Madison St., Suite 375, Denver, CO 80206; telephone: (303)-320-4411.

Publications

Megabrain Report: The Journal of Optimal Performance, Michael Hutchison, Editor., P.O. Box 65676, Los Angeles, CA 90065; telephone: (800)-475-6463. $48/year, quarterly; single issues, $15.

Smart Drug News: The Newsletter of the Cognitive Enhancement Research Institute. Published by CERI, P.O. Box 4029, Menlo Park, CA 94026; $40/year, 10 issues.

Brain-Building Electronic Devices and Nutrients

Tools for Exploration, 4460 Redwood Highway, Suite 2, San Rafael, CA 94903; telephone: (800)-456-9887. Over 1,000 products, books, and tapes in the field of brain wave technology for enhancing energy, brain power, consciousness, and health.

Life Extension Foundation, P.O. Box 229120, Hollywood, FL 33022; telephone: (800)-841-5433. For life extension nutrients and brain smart drugs.

Flower Essences

Flower Essence Services, P.O. Box 459, Nevada City, CA 95959; telephone: (800)-548-0075. For books, articles, flower remedies, and clinical referrals.

Behavioral Optometry

Optometric Extension Program Foundation and Vision Extension, Inc., 2912 South Daimler Street, Suite 100, Santa Ana, CA 92705; telephone: (714)-250-0846. Journals, pamphlets, vision products, seminars, training, and information on behavioral optometry and practitioner referrals.

ANSWERS TO PUZZLES

BRAIN BUILDERS! Workout #14, *Unscramble and Evict*. Lincoln. Cadillac. jaguar. *pheasant*. Rolls Royce. Mercedes. Lexus. These are all cars, but pheasant is a bird. Evict pheasant.

BRAIN BUILDERS! Workout #16, *Short-Term Memory Calisthenics*. Neurotransmitter.

BRAIN BUILDERS! Workout #18, *Brain Power Word Making*. Answers: *endorphin*, *Alzheimer's*, *dopamine*, *synapse*.

BRAIN BUILDERS! Workout #19, *Number Play*. The middle digit of these pairs is the sum of the first and third numbers. This is not the case with 276. It's also true that except for 276, the digit units are made of two odd numbers and one even. Thanks to Monique Le Poncin for this exercise.

INDEX

A

O

P

W

X

Y

Z